Microbiology for Health Careers

Sixth Edition

Lynne I. Grover-Lakomia

Elizabeth Fong

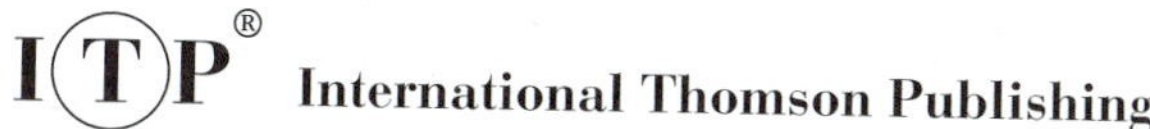

Albany • Bonn • Boston • Cincinnati • Detroit • London • Madrid
Melbourne • Mexico City • New York • Pacific Grove • Paris • San Francisco
Singapore • Tokyo • Toronto • Washington

NOTICE TO THE READER

Cover Design: Bill Finnerty

Delmar Staff:
Publisher: Susan Simpfenderfer
Acquisitions Editor: Marlene McHugh Pratt
Production Manager: Linda Helfrich
Project Editor: William Trudell
Art/Design Coordinator: Rich Killar
Editorial Assistant: Maria Perretta

an International Thomson Publishing company **I(T)P®**

The ITP logo is a trademark under license
Printed in the United States of America

For more information contact:

Delmar Publishers
3 Columbia Circle, Box 15015
Albany, New York 12212-5015

International Thomson Publishing Europe
Berkshire House
168-173 High Holborn
London, WC1V7AA
United Kingdom

Nelson ITP, Australia
102 Dodds Street
South Melbourne,
Victoria, 3205 Australia

Nelson Canada
1120 Birchmont Road
Scarborough, Ontario
M1K 5G4, Canada

International Thomson Publishing France
Tour Maine-Montparnasse
33 Avenue du Maine
75755 Paris Cedex 15, France

International Thomson Editores
Seneca 53
Colonia Polanco
11560 Mexico D.F. Mexico

International Thomson Publishing GmbH
Königswinterer Straße 418
53227 Bonn
Germany

International Thomson Publishing Asia
60 Albert Street #15-01
Albert Complex
Singapore 189969

International Thomson Publishing Japan
Hirakawa-cho Kyowa Building, 3F
2-2-1 Hirakawa-cho, Chiyoda-ku,
Tokyo 102, Japan

ITE Spain/ Paraninfo
Calle Magallanes, 25
28015-Madrid, Espana

5 6 7 8 9 10 XXX 03 02

Library of Congress Cataloging-in-Publication Data

Grover-Lakomia, Lynne I.
Microbiology for health careers / Lynne I. Grover-Lakomia, Elizabeth Fong. -- 6th ed.
p. cm.
Includes bibliographical references and index.
ISBN 0-7668-0917-X
1. Medical microbiology. 2. Allied health personnel. I. Fong, Elizabeth, 1947- II. Fong, Elizabeth, 1947- Microbiology for health careers. III. Fong, Elizabeth, 1947- Microbiology for health careers. III. Title.

QR46.G76 1999
616'.01---dc21

98-53502
CIP

CONTENTS

PREFACE

Microbiology for Health Careers is an introductory text designed for allied health students studying at the high school, vocational, and community college level and appropriate for a variety of programs, including medical laboratory technology, medical assisting, dental assisting, respiratory therapy, radiography, and licensed practical nursing.

ORGANIZATION

The text contains 21 chapters, subdivided into 5 sections. Section I, The World of Microorganisms, provides a general overview of microbiology, including an overview of the microscope, basic chemistry, and bacterial growth. Section II, Structure and Behavior of Microorganisms, introduces students to cellular structure, protists, fungi, parasites, bacteria, rickettsias, chlamydias, mycoplasmas, and microbiological techniques. Section III, Infection and Immunity explores infection by microorganisms, the body defenses, immunity, and vaccines. Section IV, Methods of Destruction of Microbiological Material discusses the physical, chemical and chemotherapeutic agents used to destroy harmful microorganisms. Section V, Public Health Microbiology, includes chapters on controlling pathogens, and health and safety measures practiced in health care facilities.

Key words are defined in a glossary at the back of the book. The 5 appendices include additional reference material for the students, such as a review of communicable diseases and culture media, staining solutions and slide preparation techniques.

Chapter Features

Each chapter includes the following learning aids to augment student learning: objectives, key words, chapter summaries, study and discussion questions, and review questions. Each of the 5 sections concludes with a comprehensive Achievement Review to test students on what they have just learned.

Procedures containing step-by-step instructions for performing some of the most common microbiology laboratory procedures also appear throughout the text as appropriate. The laboratory activities have been designed with the physician's office laboratory (PAL) or small, private laboratory in mind. If your students are headed for a large hospital or reference laboratory, additional background information on using complex and automated procedures is recommended. An appendix detailing techniques for the collection of specimens performed in physicians' offices, outpatient laboratories, as well as inpatient facilities, is also included.

NEW FOR THE REVISION

The sixth edition of this text has been revised and updated to include current information on human immunodeficiency virus (HIV), hepatitis B (HBV), and hepatitis C. Ideas and suggestions from reviewers have resulted in numerous changes that will better prepare allied health students to perform microbiological procedures, as well as increase their knowledge of important clinical infections especially antibiotic resistant microorganisms and those bacteria the cause necrotizing fasciitis.

Universal Standards, formerly called Universal Precautions, and the OSHA Bloodbourne Pathogen Rule are emphasized throughout the text. The chapters have been reorganized since the last edition to group similar subjects together in one section, rather than dispensing information on the same topics throughout the text. This makes material easier to locate for students. Common microbiology laboratory procedures now appear in procedure boxes to make them easier to use in the lab setting. Summaries have been added to each chapter to help students identify and review key concepts.

I have maintained the metric review appendix because health care students must have an understanding and concept of how metric measurements compare to our standard of measuring. The student must also understand that laboratory measurements are made in very small units, indicating a need for careful attention to detail.

Each chapter begins with a list of key words defined in a comprehensive glossary as well as a chapter summary and a variety of review questions that can be used as an assignment, a self-test or a unit examination.

SUPPLEMENTS

An Instructor's Manual accompanies this text. It provides answers to the review questions found in each text chapter, and also includes laboratory activities needed to identify some of the more common microbiological infections so that students can use investigative flow chart techniques to identify some of the organisms by name.

ACKNOWLEDGMENTS

The author would like to express a sincere appreciation to the editorial staff at Delmar Publishers, and a special thanks to Jill Rembetski for her guidance and patience with me as we worked through the changes together. To my husband, Tom, who has sacrificed our precious time together, I am blessed to have a partner with such patience, I thank you with all my heart.

A special thanks to the following reviewers who critiqued the manuscript. This edition would not have been possible without your valued input.

Paula T. Cantwell, BS, RN, BSN
Assistant Professor
New England Institute of Technology
Warwick, RI

Tese Gorszwick, MT (ASCP), CPT (ASPT)
Instructor, Health Occupations
Oceanside Unified School District
Oceanside, CA

Connie Krebs, CMA-C, BGS
Instructor/Coordinator
Medical Assistant Program
Fort Hayes Metropolitan Education Center
Columbus, OH

Catherine A. Lencioni, MS, MT (ASCP)
Assistant Professor/Director
Medical Laboratory Technician Program
Harrisburg Area Community College
Harrisburg, PA

Debra L. Privett, BA, CLA (ASCP), MLT, CMA
Medical Assisting Instructor
Duluth Business University
Duluth, MN

—Lynne I. Grover-Lakomia

ABOUT THE AUTHOR

This revised and updated version of *Microbiology for Health Careers* was written by Lynne-Grover Lakomia, BS, MA MT(ASCP), CLS(NCA), RT(CSLT), MT(AMT) who received her initial training and microbiology bench experience in North Bay and Kitchener Ontario, followed by some many years of microbiology and supervisory work in the United States. Lynne is recently retired from her position as a program coordinator of the Clinical Laboratory Assistant program at Fort Hayes Metropolitan Education Center, Columbus, Ohio, and keeps active writing text material and serving as a microbiologist and clinical operations officer in the United States Army Reserve at William Beaumont Army Medical center. Lynne has taught chemistry, physics and biology in the city school system and also holds the rank of colonel in the United States Army Reserve, with clinical experience throughout the U.S., as well as teaching experience at the Army Medical Department Center and School, located at Fort Sam Houston, Texas.

SECTION 1 THE WORLD OF MICROORGANISMS

CHAPTER 1 *The Value of Microbiology*

OBJECTIVES

After completing this chapter, you will be able to:

- define microbiology.
- describe the contributions of scientists to the conquest of disease.
- list other areas of study in the science of microbiology.
- identify basic health care procedures used to prevent and control disease.

KEY WORDS

abiogenesis
animalcules
antiseptic
aseptic
attenuate
bacteria
bacteriophage
biochemist
biogenesis
biology
botanist
contagious
disinfection
emerging pathogens
endospore
epidemiology
exobiology
feline
fermentation
fungus
germ theory
hypothesis
immune
immunology
infusion
intradermal
Koch's postulates
labile
microbes
microbiology
microorganisms
microscope
mutagenic
optics
parasites
pasteurization

KEY WORDS (cont.)

pathogen
pathologist
pericarditis
postmortem
prognosis
puerperal fever
saprophytic
sepsis
turbid
vaccine
vaporization
vector
virologist
virulence
viruses

THE SCIENCE OF MICROBIOLOGY

The modern science of microbiology began about 100 years ago. The word **microbiology** is derived from the Greek *micros,* meaning "small," *bios,* meaning "life," and *logy,* meaning "the study of." Microbiology is the branch of **biology** (the study of living things) that deals with simple life forms, usually single celled, that cannot be seen with the naked eye. These minute living organisms are referred to as **microbes** or **microorganisms** because they can be seen only through a **microscope** (an instrument fitted with a powerful magnifying lens).

The term *microbiology* encompasses the study of all microbes, including **bacteria** (bacteriology), **fungi** (mycology), **parasites** (parasitology), and **viruses** (virology). The study of microorganisms and how they affect living things is what microbiology is all about. A time line of microbiology appears in Figure 1–1.

MILESTONES IN THE DEVELOPMENT OF THE SCIENCE OF MICROBIOLOGY

The first microbes recognized were bacteria discovered more than 200 years before microbiology became a recognized science. The discovery was made in 1667 by Anton van Leeuwenhoek, a Dutch lensgrinder. He was amazed to discover tiny forms of life in a drop of water, which he was examining through a magnifying lens. Until that time, people had no idea that these microscopic organisms existed and could affect their lives in so many ways.

Anton van Leeuwenhoek (1632–1723)

Van Leeuwenhoek, by trade, was a Dutch drapery merchant. Although he had no formal scientific education, he had a keen knowledge and understanding of the art of lens grinding and **optics.** His highly inquisitive mind led him to examine a diverse assortment of materials. These include blood, suspensions of feces and pepper water, semen, urine, and water from gutters, lakes, rivers, wells, and the sea. Through van Leeuwenhoek's meticulous grinding of a single lens, his simple microscopes had a maximum magnification of 300 times.

1667 Leeuwenhoek— microscope	1713–1781 Needham— hay infusions	1729–1799 Spallanzani— spontaneous generation	1749–1823 Jenner— small pox	1822–1895 Pasteur— germ theory, rabies, etc.
1820–1893 Tyndall— spores and tyndallization	1827–1912 Lister— aseptic surgery	1843–1910 Koch— anthrax, tuberculosis, diptheria, typhoid	1843–1910 Petri— petri dishes to grow bacteria	1851–1931 Beijerinck— tobacco mosaic virus
1854–1915 Ehrlich— salvarsan cure for syphilis	1877–1977 Schick— diphtheria skin test	1895–1981 Lancefield— streptococcus typing	1921–1928 Dicks— scarlet fever test	1928 Fleming— penicillin
1935 Stanley— grew tobacco, polio viruses	1930s Electron microscope	1950s Salk and Sabin— polio vaccine	1960 Feline leukemia virus	1956 Krugman— hepatitis and gamma globulin
1970 Donor blood testing for hepatitis Australia antigen	1976 Blumburg— hepatitis B virus	1981 Merck Sharp & Dohme licensed to sell hepatitis B virus vaccine	1979 Gallo— human T–cell lymphoma virus	1987 Liebowich and Montagnier— human immunodeficiency virus
1990 Introduction of Hib vaccinations to prevent Haemophilus meningitis in children	1990–present Ongoing research to find a cure and vaccine for HIV	1995 Multiple cocktails of drugs show AIDS virus counts decreasing T-cell count up and patients in longer remissions Chicken pox vaccine is introduced	1998 Renewed hope for a breast cancer cure is on the horizon	

Figure 1–1 Time line of microbiology milestones

With these new microscopes, van Leeuwenhoek was able to see tiny living organisms in his simple materials. He called them "animalcules" in a series of letters he wrote to the Royal Society of London over a span of 50 years. In these letters, he recorded his observations with much painstaking accuracy and objectivity. In a letter dated 1683, and another in 1692, he enclosed diagrams that clearly showed the three major shapes of bacteria, which included bacilli (rod shaped), cocci (spherical

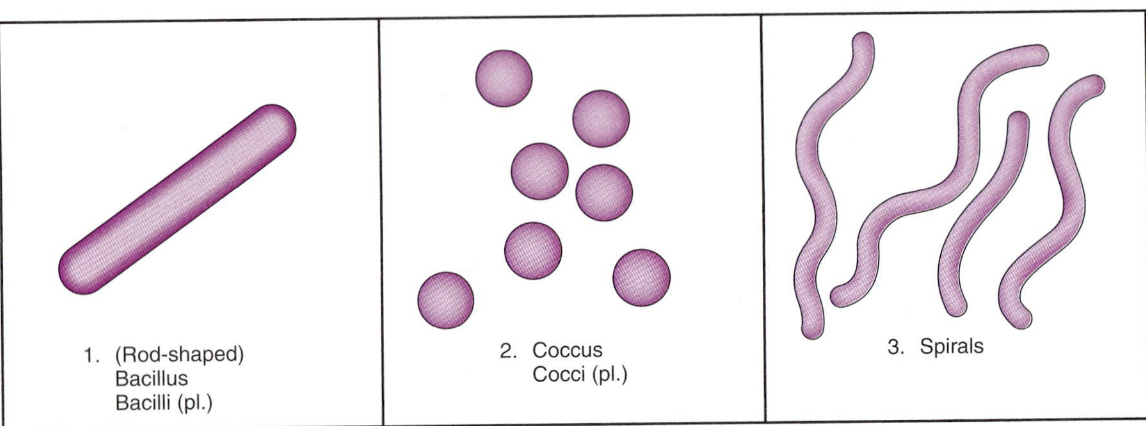

Figure 1–2 Three major shapes of bacteria

shaped), and spiral-shaped bacteria (Figure 1–2). For these discoveries he is known as the "Father of Microbiology."

After van Leeuwenhoek's death, no other individual came close to the precision of grinding a lens that could magnify up to 300 times. He did not pass on his much guarded technique to his children or to an apprentice. When he died, van Leeuwenhoek had over 400 microscopes, one for each new specimen he examined. However, only a few of these microscopes remain. The others have mysteriously disappeared. Despite the fact that he discovered microorganisms, van Leeuwenhoek did not relate them to their origin or to the cause of disease.

Spontaneous Generation

Although van Leeuwenhoek did not speculate upon the origin of microorganisms, other people did have theories. For a period of 200 years, from 1650 to 1850, the theory of spontaneous generation or **abiogenesis** was the most widely accepted explanation for the origin of microbes. Spontaneous generation states that life can suddenly or spontaneously arise from decomposing nonliving matter. This "doctrine" was apparently supported by some of the greatest and clearest scientific minds of the period. Various cases were cited for spontaneous generation: decaying meat gave rise to maggots (fly larvae); sweat-laden shirts, stored with wheat in a dark area, gave rise to mice; and hairs from a horse's tail, when placed in water, produced worms!

During the time that this doctrine was popular, two notable scientists conducted experiments to disprove it. One was Francesco Redi, an Italian biologist, physician, and poet. His experiment was simple in design, but classic. He merely set up three jars of decaying meat, one covered with gauze, the second with parchment paper, and the third left uncovered. Flies were attracted to the first two jars but could not land on the meat. Flies did land on the meat in the third uncovered jar, and eventually maggots developed. However, the other two jars did not give rise to maggots. Redi concluded that decaying meat does not give rise to maggots. Flies must land on the decaying meat and deposit their eggs. Later these eggs hatch and give rise to maggots.

Despite Redi's conclusion, other scientists quickly suggested that the gauze could not keep out microorganisms and that organic matter could give rise to microbes. Supporters of spontaneous generation proposed a new variation. Even though flies, mice, and worms could not arise from organic matter, living microbes could come from broth, hay **infusions,** rainwater, and so forth.

Lazzaro Spallanzani (1729–1799)

In 1767, still not convinced that life arises spontaneously from decomposing dead matter, Father Lazzaro Spallanzani conducted experiments to dispute the microlevel theory of spontaneous generation. He boiled meat broth in a flask and then sealed the neck of the flask by melting its glass neck. Thus, no microbes were allowed to enter and develop. However, if the neck was broken, the broth eventually became **turbid** or cloudy with the growth of **"animalcules,"** or microbes carried by contaminated air into the broth.

These conclusions were vigorously disputed by defenders of the theory of spontaneous generation, who argued that boiling the flask destroyed the life in it, and by sealing the flask the "vital life force" was prevented from entering the flask and giving rise to life. John Needham (1713–1781), a Welshman and harsh critic of Spallanzani's, stood by his own infusion experiments of 1748 which naturally supported the spontaneous generation theory. He had used cork stoppers to close his bottles. The cork not only allowed the oxygen, now referred to as the "vital principle" to enter, but also microbes in the air could easily pass through the minute vacuoles described as cells by Robert Hooke some 80 years before. Because of the necessity of oxygen for growth of many microorganisms, the doctrine of spontaneous generation prevailed for another hundred years until experiments by Louis Pasteur and John Tyndall disproved the doctrine once and for all.

Edward Jenner (1749–1823)

May of 1796 heralded one of the greatest contributions to preventive medicine, when Jenner, having been impressed by the fact that milkmaids in Gloucestershire, England, who had contracted cowpox while milking cows, became immune to the ravages of smallpox. He tested his theory by transferring a small amount of the material from a cowpox pustule to the arm of an uninfected young boy. Six weeks later the boy was inoculated with smallpox and the disease failed to develop. By 1798 some 6000 persons had been inoculated with cowpox to prevent smallpox. The word *vaccination* (from the Latin *vacca* meaning "cow") was first used by Louis Pasteur out of respect for Jenner's work.

Louis Pasteur (1822–1895)

Pasteur's work during the years 1861 through 1885 really began the era of modern bacteriology. In 1862, Pasteur, a French **biochemist** and physicist, devised several very simple but clever experiments. In one series of experiments he put beef broth into a long-necked flask. He then melted the neck and drew it out into an S shape, creating a swan-necked flask. After that, he boiled the flask. As the flask was being boiled, **vaporization** pushed the air out of the flask through the opening at the end of the swan neck. The flask was cooled and, following that, air was pulled back into it. As the air entered, it passed over water condensation in the neck. The moisture droplets and the bend of the swan neck managed to trap any airborne microorganisms and dust particles, thus keeping the broth sterile. Air, or the "vital principle," was still able to reach the broth, but the broth remained clear. If the flask was tilted, and the broth touched the bend of the neck and then ran back into the flask, the broth later became turbid. At the Pasteur Institute in Paris, some of Pasteur's original sterile flasks were sealed to prevent evaporation, and they are sterile to the present day (Figure 1–3).

In a second round of experiments, Pasteur used cotton as plugs for his sterilized broth-laden flasks. The cotton plugs acted like filters, trapping the airborne microbes and dust particles. He then, microscopically, examined these trapped microorganisms and found them to be similar to the ones found in many infusions. Therefore, if a cotton plug was dropped into a sterile flask, the broth would soon be turbid.

As a result of these two simple but very conclusive experiments, Pasteur showed that life comes from life and is self-producing, rather than spontaneous. Thus, the theory of **biogenesis,** that life comes from preexisting life, overthrew the theory of abiogenesis.

Pasteur also made other milestone contributions. He developed the **germ theory of fermentation**—that is, the idea that microorganisms are responsible for the fermentation of sugars—while examining reasons for the excessive spoilage of beer and wine in the brewing industry. During the process of **fermentation,** yeast will ferment the sugar in grapes to produce ethyl alcohol. If a bacterium such as *Acetobacter* happens to contaminate the beer or wine cask, the alcohol is changed to acetic acid (vinegar). This contamination alters the taste and ruins the beer or wine. Pasteur devised a method to destroy the contaminating bacteria in beer and wine by heating them to between 50°C to 60°C (122°F to 140°F). This technique, called **pasteurization,** has been adapted for the dairy industry to destroy lactic acid–forming bacteria which cause milk to sour. Milk is heated to 63°C (145.4°F) for 30 minutes, or to 72°C (161.6°F) for 15 seconds.

Using the germ theory of fermentation, Pasteur developed the germ theory of disease. The theory states that specific microorganisms called bacteria are the cause of specific diseases in both humans and animals. Pasteur developed specific **vaccines** against anthrax in sheep, chicken pox, cholera, and rabies. These vaccines were made from a weakened or **attenuated** pathogen (disease-causing agent). Upon injection into animals or humans, it would not cause the disease to develop but, instead, would cause them to become **immune** to the disease. When Pasteur isolated the rabies virus from the brain and spinal cord of a rabid dog, he weakened the virus by transferring it from rabbit to rabbit. Using this attenuated virus, he perfected a method of vaccination against rabies called the Pasteur treatment. Because of Pasteur's exhaustive work on bacteria and vaccines, he is known as the "father of bacteriology and immunology." All of Pasteur's experiments set a precedent for the development and appreciation of sound scientific methods for the study of the characteristics of microorganisms.

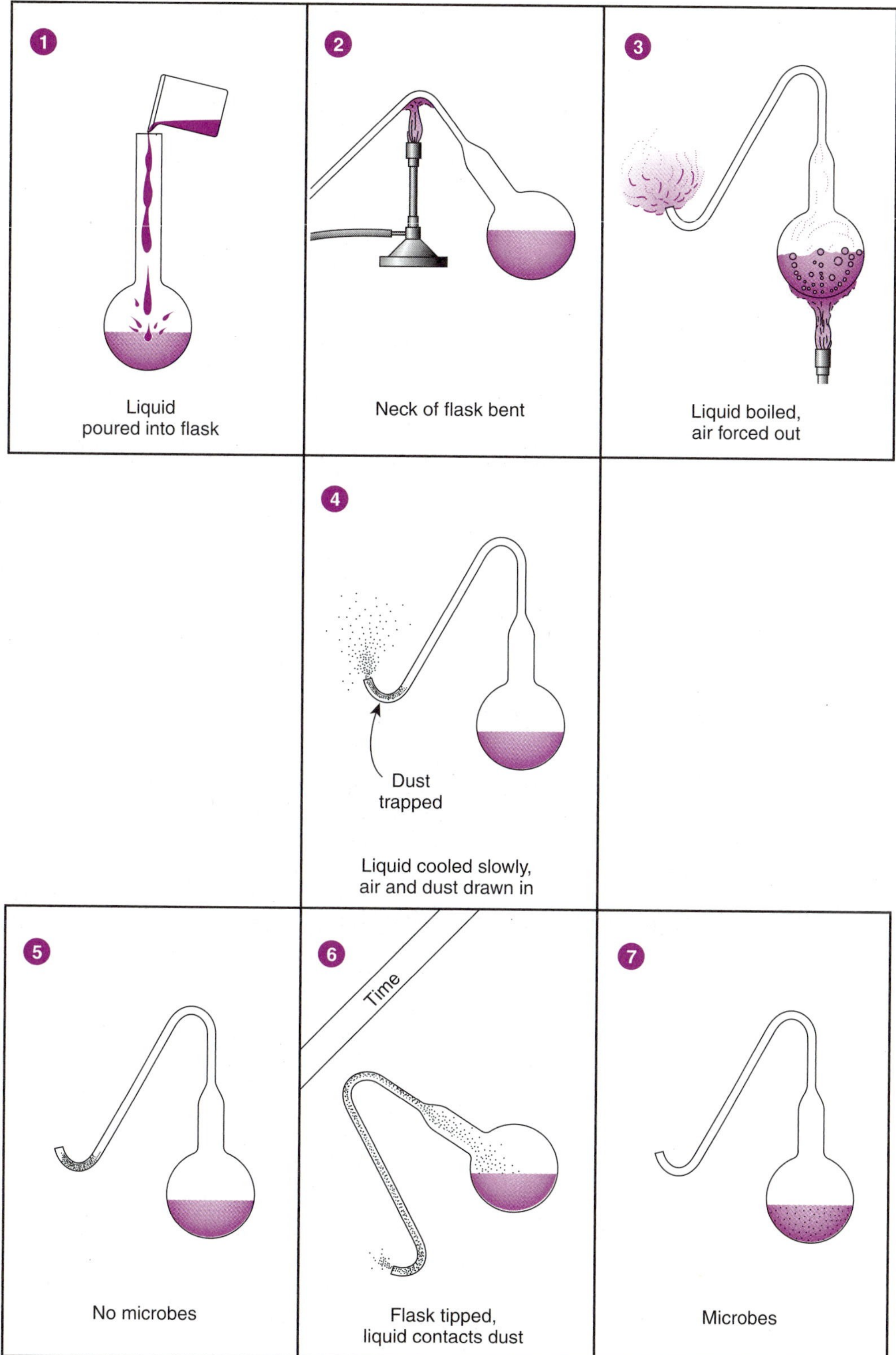

Figure 1–3 Louis Pasteur's swan-necked flask experiment, disproving the theory of spontaneous generation

Oliver Wendell Holmes (1809–1894) and Ignaz Philipp Semmelweis (1818–1865)

Oliver Wendell Holmes, a well-known American physician, published in the *New England Journal of Medicine* in 1843 that childbed fever (puerperal sepsis), a highly **contagious** disease, might be spread by the hands of doctors and nurses who went from one patient to another.

Sometime later, Ignaz Philipp Semmelweis, a Hungarian obstetrician, noted that death rates of patients being visited by physicians and medical students who had come directly from the morgue or autopsy room were much higher. After observing a **post-mortem** on a pathologist who had died of an infection complicating a dissection wound, Semmelweis saw that the disease changes were similar to those present in women who died of puerperal fever. He rightly concluded that this disease was infectious. To support his **hypothesis** he established the first real safety precautions in a hospital. On his wards all hands had to be carefully cleansed before a patient was examined, and the rooms were to be kept scrupulously clean. The mortality rate on his wards dropped dramatically; in 1847 he reported that the cause of **puerperal fever** could be found in blood poisoning. Some years later Joseph Lister would expand on this idea of a clean environment to stave off sepsis, the presence of multiplying infectious bacteria in the bloodstream.

John Tyndall (1820–1893)

As convincing as Pasteur's experiments were in disproving the doctrine of spontaneous generation, there were still a few disclaimers. Some scientists tried to duplicate Pasteur's work and were unsuccessful, because different laboratories came up with different results. Finally, in 1876, John Tyndall, an English physicist, performed a series of experiments to point out the inconsistencies between the various laboratories. In duplicating Pasteur's experiments, he discovered that there were two different types of bacteria: the heat-sensitive or **labile** form (vegetative cell) easily destroyed by boiling, and the heat-resistant type called an **endospore.** He developed a technique to kill all heat-resistant endospores. Tyndall boiled a hay infusion for 1 minute. Afterward, upon cooling, the endospores would germinate into heat-labile vegetative cells. Then he boiled the hay infusion again. The alternate process of heating and cooling was repeated five separate times to kill all the endospores. This technique is now called the fractional sterilization process or *Tyndallization.*

Lord Joseph Lister (1827–1912)

In 1865, Lord Joseph Lister applied Pasteur's germ theory of disease to his surgical practice. Lister speculated that if microorganisms could fall upon a nutrient broth and grow there, they could do the same on an open surgical wound. When this happened, surgical **sepsis** would occur, which most often led to surgical deaths. To counteract this, Lister used carbolic acid (phenol) in the washing or **disinfection** of his hands and surgical tools. He even sprayed a fine mist into the air around his patients in the operating room. After

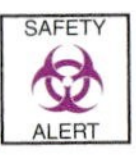

the operation he used phenol on the dressings he applied to his patient's surgical wounds. As a result of this revolutionary **antiseptic** surgery, the fatality rate of his surgical patients was very low. Today, surgeons use the **aseptic** method, in which surgical instruments and materials are sterilized prior to their use. Thanks to Lister's methods, millions of lives have been saved by reducing infection after surgery.

Robert Koch (1843–1910)

In the 1860s, a German doctor named Robert Koch developed an elaborate technique of isolating and identifying specific **pathogens** that cause specific diseases. Koch, his associates, and his students were pioneers in techniques of isolating organisms in pure culture, staining them, and producing animal inoculations, all of which are essential to microbial study. For example, one of his associates, Julius Petri, was responsible for the development of the now famous petri dish.

Koch was the first to isolate the bacterium that causes anthrax in sheep. He did this by taking blood from sheep that had died of anthrax and then growing these bacteria in pure culture. (In a pure culture only one type of bacterium is present.) In turn, these bacteria were injected into other healthy animals to see if anthrax would develop. From these animals showing symptoms of anthrax, Koch isolated and cultured bacteria identical to the ones found in the sheep that died of anthrax. This proved that the organism, when cultured, caused the disease anthrax. In 1884 he expounded his principles relating to the germ theory of disease with such clarity that the rules establishing a specific organism as the cause of a specific disease came to be known as **Koch's postulates.** They are

1. The causative agent must be present in every case of the disease and cannot be present in healthy animals.
2. The pathogen must be isolated from the diseased host and then grown in pure culture.
3. The same disease must be reproduced in healthy animals that have been injected with organisms from the pure culture.
4. The same pathogen must then be recovered from the artificially infected animals and that same pathogen reisolated in pure culture.

Upon the establishment of these postulates, Koch discovered in rapid succession the causative agents to such dreaded human diseases as tuberculosis, diphtheria, typhoid fever, cholera, and gonorrhea.

It was through the tireless and brilliant works of Pasteur, Lister, and Koch that the study of microbiology became a recognized bona fide science. France recognized Pasteur by establishing the Pasteur Institute in Paris in 1888. Germany founded a special Institute for Infective Diseases at the University of Berlin for Koch, where he became its professor of hygiene and its director. These two institutes attracted scholars and students from all over the world. In turn, these students, armed with their newfound knowledge and enthusiasm, returned to their countries and made important contributions of their own. More microorganisms were isolated as causative agents of specific diseases. The flurry of activity caused by these scientists marked the end of the nineteenth century as the "Golden Age of Bacteriology."

TWENTIETH-CENTURY MICROBIOLOGY MILESTONES

Besides the dawn of the discovery of antibiotic therapy and the beginning of the science of **immunology,** the twentieth century will long be remembered as the Age of Virology. Paul Ehrlich (1854–1915), a German scientist, discovered the "magic bullet" salvarsan—a chemical compound of arsenic that would cure syphilis. Later, Sir Alexander Fleming's accidental discovery of penicillin from the green mold (fungus) *Penicillium notatum* in 1928 would open the door to the discovery of many antibiotics from different fungi. Penicillin, along with its many derivatives, is still one of the most widely prescribed antibiotics.

Between 1921 and 1927, two American physicians, Gladys and George Dick, developed a test to determine whether a person is susceptible to scarlet fever. Their work linked the disease to the hemolytic streptococci. The resulting Dick test involved the **intradermal** (under the skin) injection of a minute amount of the scarlet fever toxin, produced by the *Streptococcus* organism and later observing for inflammation. Rebecca Craighill Lancefield (1895–1981) developed the serological typing techniques for the differentiation of the streptococcal groups still widely used today.

Around the turn of the century former students and associates of Louis Pasteur discovered toxins to diphtheria and tetanus, which led to the development of vaccines to provide immunity to these dreaded diseases. Béla Schick (1877–1977) introduced the Schick skin test for susceptibility to diphtheria, which demonstrates immunity to the disease.

Martinus Willem Beijerinck (1851–1931)

In 1898 the first virus that caused tobacco mosaic disease was recognized by Martinus Willem Beijerinck, a Dutch **botanist.** This virus, much smaller than any other infectious agent was purified in crystalline form by Beijerinck. To study the virus it was necessary to process over a ton of infected tobacco to yield just 1 tablespoon of the virus crystals. This feat was accomplished in 1935 by Wendell Meredith Stanley, a biochemist and **virologist** at the University of California. His laboratory would later also crystallize the poliomyelitis virus.

The advent of the electron microscope during the 1930s allowed virus hunters finally to see the culprits. Bacteria, measured in microns or micrometers, are approximately one twenty-five-thousandth of an inch (1/25,400). Virus particles on the other hand, are so small they can be measured only in nanometers. A nanometer is one-thousandth (1/1000) of a micrometer or 1/25,400,000 of an inch.

Yellow Fever.

Other early virologists were to see polio, influenza, smallpox, cowpox papilloma, and **bacteriophages** (viruses produced by bacteria) for the first time. Major Walter Reed, General William C. Gorgas, and Surgeon General George M. Sternberg would develop the Yellow Fever Commission to find and eradicate the cause of this virus that killed so many people during the building of the Panama Canal. General Sternberg, no stranger to virus research, developed a neutralization test, which is a key tool in identifying different types of viruses causing influenza and poliomyelitis and in testing the potency of antibodies produced by the vaccines against these two diseases.

Polio. Post–World War II brought active research into some of the most dreaded diseases. By 1949, viruses were being grown in test cultures of living tissue. Poliomyelitis or infantile paralysis was arrested with the development of vaccines by Dr. Jonas Salk and Dr. Albert Sabin. Soon a measles vaccine was also produced. Several kinds of cancer were linked to viral causes. Today a vaccine is routine for the **feline** leukemia virus, which was first discovered in 1960.

Chicken pox. A new addition to the list of childhood immunizations is the varicella vaccine for the prevention of chicken pox. Scientists have been working on an effective vaccine for many years and finally the FDA approved it in 1995; however, much controversy remains among the experts as to whether infants, children, and even nonpreviously infected adults should receive the vaccine. Some say the disease is not serious enough to warrant a vaccine, which is true in most children but not in adults who usually become quite ill with the disease. Others are not yet convinced of the effectiveness or safety of the vaccine in which only 7 years of follow-up studies have been completed to date. The National Vaccination Information Center believes this vaccine can backfire. It is effective for about 10 years, after which time the individuals vaccinated will soon become adults, further increasing their risk of catching the disease. Time and more research will determine the fate of this vaccine.

Haemophilus influenza type B. The vaccine haemophilus influenza type B (Hib) has been available for over 5 years now and is considered a must as part of all infant and children's immunization history. It is routinely given to infants at 2, 4, and 6 months of age as a prevention against the bacterium *Haemophilus influenzae B.* This organism is known to cause life-threatening diseases, particularly meningitis in children under the age of 6 years. It also causes pneumonia, **pericarditis** (inflammation around the heart), and osteomyelitis. Because this bacteria is spread in respiratory secretions by direct person-to-person contact, a vaccine seemed the best solution to prevention of spread of this disease.

Hepatitis. Today, medical authorities recognize not only hepatitis A, B, and C, but it has also become the alphabet soup disease with hepatitis D, E, F, and G, identifiable. Cures are not on the horizon, but with good hygiene, not sharing needles, education, and testing of the blood and vaccines, hepatitis can be controlled. Today, infants and children at the elementary and middle school levels are now being vaccinated against hepatitis B. Hepatitis C, D, E, F, and G are now in the forefront of researchers' activities, with hepatitis C being of the most concern, for it is known to be transmitted by blood-to-blood contact. Often referred to as the stealth disease, hepatitis C comes on without any warning. There is no cure at this time, but researchers have found that combination therapy with ribaviron, which seems to interfere with the virus' ability to replicate, and interferon alpha-2b, which boosts the immune's system's ability to fight the disease, have shown to be more effective than with interferon alone.

AIDS. Today Drs. Luc Montagnier and Robert Gallo, having been given joint credit for the discovery of the HIV virus that causes AIDS, continue their research efforts into producing a vaccine for human immunodeficiency virus (HIV). Research into the cause and successful treatment for AIDS has come a long way since its beginnings in the mid-1980s. Better medications prolonging the quality of life are being used. Patients are indeed living longer, but the sad fact is that this disease still does not have a definitive cure or vaccine to prevent the disease. AIDS is now recognized universally as a disease that strikes not only the homosexual populations and I.V. drug users, but also all groups—male or female, teens and adults, nondrug users, and newborns of infected mothers. It is distributed worldwide, with several strains now identifiable.

Other milestones. One of the most important areas of concern today is the vast numbers of **emerging pathogens** now being recognized. Once thought to be mere saprophytes found throughout the environment and occasionally in water, ventilation systems, and other unsuspecting areas, these microorganisms are now recognized as having developed into a number of potentially lethal microorganisms. These microorganisms may be found as normal flora or as easy-to-treat pathogens in the normal population, but in patients who are immunocompromised (such as when a person develops full-blown AIDS), these organisms can lead to death. Some of these emerging pathogens include the fungus *Candida albicans,* other **saprophytic** *Candida* species, and *Coccidioides immitis,* a soil fungus, all of which can cause meningitis, kidney disease, and pneumonia. Parasites found in water such as *Cryptosporidia,* which was responsible for an intestinal outbreak in Milwaukee, Wisconsin, and viruses such as *Herpes simplex* I can also have devastating effects for the immunocompromised. Tuberculosis, once almost eliminated, is now back with a vengeance and even more resistant to traditional therapies. Nonhuman mycobacterium species *(m. avium)* are now pathogenic to some. It is a challenge for our researchers to find adequate treatments that will eliminate rogue microorganisms. Microbiology into the twenty-first century will address the priority issues of vaccines, treatments, and cures.

OTHER AREAS OF MICROBIOLOGY

At present, the knowledge of the origin, behavior, and control of microorganisms can be applied to other specialized fields that affect our daily lives. These areas range from aquatic microbiology to veterinary microbiology.

Aquatic Microbiology

Aquatic microbiology studies the microorganisms found in marine (seawater) and fresh water. For instance, the teeming microbe population found in marine water is an essential component of many food cycles that provide nutrition for sea life. Human beings are becoming increasingly dependent upon the sea for many of its products in the areas of nutrition, health, and industry.

Agricultural Microbiology

Agricultural microbiology includes dairy and food microbiology. A dairy microbiologist is concerned with the proper pasteurization, processing, and grading of milk and milk products. These processes ensure that the dairy product is safe for human consumption and is free from contamination and spoilage.

The food microbiologist ensures that food is safe for human ingestion by carefully monitoring the processing, cooking, storage, and serving of food. These actions help to minimize the danger of contaminated food as well as food poisoning to humans. By rigid meat inspections, and careful control of other food and material additives, the monitoring process ensures that high-quality food products reach the consumer. Proper environmental and personal sanitation controls in food processing plants as well as enforcements of local, state, and federal health laws contribute to the quality control of the food product that ends up on the grocers' shelves.

Environmental Microbiology

Environmental microbiology is in itself a diverse field of interest. It includes air, soil, sewage, and water microbiology.

In air microbiology, air is monitored to see what kinds and numbers of microorganisms are present and how they are carried through the air. The monitoring is important because many diseases can be caused by airborne microbes that cling to dust and water droplets.

Soil microbiology studies the types and numbers of microorganisms found in the soil. This field of study is essential because microbes are responsible for soil fertility, plant maintenance, and recycling of dead organic matter (dead animals and plants) into inorganic elements.

Water and sewage microbiology is concerned with the control of disease-causing microbes found in drinking water and sewage, and is achieved through a process of mechanical filtration and chemical treatment of water. Sewage treatment involves the elimination of disease-causing and odor-causing microorganisms. Thus, water and sewage microbiology is essential to the health of humans as well as fish and other aquatic life.

Industrial Microbiology

There are countless products in daily use that are produced by the chemical action of microbes. These include alcohol, beer, wine, antibiotics, enzymes, organic acids, medicines, and vitamins. Industrial microbiologists "exploit" these little microbes to produce essential products at maximum volume with minimum cost.

Many animal and plant diseases are carried by insect carriers or **vectors.** The control and extermination of such insects is the goal of insect microbiology. In the past, potent insecticides and pesticides were used; however, they have had their ecological and environmental consequences. Continued research will find more ecologically safe biological methods that will not harm animals, birds, fish, humans, or beneficial insects.

Space Microbiology or Exobiology

Exobiology is a developing field of microbiology that began when earth scientists launched the first space satellite. A space microbiologist investigates the possibility of microbial life in outer space and on other planetary bodies (extraterrestrial life). Exobiology also deals with the prevention of contamination of earth microbes in outer space and on other planets through our astronauts and spacecrafts and vice versa.

Medical Microbiology

Medical microbiology is the study of bacteria, viruses, fungi, parasites, and other microorganisms that may cause disease (pathogens) or be infectious to humans or animals. Microorganisms are examined for their growth characteristics, similarities and differences, reaction to antibiotics, **epidemiology,** and biochemical reactions. Patterns for their disease potential, **virulence,** and **mutagenic** abilities can be helpful in predicting or determining a patient's **prognosis.** Some of the most common saprophytic microorganisms found in the air, soil, and in our bodies can cause life-threatening illnesses to one whose immune system has been compromised by HIV, toxic chemotherapy, malignancies, and other immune disorders. In addition to the identification and susceptibility of microorganisms, medical microbiology also includes the development of safe and effective methods to prevent, control, and cure diseases. The organisms studied in this textbook are mainly those with medical microbiological significance.

Veterinary Microbiology

Veterinary microbiology studies the transmission and spread and control of diseases between animals and from animals to humans. It also studies the care and breeding of livestock for human nutrition and the care of pets.

PREVENTING INFECTION

The majority of microorganisms are harmless. In fact, many are essential for life to continue on earth. However, some microorganisms are pathogenic, that is, they are harmful or cause disease.

A person with low physical resistance is especially prone to pathogenic microbial invasion. Microorganisms may cause either mild or severe disturbances in the human body. Health professionals have the responsibility to do everything possible to protect their patients. They must, therefore, be aware of the constant presence and characteristics of microorganisms.

It is vital to know how to provide proper health care. Some important health care procedures include proper handwashing, changing bed linen, sterilizing equipment, and disinfecting thermometers.

Prevention and control of disease is the responsibility of every member of the health care team. Microorganisms can cause wound infections and intestinal disorders, as well as diseases such as tuberculosis. The health specialist sets an example by keeping the surroundings clean and safe, whether in the clinic, hospital, or home.

Directly and indirectly, patients and others can be taught to practice good hygienic measures. Good hygiene contributes to the health of both the individual and the community. The best way to prevent the spread of disease is to practice good handwashing techniques:

1. Use continuously running warm water.
2. Use a generous amount of soap.
3. Apply the soap and rub hands together with vigor.
4. Count slowly to ten, or time 10 seconds on a clock.
5. Be sure to clean under and around the nails, and do not forget to wash thumbs.
6. Keeping hands pointed down, rinse well with warm water.
7. Using paper towels or clean terry cloth towels, dry hands well.
8. Turn water off with a paper towel, so as not to recontaminate the hands.

SUMMARY

In this chapter we examine the historical aspects of the development of microbiology as a science today. We discuss the milestones of the earliest pioneers who recognized that disease must be caused by some external foreign force that invaded the body and who contributed to the development in the eradication, control, and treatment of microbiological infections. Bacteria were first recognized following the crude development of a microscope by Anton Leeuwenhoek. Spontaneous generation was finally disproved by Louis Pasteur and John Tyndall some 100 years after scientists failed to give credit to Francesco Redi's decaying meat experiment. Vaccinations to prevent disease were first developed by Edward Jenner, who successfully developed the smallpox vaccine. Louis Pasteur, the "father of bacteriology," ushered in the era of the science of bacteriology with numerous experiments and discoveries, including pasteurization and vaccines for cholera, rabies, anthrax, and chicken pox. The concepts of cleanliness, sterility, and handwashing were finally recognized as the most important indicators to the prevention and spreading of disease following Lord Joseph Lister's application of Pasteur's germ theory of disease to his surgical practice. He correctly surmised that if bacteria come from the environment, then they could easily be responsible for infections in wounds following surgery. By washing his hands and instruments in carbolic acid or phenol, spraying the air with a mist of phenol, and applying the same to surgical dressing, he discovered the fatality rate of his patients decreased phenomenally. Thus began the era of aseptic surgery. Robert Koch's postulates became a guiding principle for microbiologists. The twentieth century saw the dawn of the science of immunology with many vaccinations, immunizations, and antibiotics being developed. First among the antibiotics was penicillin, to be followed over the years by many others. Viruses were identified first with the tobacco mosaic virus and the development of the electron microscope. Vaccines for polio, yellow fever, diphtheria, hepatitis, measles, mumps, rubella, and many others were developed. Scientists are closer today in the development of a vaccine for the virus that causes AIDS. The dawn of the twenty-first century brings hope of a cure for this insidious disease.

STUDY AND DISCUSSION

- Individually, or in small groups, prepare a report about one or more of the scientists discussed in this chapter. Show how his or her contribution has helped people.
- Explore and discuss these other areas in microbiology: immunology, virology, mycology, phycology, protozoology, and microbial genetics.
- Discuss the steps taken by members of the health care team in a hospital to prevent infection. How can these steps be used outside the hospital environment?
- Find a newspaper or magazine article that deals with microorganisms, and discuss it with the class.

REVIEW QUESTIONS

A. General Questions: Provide complete answers to each of the following.

1. What is microbiology?

2. Discuss Anton van Leeuwenhoek's role in the development of microbiology and why he is called the "Father of Microbiology."

3. What is the theory of spontaneous generation? What is another term for it?

4. Briefly explain how Redi and Spallanzani tried to disprove the theory of spontaneous generation.

5. Discuss why Louis Pasteur and John Tyndall were finally successful at disproving the theory of spontaneous generation.

6. Explain how pasteurization prevents beer, wine, and milk from spoiling.

7. State and explain the germ theory of disease.

8. What is meant by the term *attenuated pathogen?*

9. What is meant by a heat-labile bacterium?

10. What is the difference between antiseptic surgery and aseptic surgery?

11. List all the important points in Koch's postulates.

12. What contribution did Sir Alexander Fleming make to the conquest of disease?

13. Explain the job of dairy and food microbiologists. Explain why their jobs are so important to our well-being.

14. What are some of the products an industrial microbiologist produces for our daily use?

15. What is the newest field of microbiology and what does it study?

16. List three things you as a health care professional can do to prevent and control the spread of disease.

B. Matching Questions: Match the names in Column I with the contributions in Column II.

Column I		Column II
_______	1. Gladys and George Dick	a. Germ theory of disease
_______	2. Dr. Jonas Salk	b. Polio vaccination
_______	3. Sir Alexander Fleming	c. Microscopic organisms
_______	4. Louis Pasteur	d. Penicillin
_______	5. Albert Sabin	e. Scarlet fever test
_______	6. Anton van Leeuwenhoek	f. Oral polio vaccine
_______	7. Robert Koch	g. Isolation of tuberculosis microorganisms
_______	8. Béla Schick	h. Yellow fever virus
_______	9. Martinus Beijerinck	i. Tobacco mosaic virus
_______	10. Major Walter Reed	j. Diphtheria
_______	11. Luc Montagnier/Robert Gallo	k. HIV

C. Multiple Choice Questions: Select the letter of the choice that best answers the question.

1. The study of all tiny or minute organisms is _______ .
   a. bacteriology
   b. microbiology
   c. virology
   d. parasitology
   e. mycology

2. The first microscope was made by _______ .
   a. Anton van Leeuwenhoek
   b. Robert Hooke
   c. Lazzaro Spallanzani
   d. John Tyndall
3. Supporters of the theory of spontaneous generation included:
   a. Spallanzani
   b. Redi
   c. Pasteur
   d. Needham
4. Mycology is the study of _______ .
   a. birds
   b. fungi
   c. parasites
   d. viruses
5. A bacillus is a _______-shaped organism.
   a. spheroid
   b. club
   c. rod
   d. spiral
6. Edward Jenner discovered a cure for _______ .
   a. rabies
   b. smallpox
   c. anthrax
   d. syphilis
7. _______ was the first to introduce disinfectants to the operating room.
   a. Robert Koch
   b. John Tyndall
   c. Joseph Lister
   d. Louis Pasteur
8. The idea of proper handwashing techniques in a hospital environment was introduced _______ .
   a. as a result of the AIDS and hepatitis concerns
   b. by the new OSHA rules on bloodborne pathogens
   c. by Lord Joseph Lister
   d. by a Hungarian obstetrician some 150 years ago.
9. The first cure for syphilis was _______ .
   a. penicillin
   b. salvarsan
   c. sulfonamide
   d. streptomycin
10. The Dick test was developed for susceptibility to _______ .
    a. scarlet fever
    b. strep throat
    c. yellow fever
    d. diphtheria
11. The oral polio vaccine was developed by _______ .
    a. Jonas Salk
    b. Albert Schweitzer
    c. Albert Sabin
    d. Walter Reed
12. Yellow jaundice is _______ .
    a. hepatitis
    b. yellow fever
    c. encephalitis
    d. infantile paralysis
13. The bloodborne pathogen of most concern to health care workers is _______ .
    a. hepatitis A
    b. hepatitis B
    c. malaria
    d. both a and b

D. Fill in the Blank: From the following list of terms, fill in the blanks with the correct choice.

virulence	attenuate	bacteriophage
leukemia	puerperal fever	pasteurization
disinfection	Streptococcus	environmental
petri	industrial	agricultural
saprophyte	anthrax	contagious

1. The heating of milk to destroy pathogenic organisms is known as _______ .
2. _______ is a malignant disease of the white blood cells.
3. A _______ is a virus that attacks only bacteria.
4. A disease that often killed new mothers after delivery was called _______ , and the culprit organism was a _______ .
5. Killing pathogens by chemical or physical means is called _______ .
6. The severity of a disease can be measured by the _______ of the organism causing the illness.
7. To weaken or dilute the degree of pathogenicity of a microorganism by chemical or physical means is to _______ it.
8. A special plate or dish used to hold culture media upon which bacteria grow is a _______ dish.
9. _______ microbiologists are concerned with microorganisms found in air, soil, and sewage.
10. _______ microbiologists are concerned with microorganisms found in meats, dairy products, and canneries.
11. _______ microbiologists are concerned with microorganisms found in medicines, vitamins, and beer.
12. An organism that gets its nutrients from another but does it no harm is called a _______ .
13. A disease of cattle that is also extremely harmful to humans is _______ .
14. A disease is _______ when it can be passed from one person to another.

CHAPTER

2

The Microscope

OBJECTIVES

After completing this chapter, you will be able to:

- identify the parts of the compound microscope and describe their functions.
- demonstrate use of the microscope by focusing on a prepared slide or object.

KEY WORDS

binocular microscope
brightfield microscope
compound microscope
darkfield microscope
electron microscope
fixation
millimeter
monocular microscope
objective lens
ocular lens
oil-immersion objective
organelle
parfocal
phase-contrast microscopy
resolution
stain
turret

THE MICROSCOPE

The microscope, an instrument used to magnify objects hundreds and even thousands of times, is one of the most important diagnostic tools used by the microbiologist. The earliest microscopes were very simple as compared with those used today. The first, used by Anton van Leeuwenhoek, was merely a single piece of ground glass fixed between two perforated metal plates. Today, microscopes can be so complex that microscopic material magnified thousands of times can be photographed in detail, projected onto video screens, and even videotaped for future use. **Electron microscopes** utilizing beams of electrons encased in a vacuum tube can detail the smallest **organelles** within a single cell and magnify the tiniest of viruses, once thought to be the invisible microbes because of their size.

The binocular compound (ocular as well as objective lens to magnify the object) light or **brightfield microscope** (one whose light source illuminates the object from below) is the one most commonly found in microbiology laboratories today. Other useful microscopes include the **darkfield microscope,** in which the background is dark so that unstained organisms such as the spirochete can be seen; the fluorescent microscope, which enhances materials stained with fluorescent dyes; and phase-contrast microscopes, which allow observation of dense structures in living organisms such as platelets—the clotting elements found in blood.

THE COMPOUND MICROSCOPE

Today's **compound microscope** (Figure 2–1) has a two-lens system of magnification. One, often called the **ocular lens,** is in the eyepiece. The other lens, through which the object is viewed, is called the **objective lens.**

The optical parts of the modern compound light microscope are the ocular lens mounted in the eyepiece and two or three objective lenses. Depending on the microscope, the ocular lens can be just one ocular lens mounted in one eyepiece housing, which is called the **monocular microscope.** Two ocular lenses each mounted in separate eyepiece housings together are called a **binocular microscope.** The ocular lens in the eyepiece gen-

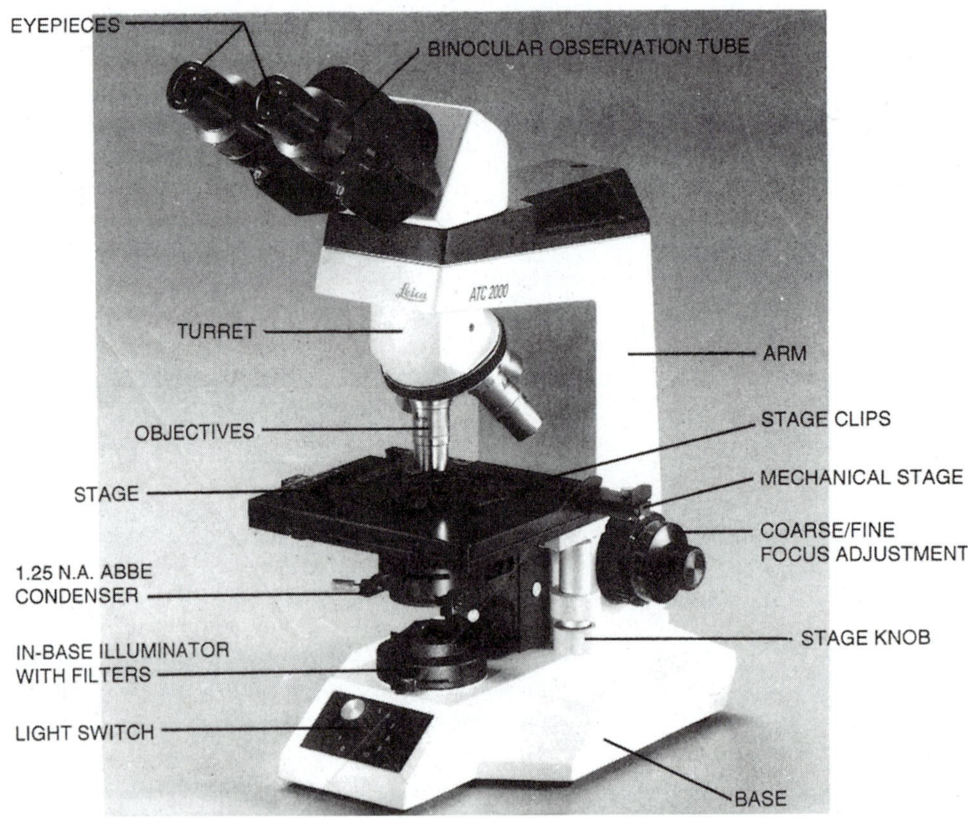

Figure 2–1 ATC 2000 Advanced compound microscope (*Courtesy of Leica Inc., Buffalo, New York*)

erally has a magnification of 10X (10 times). "X" means the power or times the actual (normal) size of a specimen is being viewed.

The objective lenses are usually mounted on a rotating wheel called a **turret** or revolving nosepiece. A low-power objective lens, high-power objective lens, and an oil-immersion lens are mounted beneath the turret. The objective lenses can be rotated depending on the total magnification desired and the object being viewed. The low-power objective has the shortest length and is generally used to locate microbes to be studied. It gives a magnification of 10X. Together, the ocular lens and the low-power objective lens give the specimen a total magnification of 100 times (100X), (10X × 10X = 100X). In other words, the ocular lens in the eyepiece (10X) times the low-power objective (10X) cause the specimen to appear enlarged 100 times (100X) its normal size.

Eyepiece magnification does not change; however, objective magnification may change, depending on the objective being used. A high-power objective, for instance, usually has a magnification power of 45 times (45X). Therefore, if a high-power objective is used, the total magnification power is 45X times 10X = 450X. Once located and brought into clear view using the 10X objective, this higher magnification then allows the microbiologist to study some of the larger microorganisms such as protozoa (one-celled animals) in greater detail.

To view bacteria clearly, an even greater magnification is preferred. In such cases, the **oil-immersion objective** is used (Figure 2–2). Its total magnification is 950X or 1000X. Microbiologists prefer this objective for viewing bacteriological material because of the enhanced color and clarity of stained material and because the oil-immersion objective gives a higher magnification than any other lens. When in use it requires the greatest care and attention, because it comes very close to the specimen. When the oil-immersion lens is fully focused, the distance between it and the cover slip is only a fraction of a **millimeter** (Table 2–1). At such a high magnification (1000X for an oil-immersion lens), much more light is needed. Thus, procedures must be taken to avoid the loss and scattering of light in the air space between the coverslip and the objective lens. A drop of immersion oil is used to help concentrate the light; otherwise the image will be too dark and blurred. A drop of immersion oil (cedar or mineral oil) is placed directly on the slide or on the tiny coverslip covering the specimen. Then the oil-immersion objective is very carefully rotated onto the oil. (The objective should never touch the coverslip or slide.) Then focus is away from the coverslip, as with any other lens. This prevents the coverslip, slide, and objective lens from breaking. The oil-immersion lens has greater light-gathering power and greater resolution than regular powerful lenses. Thus, the image viewed through a compound light microscope using an oil-immersion objective is much brighter and sharper than in a microscope using an objective of the same power but not designed for oil immersion.

There is, of course, more to a compound microscope than the lenses or optical parts. The compound microscope also has several mechanical parts and an illuminating or light source system. The mechanical parts include the body tube, revolving nosepiece (housing the low-power, high-power, and oil-immersion objectives), stage clips or mechanical stage, arm, base, and the coarse and fine adjustment knobs. Depending on the design of the microscope, the coarse and fine adjustment knobs can do one of two things. They can raise and lower the stage or the body tube and nosepiece. The coarse adjustment knob

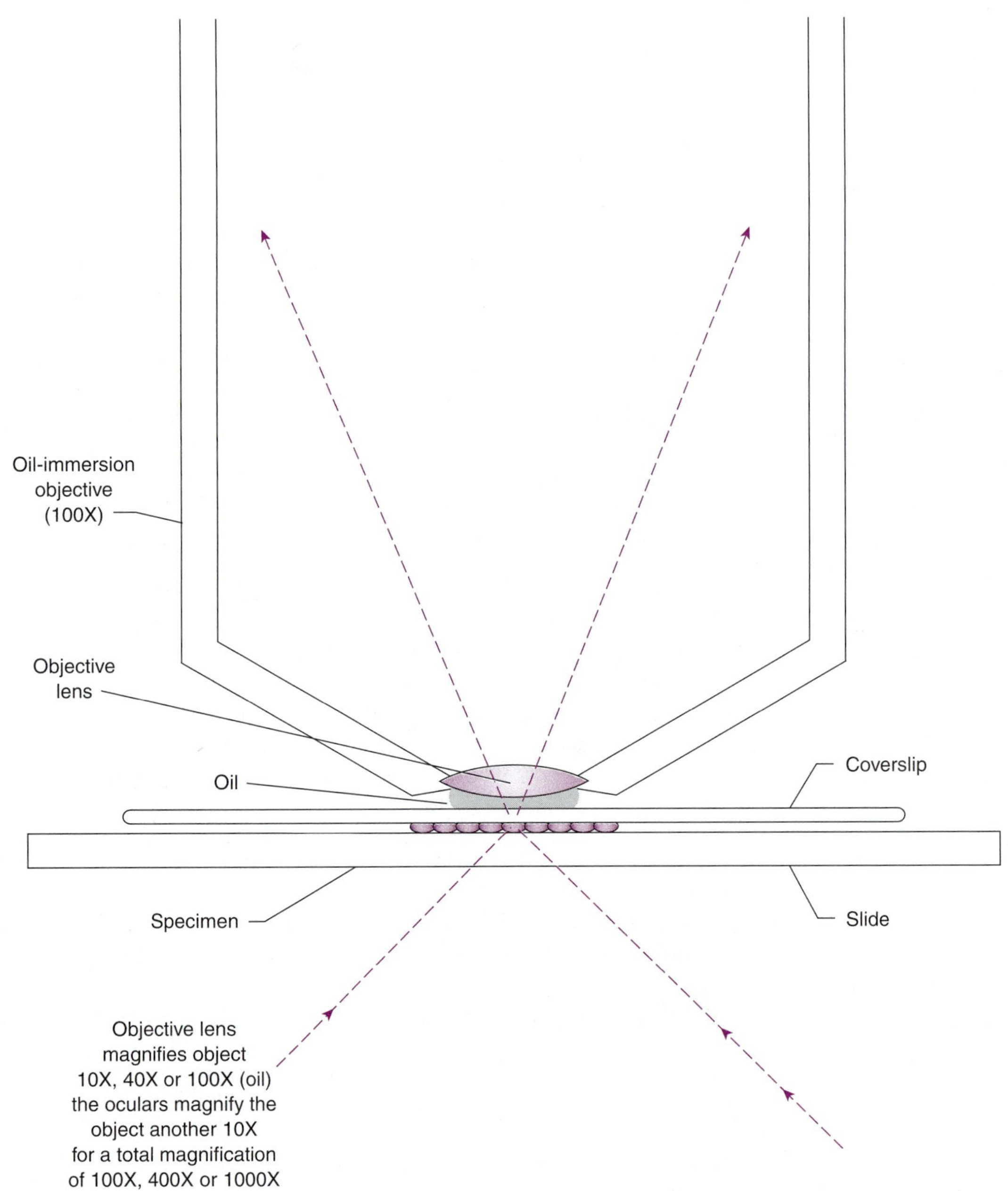

Figure 2–2 Oil-immersion objective

Table 2–1 Units of Length in the Metric System and Math for Review

1 meter = 39.37 inches
1 centimeter (cm) = 1/100 or 0.01 or 10^{-2} meter
1 millimeter (mm) = 1/1000 or 0.001 or 10^{-3} meter
1 micrometer (μm) or micron (μ) = 1/1,000,000 or 0.000001 or 10^{-6} meters
1 nanometer (nm) = 1/1,000,000,000 or 0.000000001 or 10^{-9} meter
angstrom (Å) = 1,10,000,000,000 or 0.0000000001 meter or 10^{-10} meter

2.54 cm = 1 inch
100 cm = 1 meter ($10^2 = 100$)
1000 mm = 1 meter ($10^3 = 1000$)
1,000,000 micrometers = 1 meter ($10^6 = 1{,}000{,}000$)
or 1 micrometer = 10^{-6} meter
and 1 nanometer = 10^{-9} meter

terms: centi = hundredths
milli = thousandths
micro = millionths
nano = billionths

$$\frac{1 \text{ in}}{1 \text{ m}} = \frac{2.54 \text{ cm}}{100 \text{ cm}}$$

$$1 \text{ in} = \frac{2.54 \text{ cm} \times 1 \text{ m}}{100 \text{ cm}} = 2.54 \times 10^{-2} \text{ meter}$$

Therefore, if 1 inch = 2.54×10^{-2} meter, or 0.0254 meter,
and 10^6 micrometers = 1 meter,

$$\text{then } 1 \text{ inch} = 0.0254 \text{ meter} \times \frac{10^6 \text{ micrometers}}{1 \text{ meter}}$$

and 1 inch = 25,400 micrometers.
Dividing both sides by 25,400,

$$\frac{1 \text{ inch}}{25{,}400} = \frac{25{,}400 \text{ micrometers}}{25{,}400}$$

Thus, 1 micrometer = 1/25,400 inch
and 1 nanometer = 1/25,400,000 inch.

moves the microscope part over a greater vertical distance, bringing the specimen into approximate focus. The fine adjustment knob lowers and raises the microscope part very slowly for finer focusing and resolution.

Most people can easily separate two tiny objects or points lying as close together as 0.03 millimeter without the aid of a magnifier (1 millimeter equals 1/25 of an inch). Any closer than 0.03 millimeter the two objects are usually seen as one object. The ability of a lens to clearly distinguish between two such objects is referred to as its resolving power or

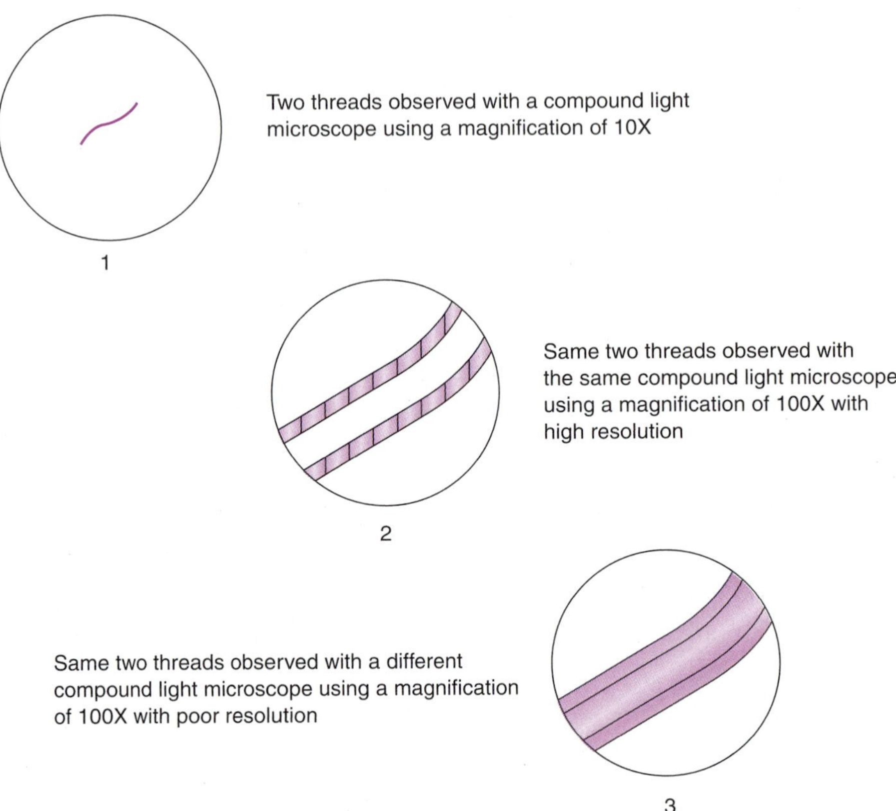

Figure 2–3 Magnification and resolution

resolution. The resolution makes objects more clear, while the magnification enlarges objects. The microscope allows the human eye to distinguish between two objects as close as 0.0002 millimeter. It is useless to increase the magnification without also increasing the microscope's clarity or resolution. Without excellent resolution, details of the enlarged object are not distinguishable (Figure 2–3).

The illuminating system of the compound microscope is made up of a built-in lamp, a condenser lens, and the diaphragm. The lamp sends light through the opening in the stage, then through the specimen and the objective lens, and finally to the eye, which receives the magnified image. The Abbe condenser is a lens or a system of lenses found under the central opening in the stage. It is designed to gather and concentrate the light that comes from the built-in lamps. Thus, the Abbe condenser will direct the light upward through the opening in the stage and then through the specimen. The condenser also houses the iris diaphragm, which regulates the amount of light entering the objective just as the human iris regulates the amount of light entering a person's eye. A lever or a rotating knob is used to operate the diaphragm. A separate adjustment knob is used to lower or raise the Abbe condenser. Lowering the condenser lens lessens the amount of light reaching the specimen, which is generally a disadvantage in microbiological work. It is best to keep the condenser lens fully raised. Any adjustment in the light intensity can be done using the iris diaphragm. The greater the magnification, the greater the amount of light needed.

Magnification is only one of the key elements of microscopy. Even magnified under the compound microscope most organisms appear almost structureless and transparent. To enhance and distinguish the fine details and structures of a specimen to be examined microscopically the specimen is processed through a series of chemical procedures called **fixation** and staining. Fixing (or adhering the material or stain onto the slide or specimen so it will not wash away) causes little damage to the cellular structures of a microorganism. After being chemically treated or heat fixed, the microorganism can be **stained** (dyed) with various types of dyes to make all the structures stand out vividly and to give contrast.

Proper use of the microscope aids in the understanding of microbiology. The world under the microscope can be interesting, exciting, and educational. It is therefore recommended that you do the activities at the end of this chapter, and use them as part of this material.

OTHER KINDS OF MICROSCOPES

Other microscopes are also used by research microbiologists. Several kinds include the darkfield, phase-contrast, and electron microscopes. The darkfield microscope has its source of illumination at the side of the specimen. Thus, the only light reaching the objective is that reflected from the specimen, which makes the specimen appear as a bright object against a dark field or background. In **phase-contrast microscopy,** the microorganisms are observed alive with very sharp contrast; thus, fixation and staining are not needed.

Scanning Electron Microscope. (SEM)

The development of the scanning electron microscope (SEM) brought new areas of study in the medical sciences, because it allows examination of specimens in the greatest of detail (see Figure 2–4). Specimens can be magnified up to 250,000 times and more. As in any microscope, the concept is to gain magnification and clarity of an object. An optical microscope uses lenses to bend the light waves, and the lenses are then adjusted to focus the specimen. In the SEM, electromagnets are used to bend an electron beam, which scans over the area to be magnified and transfers the image to a television screen. By scanning with an electron beam that has been generated and focused by the operation of the microscope, the image is formed in much the same way as in a television. The electron beam stops at 1000 points as it scans across the sample and 1000 lines as it scans down the sample. This produces 1 million points of information. The signal is then transferred to the TV screen. When using electromagnets, the observer has more control over the magnification that is obtained, and the electron beam provides much greater clarity in the image being produced. The SEM allows increased depth of focus compared with the binocular optical microscope in that it can produce an image that is a good representation of a three-dimensional sample (see Figure 2–5).

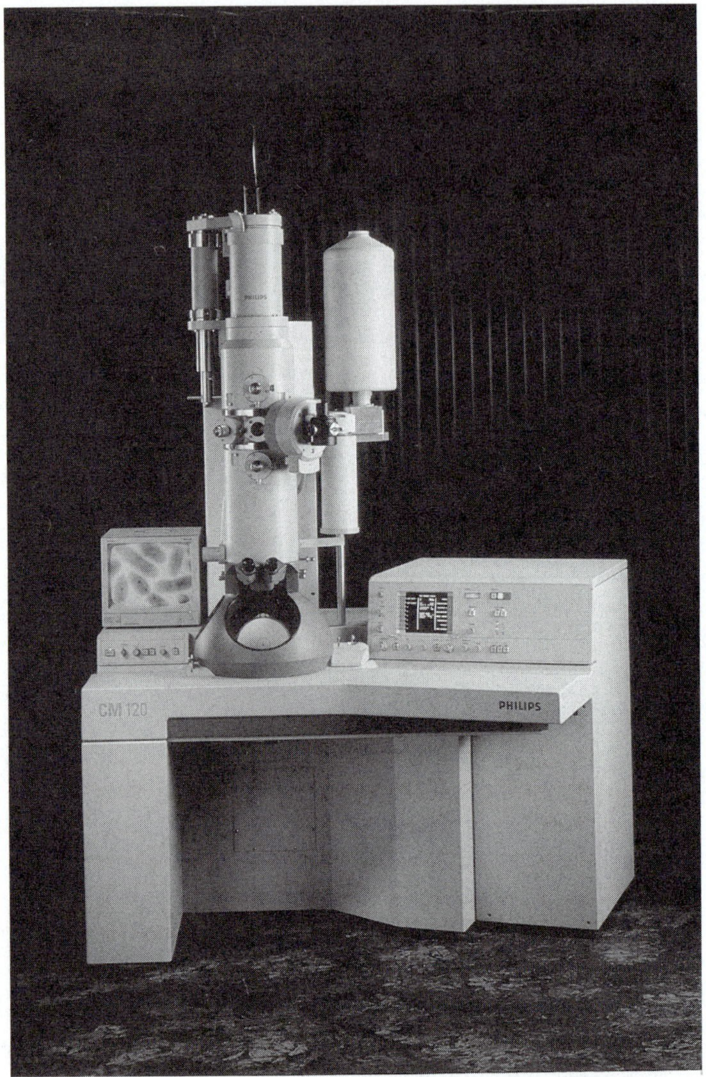

Figure 2–4 S440 Scanning electron microscope (*Courtesy of Leica Inc.*)

STUDY AND DISCUSSION

- Sketch a diagram of a compound microscope and label each part.
- To gain skill in the use of the microscope, follow the procedure outlined here. Use Figure 2–4 for reference. Before handling the microscope, read the procedure and think through the steps. Then proceed with the instructions.

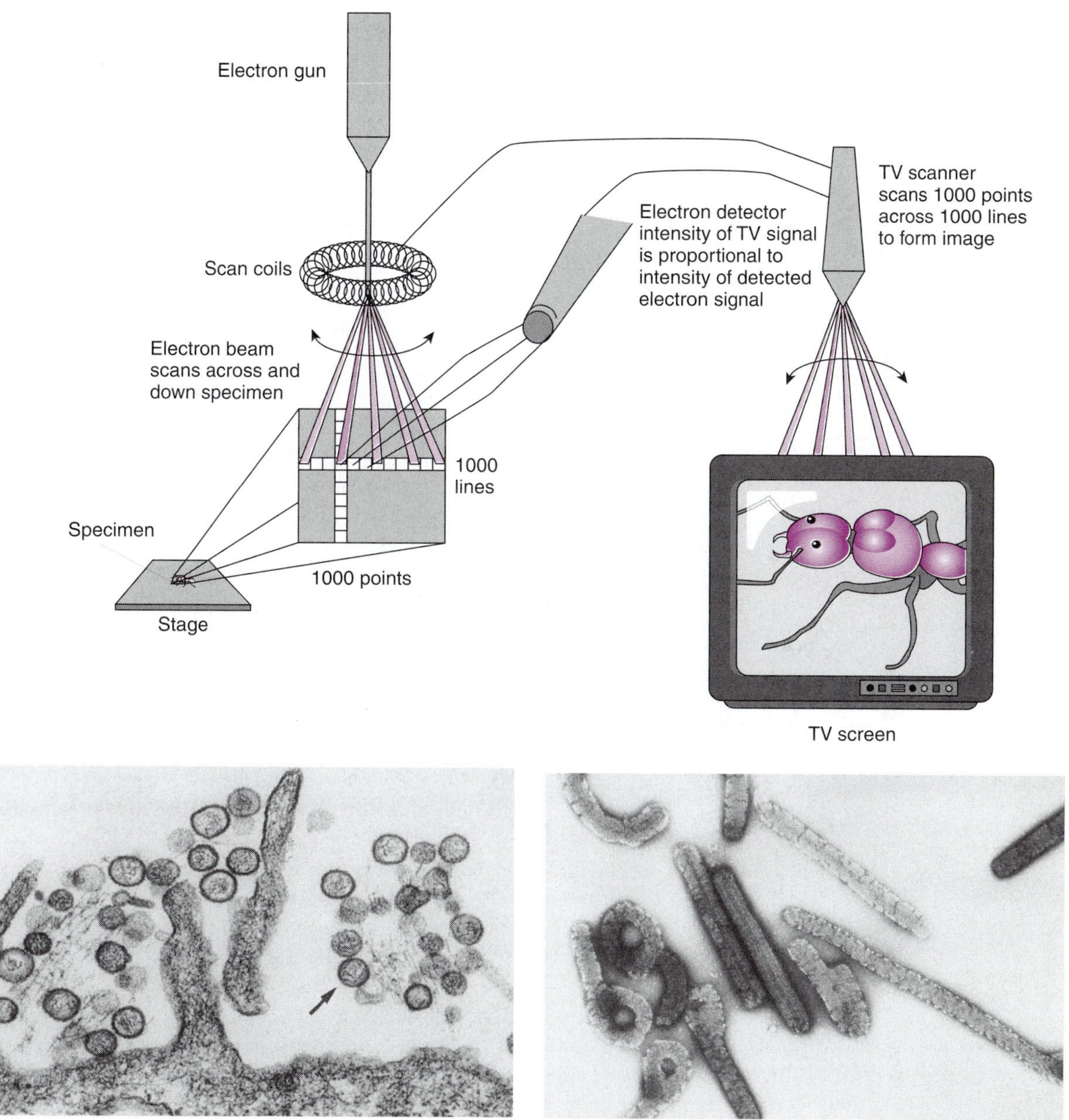

Figure 2–5 (Top) how a scanning electron microscope (SEM) image is produced; (bottom) electron micrographs of (left) hautavirus and (right) ebola virus (*Courtesy of the Centers for Disease Control, Atlanta, Georgia*)

Procedure 2–1 Use and Care of the Microscope

Equipment and Materials Needed

Compound light microscope
Lens paper
Microscope lamp (optional)
Glass slide (optional)
Coverslip (optional)
Small bottle of immersion (cedar or mineral) oil
Water (optional)
Dropper (optional)
Prepared letter "e" slide or any letter slide, prepared slides of bacteria, a sample of human hair, a textile fiber, or any other appropriate specimen
Small bottle of iodine or methylene blue stain

Care and Cautions in Handling the Microscope

1. Always use both hands when carrying the microscope—one hand holding the arm and the other supporting the base (as seen in Figure 2–6).
2. Before starting any laboratory exercise, carefully examine your microscope and report any damage to your instructor.
3. Use clean, dry lens paper to clean off the oculars, objectives, condenser lens, and mirror.
4. Pay close attention to the instructor's directions for operation of your particular microscopes. For some types of microscopes the coarse and fine adjustment knobs bring the stage to the objective lens. On others, the whole body tube is lowered to bring the objective to the stage.

Method

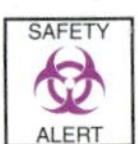

1. Wash hands using good handwashing techniques (especially if using live bacterial or microbial cultures).
2. Assemble the needed equipment and materials.
3. Go to the microscope cabinet and take the microscope assigned to you by the instructor. (*Note:* Use the proper method for carrying a microscope to and from the microscope cabinet, as shown in Figure 2–6).
4. Place the microscope on the table at a convenient height to your seated position. Make sure the arm of the microscope is facing toward your body.
5. Clean the ocular(s) and objectives with lens paper.
6. Adjust the eyepiece using the large screw located between the two eyepieces to suit your individual eye capacity.
7. Locate the coarse adjustment knob on your microscope. Rotate the knob gently and slowly, and watch the upward or downward movement of the body tube.
8. Slowly turn the coarse adjustment knob to raise the revolving nosepiece unit.
9. Turn the condenser knob to raise the condenser.

Procedures for the use of the low-dry objective:

10. Locate the low-dry* objective (10X) and rotate it into place so that it is directly over the opening in the stage.

*The term *dry,* as used in low-dry and high-dry objectives, refers to objectives not needing immersion oil.

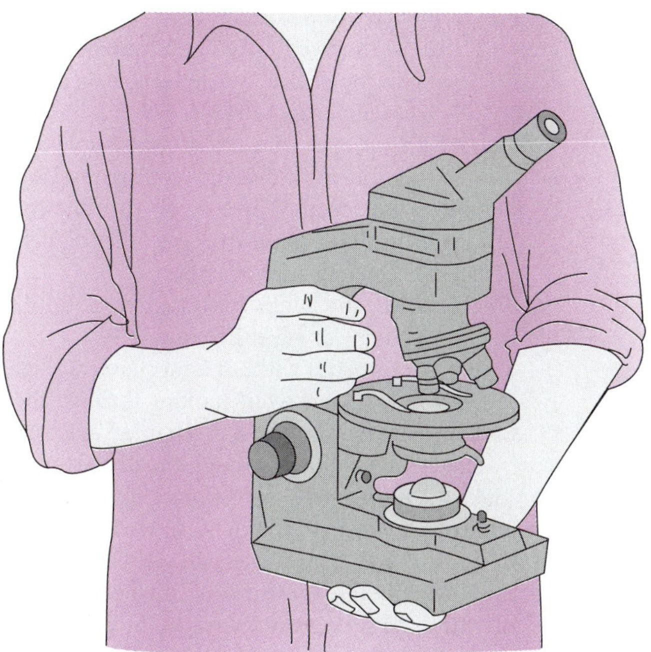

Figure 2–6 Correct method of carrying a microscope

11. For microscopes with a built-in illuminator or lamps, simply turn on the light.
12. Open the diaphragm until the maximum amount of light is coming through the condenser.
13. Gently place the letter "e" slide (or any other prepared letter slide) in the proper reading position (e) on the stage. Make sure the *e* is placed over the opening in the stage. Gently lower the two stage clips over the slide. (If prepared slides are not available, place a sample of a human hair or textile fiber on a slide. Add one drop of water to the specimen and cover with a coverslip.)
14. Locate the coarse adjustment knob.
15. Keeping your eyes on the low-power objective, rotate the coarse adjustment knob until the objective and the slide are as close to each other as possible. Then, looking through the oculars, slowly adjust the coarse adjustment knob until the object comes into focus. This sequence moves the objective away from the slide, allowing your eyes to focus the object without cracking the slide. To avoid scratching the objective lens, do not rotate the coarse adjustment too hard or too fast.
16. Observation and focusing:
    a. For monocular microscopes:
        1. Look into the ocular.
        2. Keep both eyes open. (Yes, both eyes. You will soon learn to ignore anything seen with the other eye through practice.)

b. For binocular microscopes:
   1. Adjust the two oculars horizontally to the width of your eyes. (If your microscope has a knurled collar on each ocular, you will need to adjust each ocular separately.)
   2. With a proper adjustment, you should only see a single, circular field of vision. (The *field of vision* is the bright, round area seen through the ocular(s).)

17. Look into the ocular(s) and slowly turn the coarse adjustment knob to raise the body tube until the letter *e* or any other object on the slide comes into focus.
18. Locate the fine adjustment knob.
19. Turn it slowly and gently back and forth, until the object comes into sharpest focus.
20. Scan the slide by using either step:
    a. For microscopes without a mechanical stage, move the slide in any direction with your fingers while looking through the ocular(s).
    b. For microscopes with a mechanical stage, turn the stage knobs to move the slide while looking through the ocular(s).
21. Make the following observations:
    a. Move the slide to the right. In what direction does the object move?
    b. Move the slide to the left. In what direction does the object move?
    c. Move the slide toward you. In what direction does the object move?
    d. Move the slide away from you. In what direction does the object move?
    e. Open and close the diaphragm. How does this affect the image?

    (*Note:* The low-dry objective should give you an overview of the slide and allow you to select an area for closer examination at the next higher power.)
22. In the space provided, draw a diagram of what you see through the ocular under low-power magnification.

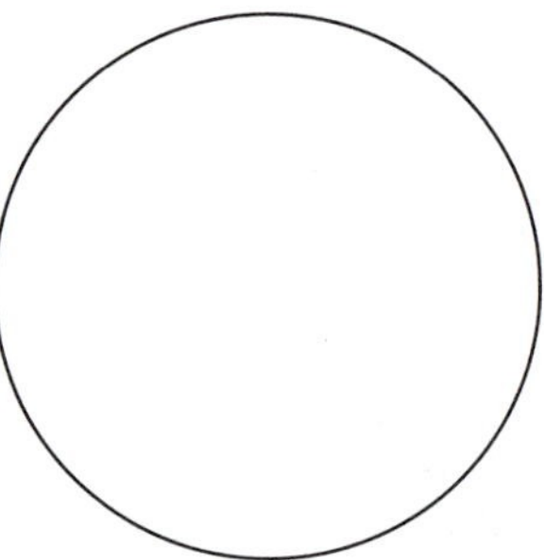

Low-power objective drawing

What is the total magnification of this view? _____

Procedures for the use of the high-dry objective:

23. Select an area you wish to study further, and place it in the center of the field. Rotate the high-dry objective into place while making sure the objective does not "crash" into the slide (Figure 2–7).
24. Look through the ocular(s). The object on the slide should be almost in sharp focus. Focus by rotating the fine adjustment knob *only.* (*Note:* Never use the coarse adjustment knob when the high-dry lens is being used.) Adjust light.

25. In the space provided, draw a diagram of what you see through the ocular under high-power magnification.

High-power objective drawing

What is the total magnification of this view? _____

26. Compare this view under the high-power objective with the one under the low-power microbiology. Explain:
    a. How the amount of light compares with that under low power. (You may need to adjust the diaphragm for better viewing.)
    b. Whether you see a larger or smaller area of the object than was seen under low power.
27. Before continuing with the use of the oil-immersion lens, further practice with the microscope is helpful. This time you will prepare a simple slide for observation.

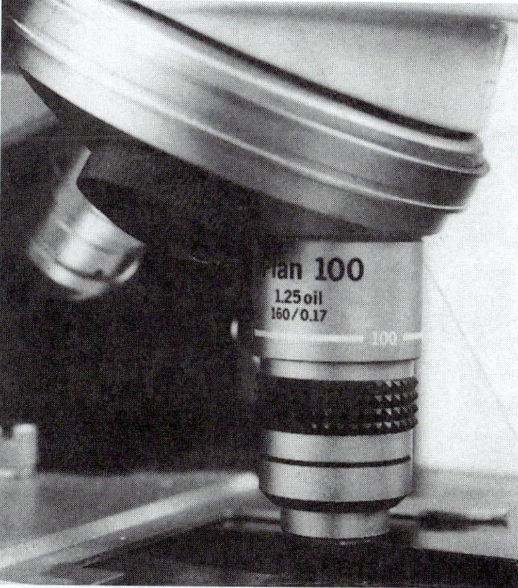

Figure 2–7 When lowering the high-dry or oil objective, use caution so the objective does not crack the slide

28. Procedure for the preparation of a cheek cell slide:
    a. Gently scrape the lining of your cheek with a clean, flat toothpick.
    b. Add a drop of water to a microscope slide, spread the material scraped from your cheek around in the water, and carefully lower a coverslip over it.
    c. Observe under both low- and high-power magnification. (Keep in mind the procedures you learned earlier on the proper use of the low- and high-dry objectives.)
    d. Draw what you see under both magnifications on a separate sheet of paper.
29. Repeat procedure 28, steps a through d, but add a drop of iodine or methylene blue stain to highlight the parts of the cell.

Procedures for the oil-immersion objective:

30. Use a commercially prepared bacterial slide.
31. Repeat procedures 5 through 25.
32. Rotate the high-dry objective a little to one side and place a drop of immersion oil directly over the stage opening.
33. Keeping your eyes on the oil-immersion objective (100X), slowly and gently rotate the 100X lens into place, making sure it does not strike the slide or stage.
34. Still keeping your eye on the 100X objective, carefully lower the body tube until the tip of the lens is immersed in the oil. (Make sure your lens does not touch the slide, as shown in Figure 2–8.)
35. Locate the fine adjustment knob.
36. Look through the ocular(s) and carefully rotate the fine adjustment knob until the specimen comes into focus. Be sure to use *only* the fine adjustment knob when

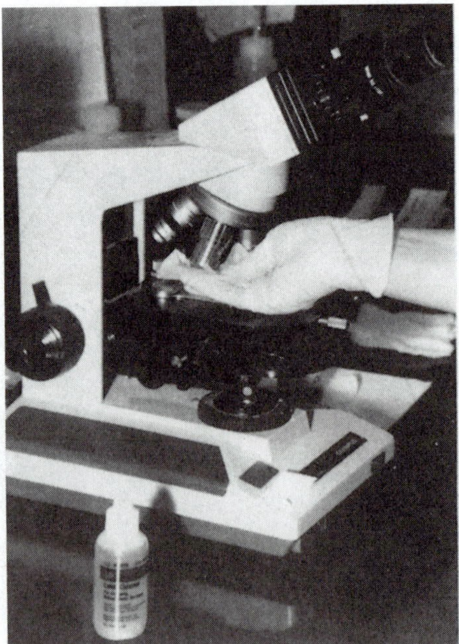

Figure 2–8 Cleaning the objective lens with lens paper and cleaner after use

focusing with the oil-immersion lens. (*Note:* The specimen should come into immediate focus, because most microscopes are **parfocal,** that is, the specimen should remain in focus even when switching from one objective to another. If your microscope is parfocal, you do not have to move the body tube.)

37. Study the image seen through the ocular(s) very carefully using the 100X lens. Make note of the following facts regarding the difference in magnification among the oil-immersion, high-dry, and low-dry objectives.
    a. The oil-immersion magnification is about 2 1/2 times greater than that of the high-dry objective.
    b. It is about 10 times that of the low-dry lens.
38. In the space provided, draw a diagram of what you see through the ocular under oil-immersion magnification.

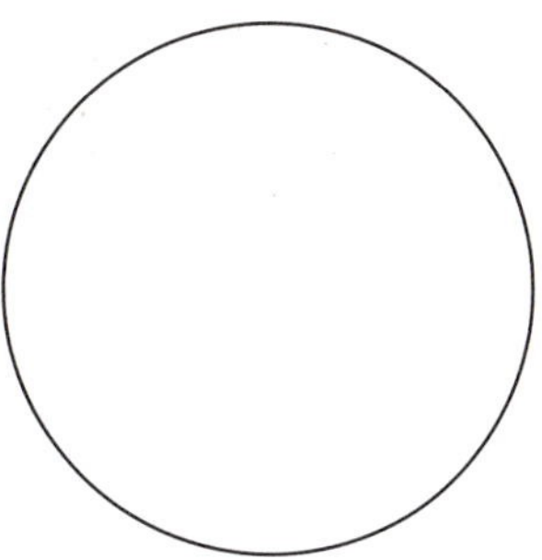

Oil-immersion objective drawing

What is the total magnification of this view? _____

39. When you have finished procedure 38, carefully lower the stage, then rotate the low-dry objective into place. (Do *not* let the high-dry lens touch the oil.)
40. At the end of each use, remove the slide, wipe the oil from the slide and the oil-immersion objective.
41. Clean the stage and the condenser with lens paper.
42. Turn off the microscope light and disconnect.
43. Drop the stage to its lowest level.
44. Rotate the low-power objective so that it is centered above the stage.
45. Unplug and wrap the cord around the base.
46. Place the dust cover over the microscope and return it to the microscope cabinet.
47. Clean the work area around you.

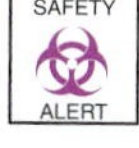

48. Do not forget to wash your hands using the good handwashing techniques described in Chapter 1. Microscopes, as with any piece of equipment, are easily contaminated.

SUMMARY

In this chapter we examine the compound microscope and the scanning electron microscope (SEM). The compound microscope is the trademark for microbiologists and discussion includes identification and uses for all parts of the microscope, and how to use the compound microscope. Two tables illustrating the metric system and a short math review are included so that the reader can attach a relationship to the size of the magnification capability of the microscope and can appreciate just how small bacterial particles are. An exercise describing the methodology for handling and using the microscope concludes this chapter.

REVIEW QUESTIONS

A. General Questions: Provide complete answers to each of the following.

1. Why do you need more light at higher powers?

2. What happens when the condenser is lowered and raised?

3. What is the difference between van Leeuwenhoek's microscope and today's modern microscope?

4. Why is a drop of oil needed when using the oil-immersion objective?

5. What would happen if you lowered the body tube without watching the objective lens?

6. What is the specific function of each of the following parts of the microscope?
   a. Illuminator

   b. Iris or disk diaphragm

c. Ocular lens

d. Low-power lens

e. High-power lens

f. Coarse adjustment control

g. Fine adjustment control

B. Multiple Choice Questions: Select the letter of the choice that best completes the sentence.

1. A binocular microscope has _____ .
   a. two eyepieces
   b. two objectives
   c. two night lights
   d. two light sources
2. The oil-immersion objective is the _____ objective.
   a. 4X
   b. 10X
   c. 40X
   d. 100X
3. The turret is located _____ .
   a. on the stage
   b. on the body tube
   c. on the base
   d. behind the light source
4. The _____ microscope receives its light source from the side.
   a. phase-contrast
   b. fluorescent
   c. electron
   d. darkfield
5. Viruses _____ be seen with a fluorescent microscope.
   a. can
   b. cannot
6. If the eyepiece is 10X and the objective is 100X, the total magnification is _____ .
   a. 110X
   b. 10X
   c. 100X
   d. 1000X
7. The _____ objective is called the oil-immersion lens.
   a. 4X
   b. 10X
   c. 100X
   d. 45X
8. Microscopes are transported _____ .
   a. with one hand on the base
   b. tucked under the arm
   c. with one hand on the body tube
   d. with one hand on the body tube and one hand on the base.
9. Scanning electron microscopes can enlarge an object
   a. 2500 times
   b. 25,000 times
   c. 2,500,000 times
   d. 250,000 times

10. In the scanning electron microscope the light source comes from _____ .
    a. an external light source
    b. an electron beam
    c. a television screen
    d. an objective lens

C. From the following list of terms, fill in the blanks with the correct choice.

Abbe condenser	phase-contrast microscopy	high-dry
electron beam	darkfield microscope	oil
diaphragm	electron microscope	scanning
resolution		

1. The ability to see objects close together with much clarity is called __________ .

2. The microscope in which the object is light against a dark background is the __________ .

3. __________ allows one to view living material.

4. The __________ houses the ___________ .

5. The 45X objective is the __________ objective.

6. The 100X objective is the__________ objective.

7. The 4X or 10X is the __________ objective.

8. The __________ allows one to view organelles.

9. The __________ scans across and down the specimen.

D. Matching Questions: Match the terms in Column I with their corresponding terms in Column II.

Column I		Column II
_______	1. Initial focus	a. 100X objective
_______	2. Requires oil	b. Stage
_______	3. Holds the slide	c. Coarse adjustment knob
_______	4. Final focus	d. Revolving nosepiece
_______	5. Lenses closest to the object	e. Body tube
_______	6. Turret	f. Eyepiece
_______	7. Holds turret	g. Fine adjustment knob
_______	8. Magnifies 10 times	h. Objectives
_______	9. Monocular	i. Lens system
_______	10. Abbe condenser	j. One eyepiece

CHAPTER 3

Basic Chemistry and Its Relationship to Microbiology

OBJECTIVES

After completing this chapter, you will be able to:

- explain the value of a formula and give at least four examples.
- describe the difference between a dilute solution and a concentrated solution.
- describe the difference between an inorganic compound and an organic compound, and list some examples of each.
- explain the difference between dehydration synthesis and hydrolysis and give an example for each reaction.
- differentiate between an amino acid group and a carboxyl group.
- differentiate between the messenger RNA molecule and the transfer RNA molecule.
- explain the process of neutralization and list the products it forms.
- explain indicators and give some examples.
- describe a pH scale and tell what it attempts to measure.
- explain why the maintenance of a specific pH is crucial to all living organisms.

KEY WORDS

acid
active site
adenosine triphosphate (ATP)
alkali
amino acid
amino group
apoenzyme
atom
base
buffer
carbohydrate
carboxyl group
chromosomes
coenzyme
compound
dehydration synthesis
disaccharide
element
enzyme
enzyme–substrate complex
formula
genes
helix
hydrocarbon
hydrolysis
hydronium ion
hydroxide
insoluble
ionize
isomer
lustrous
molecule
monosaccharide
multicellular
neutralization
nucleic acid
nucleotide
organic compound
oxidation
para-aminobenzoic acid (PABA)

KEY WORDS (cont.)

peptide bond
pH
polymer
polypeptide
polysaccharide
protein
ribose
salt
saturated
soluble
solute
solution
solvent
substrate
tincture
unicellular
unsaturated
yield

BASIC CHEMISTRY

Despite the small size of microorganisms, their ability to live and thrive has affected many areas of our daily lives. Health care professionals must have knowledge of the behavior of microbes in order to control them. The behavior and function of all microorganisms is dependent upon many biochemical processes and reactions that occur inside them. In the study of microbes at the molecular level, scientists have gained an insight into the chemical basis of life. To reach some understanding of microbiology at the molecular level, it is wise to have some knowledge of basic chemistry.

The basic chemistry in this chapter will serve as background or reference information for many microbiological ideas mentioned throughout the book. Students with a prior knowledge of chemistry will find it to be a helpful review, while others will encounter it for the first time.

Atoms

All substances, whether they are solids, liquids, or gases, consist of certain fundamental building blocks. The smallest basic particle, the **atom** is made up of negatively charged electrons, positively charged protons, and noncharged neutrons. Protons and neutrons are found in the nucleus of the atom, while the electrons orbit about the nucleus. An uncharged atom will contain the same number of protons and electrons. When electrons are gained or lost, the atom becomes charged. Gained electrons result in a negative charge and lost electrons result in a positive charge. Such gains and losses of electrons are the basis for the bonding of different kinds of atoms.

Elements

Substances containing only one kind of atom are called **elements.** Oxygen, carbon, sodium, and chlorine are examples of elements. There are some 109 elements known today. They are arranged in a periodic table according to their activity (Figure 3–1). Most of the elements are found in nature, but some are humanmade, including curium, neptonium, and plutonium. All the elements are represented by a chemical symbol or abbreviation. Sometimes the symbol comes from the first letter or two of the element—C for carbon, O for oxygen, and Ba for barium—but often the symbol is derived from the Latin

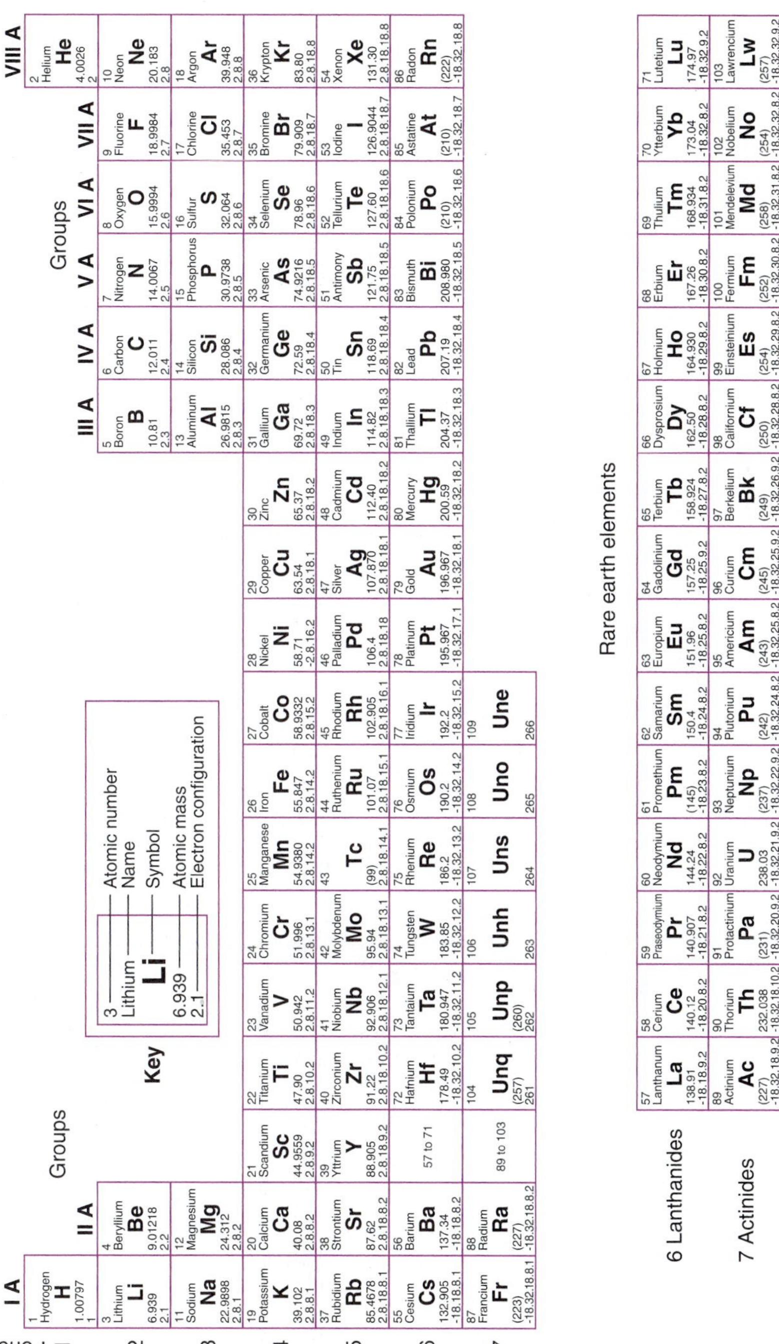

Figure 3–1 Periodic Table of the Elements

Table 3–1 Elements Found in Living Matter

Element	Symbol
Boron	B
Calcium	Ca
Carbon	C
Chlorine	Cl
Cobalt	Co
Copper	Cu
Hydrogen	H
Iron	Fe
Magnesium	Mg
Manganese	Mn
Molybdenum	Mo
Nitrogen	N
Oxygen	O
Phosphorus	P
Potassium	K
Sodium	Na
Sulfur	S
Tin	Sn
Vanadium	V
Zinc	Zn

term for the element—sodium is Na for natrium, gold is Au for aurum, and silver is Ag for argentum. Note that when a chemical symbol has two letters the second letter is always written in lower case.

Of all the elements, approximately twenty are generally found in all living things. Among these twenty elements, four comprise over 97% of all living matter. These are carbon, hydrogen, oxygen, and nitrogen. The remaining sixteen elements are found in very small quantities in living matter, and hence are called "trace elements." Table 3–1 lists these twenty elements with their chemical symbols.

Molecules

When two or more atoms are joined together, a **molecule** is formed. Molecules may be of similar atoms, such as oxygen gas (O_2), or they may be of different atoms, such as carbon dioxide (CO_2). A molecule is an unchanged or neutral particle in which two or more atoms are bonded together.

Compounds

When two or more atoms or molecules are joined in a definite proportion by weight, a **compound** is formed. A compound has different characteristics or properties from the elements that comprise the compound, because a chemical change has occurred. For example, water (H_2O) is made up of two parts (or atoms) of hydrogen and one part (or atom) of oxygen to form one molecule of the compound water. Separately, hydrogen and oxygen are gaseous elements, but when combined to form water, the resulting compound is a liquid. Common table salt is a compound made from the two elements sodium (Na) and chlorine (Cl), and it is chemically called sodium chloride (NaCl). Separately, sodium is a metallic element. It is light, silver-white, and **lustrous** (shiny) when freshly cut, but rapidly becomes dull and gray when exposed to air. Chlorine, on the other hand, is an irritating, greenish-yellow poisonous gas with a suffocating odor. However, the chemical combination of both sodium and chlorine results in sodium chloride, which is a crystalline powder that can be dissolved in water.

Just as elements are represented by symbols, compounds are represented by a **formula.** A formula shows the types of elements present and the proportion of each element present by weight. Some common formulas are H_2O (water), NaCl (common table salt), HCl (hydrogen chloride or hydrochloric acid), $NaHCO_3$ (sodium bicarbonate or baking powder), NaOH (sodium hydroxide or lye), $C_6H_{12}O_6$ (glucose or grape sugar), $C_{12}H_{22}O_{11}$ (sucrose or common table sugar), CO_2 (carbon dioxide), and CO (carbon monoxide).

A living organism, whether it is a **unicellular** (one-celled) microbe or a **multicellular** animal or plant, can be compared with a chemical factory. Most living organisms will take the twenty essential elements and change them into needed compounds for the maintenance of the organism. In many living organisms, the elements carbon, hydrogen, and oxygen are united to form **organic compounds** (compounds found in living things containing the element carbon). An example of organic compounds manufactured are **carbohydrates** such as sugars and starches.

Solutions

Most chemical processes that occur in a living cell or a microbe take place in a **solution.** A solution is a mixture formed when one substance dissolves (readily disappears) into another substance. The substance that dissolves is known as the **solute.** The substance that the solute blends into is called the **solvent.** A substance that can dissolve into a solvent is said to be **soluble.** A substance that cannot dissolve into a solvent is either **insoluble** or slightly soluble. For example, sugar is soluble in water, thus forming a sugar solution. However, starch is insoluble in water, thereby forming no solution. Water dissolves so many substances it is generally called the "universal solvent." In microbiology, a solution of alcohol and some other substance is known as a **tincture.** For instance, a solution of alcohol and iodine is called tincture of iodine. Table 3–2 gives some examples of different types of solutions.

Types of Compounds

Elements can combine in a variety of ways to form a great number of compounds. All known compounds, whether natural or synthetic, can be classified into two groups—inorganic and organic.

Table 3–2 Types of Solutions

State of Solvent and of Solution	State of Solute	Example
Gas	Gas	Air
	Liquid	Air containing moisture crystals
	Solid	Air with vapor from "moth crystals"
Liquid	Gas	Carbonated water
	Liquid	Alcohol and water
	Solid	Sugar in water
Solid	Gas	Pallidium–hydrogen alloy
	Liquid	Rubber with ether
	Solid	Coin silver

Inorganic compounds. Inorganic compounds are those that usually do not contain the element carbon, and most often include a metal as the positive ion. Two exceptions are carbon dioxide (CO_2) and calcium carbonate ($CaCO_3$). Many inorganic compounds are found in living organisms and in microbes. Table 3–3 shows a sampling of some inorganic compounds. Most are soluble in water.

Organic compounds. Organic compounds are those that always contain carbon and are found in nature or living things. Some organic compounds found in nature and containing only hydrogen and carbon are referred to as **hydrocarbons.** These substances are mainly gases such as methane (CH_4). Most organic compounds found in living things contain at least carbon, hydrogen, and oxygen. Nitrogen and phosphorus are also important ingredients in many organic compounds. Carbon has the ability to combine with other carbons as well as other elements to form a large number of organic compounds. The carbon-to-carbon linkage allows the formation of large molecules bonded together in "chains."

Table 3–3 Different Types of Inorganic Compounds

Inorganic Compound	Chemical Formula
Calcium carbonate	$CaCO_3$
Calcium phosphate	$Ca(PO_4)_2$
Hydrochloric acid	HCl
Phosphoric acid	H_3PO_4
Potassium chloride	KCl
Sulfuric acid	H_2SO_4
Sodium bicarbonate	$NaHCO_3$
Sodium chloride	$NaCL$
Water	H_2O

Table 3–4 Different Types of Organic Compounds

Organic Compound	Chemical Formula
Methane	CH_4
Ethyl alcohol	CH_3CH_2OH (C_2H_5OH)
Isopropyl alcohol	$CH_3CH_2CH_2OH$ (C_3H_7OH)
Glucose	$C_6H_{12}O_6$
Sucrose (table sugar)	$C_{12}H_{22}O_{11}$
Cholesterol	17, C, D, A, B, 3, 5, 6, HO

The molecules of organic compounds are comparatively large and very complex. By comparison, inorganic molecules are much smaller. The four main groups of organic compounds essential to life are carbohydrates, lipids, proteins, and nucleic acids (see Table 3–4).

Carbohydrates

All carbohydrates are compounds composed of the elements carbon (C), hydrogen (H), and oxygen (O). These three elements occur in the ratio of 1:2:1 or CH_2O. Carbohydrates are divided into three groups—monosaccharides, disaccharides, and polysaccharides.

Monosaccharides.

Monosaccharides (Greek *mono*, meaning "one," and *sakcharon*, meaning "sugar") are sugars that in nature cannot be broken down any further. Hence, they are also called single or simple sugars. The three types of monosaccharide sugars are glucose, fructose, and galactose. They are **isomers** of each other. Isomers are compounds that have the same formula but different structures. For example, the formula for glucose, fructose, and galactose is $C_6H_{12}O_6$, but, as seen in Figure 3–2, the structures are different.

```
      H                 H                 H   O
      |                 |                  \ //
      C=O           H-C-OH                  C
      |                 |                   |
  H-C-OH               C=O              H-C-OH
      |                 |                   |
 HO-C-H            HO-C-H              HO-C-H
      |                 |                   |
  H-C-OH            H-C-OH             HO-C-H
      |                 |                   |
  H-C-OH            H-C-OH              H-C-OH
      |                 |                   |
  H-C-OH            H-C-OH              H-C-OH
      |                 |                   |
      H                 H                   H
```

Glucose ($C_6H_{12}O_6$)	Fructose ($C_6H_{12}O_6$)	Galactose ($C_6H_{12}O_6$)

Figure 3–2 Structural Differences between Glucose, Fructose, and Galactose

Organic compounds can be illustrated by their structural formulas, which allows the reader to see exactly where on the chain the bonds are located. Hydrogen bonds have only one bonding, oxygen requires two bonds, carbon requires four bonds, and nitrogen needs three bonds. A single bar (−) denotes one or a single bond. A double bond (equivalent to two bonds) is shown as two bars (=), and a triple bond is drawn as three bars (≡). Double and triple bonds are less stable than single bonds.

$$\begin{array}{cccc} \mathrm{H}- & -\mathrm{O}- & \begin{array}{c}|\\ \diagdown\mathrm{N}\diagup\end{array} & \begin{array}{c}|\\ -\mathrm{C}-\\ |\end{array} \\ \text{1 bond} & \text{2 bonds} & \text{3 bonds} & \text{4 bonds} \end{array}$$

$$\begin{array}{cccc} \mathrm{C{=}C} & \mathrm{C{=}O} & \mathrm{N{\equiv}N} & -\mathrm{C{\equiv}C}- \end{array}$$

Double bonds Triple bonds

CH_4 may be written
$$\begin{array}{c} \mathrm{H} \\ | \\ \mathrm{H{-}C{-}H} \\ | \\ \mathrm{H} \end{array}$$

$CH_3CH_3(C_2H_6)$ may be written
$$\begin{array}{ccccc} & \mathrm{H} & & \mathrm{H} & \\ & | & & | & \\ \mathrm{H}- & \mathrm{C} & - & \mathrm{C} & -\mathrm{H} \\ & | & & | & \\ & \mathrm{H} & & \mathrm{H} & \end{array}$$

Similarly, CH_3CH_2OH (C_2H_5OH) is
$$\begin{array}{ccccc} & \mathrm{H} & & \mathrm{H} & \\ & | & & | & \\ \mathrm{H}- & \mathrm{C} & - & \mathrm{C} & -\mathrm{OH} \\ & | & & | & \\ & \mathrm{H} & & \mathrm{H} & \end{array} \quad \text{or} \quad \begin{array}{ccccc} & \mathrm{H} & & \mathrm{H} & \\ & | & & | & \\ \mathrm{H}- & \mathrm{C} & - & \mathrm{C} & -\mathrm{O}-\mathrm{H} \\ & | & & | & \\ & \mathrm{H} & & \mathrm{H} & \end{array}$$

Structural formulas may also be rotated or mirror images shown without changing the organic compound.

$$\begin{array}{ccccc} & \mathrm{H} & & \mathrm{H} & \\ & | & & | & \\ \mathrm{HO}- & \mathrm{C} & - & \mathrm{C} & -\mathrm{H} \\ & | & & | & \\ & \mathrm{H} & & \mathrm{H} & \end{array}$$ is still C_2H_5OH, ethyl alcohol (ethanol).

Glucose (dextrose or grape sugar) is a very important sugar. It is the main source of energy in cells. Glucose is carried by the bloodstream to individual cells, and is thus called "blood sugar." In the cell, glucose combines with oxygen in a chemical reaction called **oxidation,** which produces high-energy molecules of **adenosine triphosphate (ATP).** The ATP molecule provides the energy source for the cell or microbe and its many cellular or microbial activities.

Fructose is a sugar found in fruits and honey; it is the sweetest monosaccharide. It is an important isomer of glucose because, in the absence of glucose, fructose becomes involved in energy-releasing reactions.

Galactose is found in small amounts in agar, flaxseed, and milk.

Table 3–5 The Monosaccharide Composition of Sucrose, Maltose, and Lactose

Monosaccharide + Monosaccharide − Water (Dehydration Synthesis)		Disaccharide + Water (Hydrolysis)
1. Glucose + Fructose	Dehydration synthesis → / ← Hydrolysis	Sucrose + Water
2. Glucose + Glucose	Dehydration synthesis → / ← Hydrolysis	Maltose + Water
3. Glucose + Galactose	Dehydration synthesis → / ← Hydrolysis	Lactose + Water

Disaccharides. A **disaccharide** is known as a double sugar because it is formed from two monosaccharide molecules by a chemical reaction called **dehydration synthesis.** Dehydration synthesis involves the synthesis of a large molecule from small ones by the loss of a molecule of water. Table 3–5 illustrates the process of dehydration synthesis, and its opposite reaction **hydrolysis,** in which a disaccharide is broken down into two monosaccharides by the addition of water.

Examples of disaccharides are sucrose (table sugar), maltose (malt sugar), and lactose (milk sugar). Common table sugar has the formula $C_{12}H_{22}O_{11}$.

Polysaccharides. A large number of carbohydrates found in or made by living organisms and microbes are polysaccharides. **Polysaccharides** are large, complex molecules made up of hundreds to thousands of glucose* or other simple sugar molecules bonded together in one long chainlike molecule. Such a collection of many similar, repeating molecules forming a large molecule is called a **polymer** (meaning "many parts"). Examples of polysaccharide polymers are starch, cellulose, and glycogen. Under the proper conditions, polysaccharides can be broken down into disaccharides and then finally into monosaccharides.

Starch is made in plant cells, where it serves as the storage form of glucose. Cellulose is a "tough" molecule that gives the necessary rigidity and support to plant cells. It is the main carbohydrate found in cotton, paper, cellophane, and wood. Cellulose molecules are generally longer than starch molecules. Glycogen or "animal starch" is the storage form of glucose found in the liver and muscles of vertebrates. Glycogen molecules are usually shorter than starch or cellulose molecules.

*Other saccharide molecules may also form polysaccharides.

Lipids

Lipids are molecules also containing the elements carbon, hydrogen, and oxygen. Lipids are different from carbohydrates because there is proportionately much less oxygen in relation to hydrogen. For instance, the formula for castor oil is $C_{18}H_{34}O_3$. Their molecules are relatively small, and they are not grouped together as polymers. Examples of lipids are fats, oils, and waxes.

Characteristics of lipids.

At room temperature, fats are solid and oils are liquid, even though they have the same molecular structure. Lipids are much better sources of energy than carbohydrates, which simply means that for a given quantity of fat oxidized, it will **yield** (give up) more energy than does the same quantity of carbohydrate. How-

Table 3–6 Saturated versus Unsaturated Fats

Characteristic	Saturated Fats	Unsaturated Fats
Carbon bonding	Simple covalent bonds C–C	Double covalent bonds C=C
Hydrogen bonds	Fully loaded hydrogen bonds	Lacks 2 hydrogen bonds to form a double covalent bond (monounsaturated), or lacks 8 or more hydrogen bonds forming 4 or more double covalent bonds (polyunsaturated)
Room to body temperatures	Solids	Liquid or soft
Action in blood	Can block arteries	Does not block arteries
Chemical action	Long chains of neatly and tightly packed carbon-hydrogen groups that are very stable and difficult to break up, thus they travel in the circulatory system and sometimes form sticky patches on the arterial walls (plaque)	Long chains of "kinky" double bonds that easily break up and decompose. There are several types of double bonds. One, the "cis" type, is considered to be the most healthy because "cis" bonds or kinks decompose readily. Partially hydrogenated oils do not join their carbons by "cis" bonds, thus they do not readily decompose and are not as healthy
Cholesterol	Raises it	Lowers it
Examples	Butter, meat fat, dairy products, cheese, cream, processed meats (hot dogs), pastry, lard, coconut and palm oils	Polyunsaturates: vegetable, sunflower, safflower, corn, soybean, and cottonseed oils as well as fish oils Monounsaturates: canola oil, olive oil, margarine

ever, more glucose molecules are oxidized in a cell for energy than lipids, because lipids are harder to oxidize.

Lipids are found in many living organisms and they are categorized into three groups: simple lipids, compound lipids, and derived lipids.

Simple lipids contain the elements carbon, hydrogen, and oxygen. Examples are fats and oils such as butter and margarine and corn, olive, peanut, and safflower oils. Other simple lipids are waxes such as beeswax and lanolin. Simple lipids (fats and oils) contain one glycerol molecule and three fatty acid molecules. They may be **saturated** fats (when all bonds between carbon bonds are single because each carbon atom is saturated with hydrogen) or **unsaturated** fats (when two or more of the hydrogen bonds are replaced with double bonds between the carbon atoms (C=C). The more double carbon bonds in a fat the more unsaturated the fat or oil will be. Of the two types of simple lipids, unsaturated fats are easier to digest and are better for us. Table 3–6 compares saturated and unsaturated fats.

Compound lipids are composed of carbon, hydrogen, oxygen, nitrogen, and phosphorus. They include the phospholipids, which are found in cell membranes, and the glycolipids in brain and nerve cells. Compound lipids are not fats, and their amounts remain constant in the organism.

Finally, there are the derived lipids containing only carbon, hydrogen, and oxygen. They include the steroids found in the male and female sex hormones, vitamin D, cholesterol, and the fat-soluble vitamins A, E, and K. These substances are classed as lipids only because they are soluble in fat solvents. See Table 3–6.

Formation of simple lipids. The simple lipids (fats and oils) contain one glycerol ($C_3H_8O_3$) and three fatty acid molecules (C_nH_{2n+1}, C=OOH) (Figure 3–3). A lipid molecule is formed by the dehydration synthesis of one glycerol molecule and three fatty acid molecules (Figure 3–4).

Table 3–7 lists the names, formulas, and sources of some of the more common fatty acids.

Proteins

Proteins are organic compounds containing the elements carbon, hydrogen, oxygen, and nitrogen and, most times, phosphorus and sulfur. Proteins are among the most diverse and essential organic compounds found in all living organisms, including microbes. Proteins are found in every part of a living cell. They are found in the nucleus, the cellular organelles, and in the cell membrane. Proteins are an important part of the outer protein

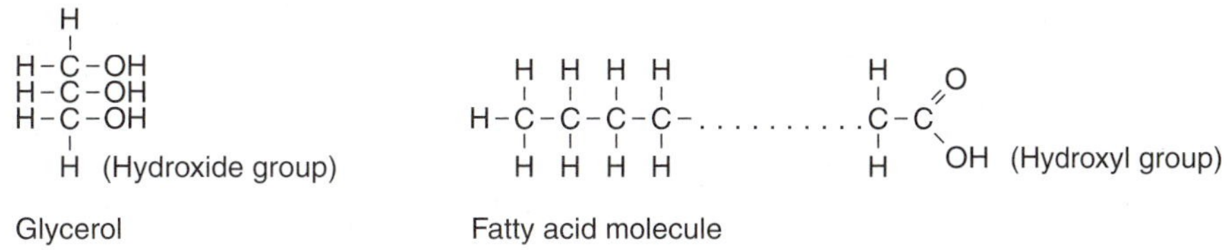

```
    H
    |
H-C-OH                H  H  H  H               H    O
H-C-OH                |  |  |  |               |   //
H-C-OH              H-C--C--C--C-. . . . . . . C-C
    |                 |  |  |  |               |   \
    H (Hydroxide group)  H  H  H  H            H    OH (Hydroxyl group)

Glycerol              Fatty acid molecule
```

Figure 3–3 Structural Formulas for Glycerol and a Fatty Acid Molecule

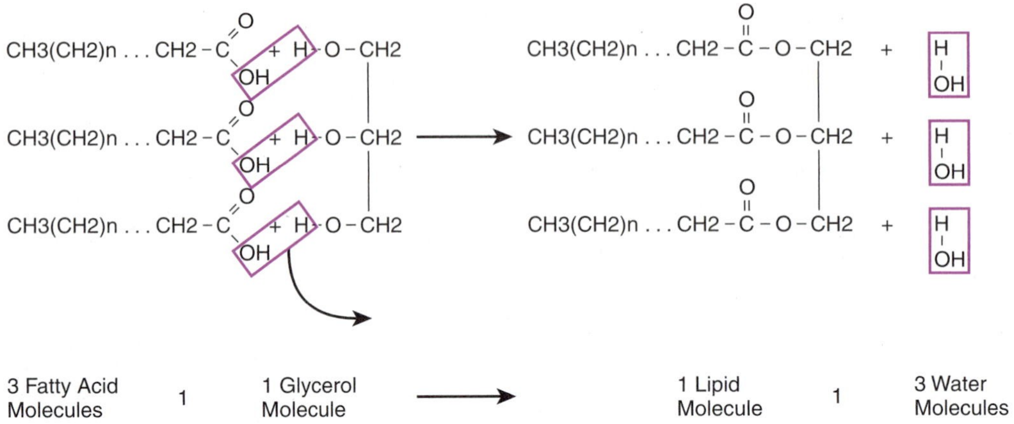

CH3(CH2)n . . . CH2 − C(=O)OH + H − O − CH2
CH3(CH2)n . . . CH2 − C(=O)OH + H − O − CH2 ⟶ CH3(CH2)n . . . CH2 − C(=O) − O − CH2 + H−OH
CH3(CH2)n . . . CH2 − C(=O)OH + H − O − CH2

CH3(CH2)n . . . CH2 − C(=O) − O − CH2 + H−OH
CH3(CH2)n . . . CH2 − C(=O) − O − CH2 + H−OH

3 Fatty Acid Molecules 1 1 Glycerol Molecule ⟶ 1 Lipid Molecule 1 3 Water Molecules

Figure 3–4 Formation of a Lipid Molecule by Dehydration Synthesis
Note that glycerol is arranged as its mirror image to facilitate bonding.

Table 3–7 Names, Formulas, and Sources of Some Common Fatty Acids

Name	Formula	Source
Butyric	C_3H_7COOH	Rancid butter
Lauric	$C_{11}H_{23}COOH$	Coconuts
Myristic	$C_{13}H_{27}COOH$	Widely found
Palmitic	$C_{15}H_{31}COOH$	Plant fat
Stearic	$C_{17}H_{35}COOH$	Animal and plant fat
Oleic	$C_{17}H_{33}COOH$	Corn oil
Linoleic	$C_{17}H_{31}COOH$	Cottonseed and soybean oils

coat of all viruses. Proteins also serve as binding and structural components of all living things. For example, large amounts of protein are found in fingernails, hair, cartilage, ligaments, tendons, and muscle.

The small molecular units that comprise the very large protein molecules are called **amino acids.** Proteins are large polymers of amino acids. There are twenty-two different amino acids that can be combined in any number and sequence to make up the various kinds of proteins.

Figure 3–5 shows the general structural formula of an amino acid. The central carbon atom indicated by number 1 is bonded or linked to four different molecular groups. At position 2, the carbon atom is bonded to an **amino group** (NH_2), and at position 3 it is bonded to a hydrogen atom. At site 4 it is bonded to a **carboxyl group** (COOH) and at site 5 to a variable side group (R).

A variable side group or "R" represents any one of the twenty-two different groups that can be placed into that position to make various amino acids. For example, if the hydrogen (H) atom is substituted for the R group, the resultant amino acid is glycine,

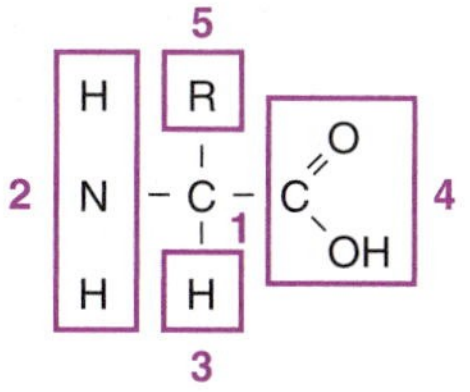

Figure 3–5 General Structural Formula of an Amino Acid

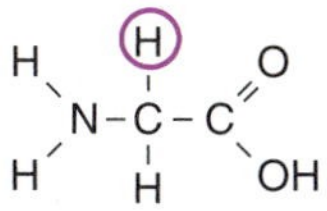

Figure 3–6 Glycine

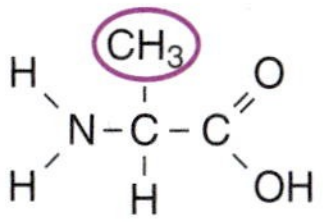

Figure 3–7 Alanine

which is the simplest amino acid. Figure 3–6 shows the structural formula of glycine. If, however, a methyl group (CH_3) is substituted, the amino acid now becomes alanine. Figure 3–7 shows the structural formula of alanine.

Table 3–8 gives a listing of the twenty naturally occurring amino acids with their three-letter symbol. Note that most of the amino acids tend to end in *-ine.*

Table 3.8 Twenty Naturally Occurring Amino Acids

Amino Acid	Symbol
Alanine	Ala
Arginine	Arg
Asparagine	Asn
Aspartic acid	Asp
Cysteine	Cys
Glutamic acid	Glu
Glutamine	Gln
Glycine	Gly
Histidine	His
Isoleucine	Ileu
Leucine	Leu
Lysine	Lys
Methionine	Met
Phenylalanine	Phe
Proline	Pro
Serine	Ser
Threonine	Thr
Tryptophan	Trp
Tyrosine	Tyr
Valine	Val

Table 3–9 Nine Essential Amino Acids

Essential Amino Acid	Symbol
Histidine	His
Isoleucine	Ileu
Leucine	Leu
Lysine	Lys
Methionine	Met
Phenylalanine	Phe
Threonine	Thr
Tryptophan	Trp
Valine	Val

Table 3–9 gives a list of the nine essential amino acids. Essential amino acids are needed by the human body, and must be ingested, because they cannot be made by the body.

Large protein molecules are constructed from any number and sequence of these amino acids. The quantity of amino acids in any given protein molecule can number from 300 to several thousand.

In the cells of living organisms and microbes, proteins are made by means of dehydration synthesis. Here, there is a linkage of specific amino acid molecules, in much the same fashion that complex carbohydrates are made from glucose molecules. In the bonding of one amino acid to another, a C–N bond forms between the carboxyl group of one amino acid and the amino group of the next amino acid. This C–N bond formed between amino acids is called a **peptide bond.** A series of amino acids linked together in this fashion is called a **polypeptide.** Figure 3–8 shows a peptide bond formed between two typical amino acids—glycine and alanine—to form a simple protein called glycylalanine.

Polypeptides with a biological function are commonly referred to as proteins. Proteins can have several structures (Figure 3–9). The primary protein structure is a sequence of amino acids in a single chain. Most polypeptides twist into a spiral shape called a **helix.** These proteins are known as secondary protein structures. Fibrous proteins such as hair and nails are secondary protein structures. When the long coil becomes folded and twisted, the characteristic three-dimensional tertiary protein structure is formed. Enzymes are typical tertiary structures. A fourth, quaternary structure exists when two or more polypeptide chains are bonded together. Hemoglobin is such a structure.

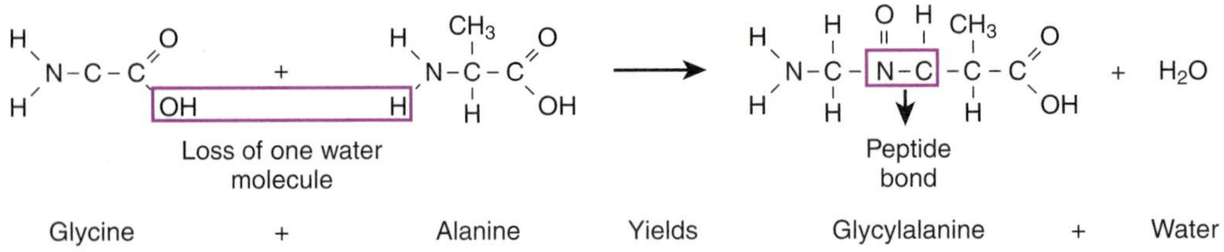

Loss of one water molecule

Peptide bond

Glycine + Alanine Yields Glycylalanine + Water (H_2O)

Figure 3–8 Formation of a protein

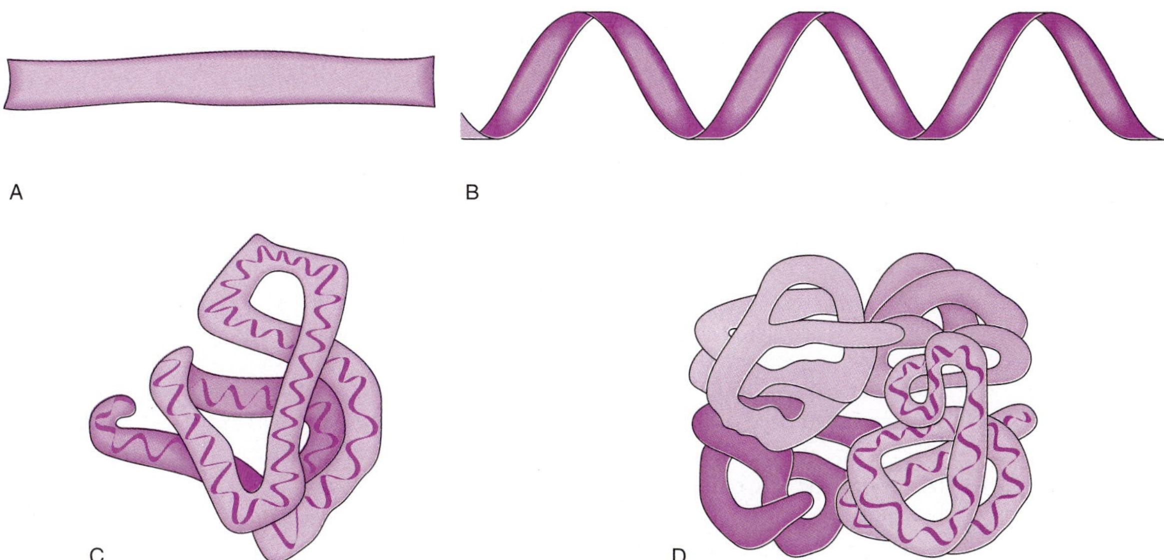

Figure 3–9 Basic protein structures: (A) primary, (B) secondary (helix), (C) tertiary, (D) quarternary

Enzymes

Enzymes are specialized protein molecules that are found in all living cells and microbes. They help with the fine control of the various chemical reactions occurring in a cell and in a microbe, so each reaction occurs at just the right moment and at the right speed. Enzymes help provide energy for the cell, assist in the making of new cell parts, and control almost every process in a cell or microbe. Because enzymes are capable of such activity, they are known as *organic catalysts.* An enzyme or organic catalyst affects the rate or speed of a chemical reaction without itself being changed. Enzymes can also be used repeatedly. An enzyme molecule is highly specific in its action.

Composition of enzymes.

Enzyme molecules are very large and complex protein molecules. Enzymes are made up of either all protein or part protein attached to a nonprotein part. The protein part of an enzyme molecule is known as an **apoenzyme,** and the nonprotein component is called the **coenzyme.** Minerals such as calcium (Ca), iron (Fe), magnesium (Mg), and copper (Cu) and vitamins such as C and B-complex serve as coenzymes.

How enzymes function.

Enzyme molecules are much larger than the molecules with which they have to interact. When an enzyme molecule reacts with another molecule, the reaction occurs only at a highly specific place on the enzyme. This localized site on the enzyme molecule is called the **active site.** Each enzyme has its own pattern on its active site; therefore, no two enzymes are alike. An enzyme reacts with a reactant whose molecular pattern fits the enzyme's molecular pattern. The molecule that the enzyme reacts with is called a **substrate** molecule. The function of an enzyme is explained by a

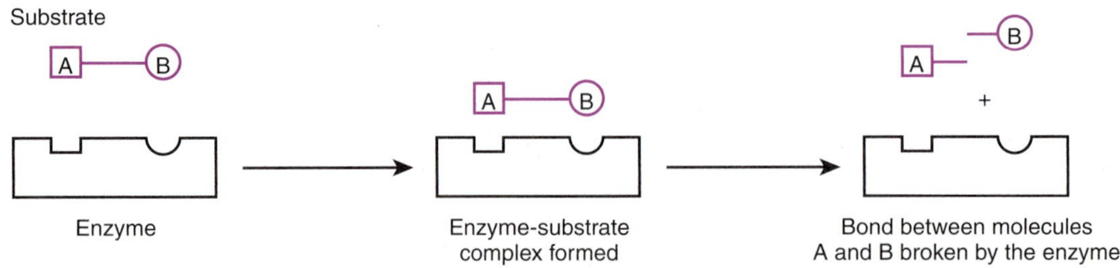

Figure 3–10 Enzyme Action

theory called the "lock-and-key" model. The relation between an enzyme molecule and its specific substrate molecule can be compared with the relation between a lock and the key that fits and turns that lock. Similarly, only a substrate molecule having a particular pattern can fit into the active site of its specific enzyme molecule. When this fit is "good," the enzyme molecule alters the substrate molecule chemically. The temporary physical binding of the enzyme molecule and the substrate molecule is called an **enzyme–substrate complex.** Enzyme activity occurs while the enzyme–substrate complex is together.

Figure 3–10 shows how an enzyme may cause a complex molecule, represented as A-B, to separate into smaller, independent molecules, A and B.

The name of an enzyme usually ends in *-ase*. The *-ase* ending is added to the stem word taken from the substrate.

Table 3–10 shows some examples of enzyme names.

Example of bacterial enzyme action. Many bacteria have an enzyme that needs a compound called **para-aminobenzoic acid (PABA).** PABA helps bacteria to synthesize a vitamin called folic acid, which the bacteria need for proper growth. Figure 3–11 shows the structural formulas of PABA and the antibiotic drug sulfanilamide. Upon close examination, both compounds structurally are much alike.

When the antibiotic sulfanilamide is given to the bacteria, instead of PABA, the sulfanilamide molecules attach themselves to the active sites of the bacteria. Thus, the active sites on the bacteria cannot attract PABA molecules and folic acid cannot be made. When this happens, the bacteria cannot grow.

Table 3–10 Examples of Some Enzymes and Their Substrates

Enzyme	Substrate
Amylase	Starch
Lactase	Lactose
Lipase	Lipids
Maltase	Maltose
Protease	Proteins
Sucrase	Sucrose

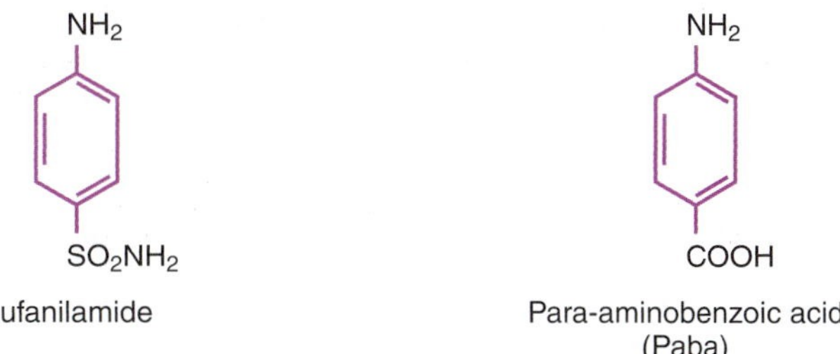

Figure 3–11 Structural Formulas of Sulfanilamide and Para-aminobenzoic Acid

When sulfanilamide is used to treat bacterial diseases, bacteria become weak, cannot grow, and are readily killed by white blood cells.

Nucleic Acids

Nucleic acids are very important organic compounds containing the elements carbon, oxygen, hydrogen, nitrogen, and phosphorus. There are two types of nucleic acids—deoxyribonucleic acid (DNA) and ribonucleic acid (RNA). DNA is involved in the process of heredity. Specific genetic information is carried in the DNA molecule, which is found in the nuclear **chromosomes** and **genes** of all cells. This genetic information tells a cell what structures it will possess and what functions and behavior it will have. The DNA molecule passes on this genetic information from cell to cell and eventually from one generation to the next. DNA can also be found in the plasma membrane, mitochondria, and chloroplasts. RNA is essential in helping a cell or microbe to synthesize proteins. Proteins are needed to help a cell or microbe to grow and repair damaged or worn-out parts. Large amounts of RNA can be found in the nucleoli, cytoplasm, and ribosomes of cells.

Structure of nucleic acids.

Nucleic acids are the largest known organic molecules. They are very-high-molecular-weight polymers made from thousands of smaller, repeating subunits called **nucleotides.** A nucleotide itself is a very complex molecule. It is composed of three different molecular groups. Figure 3–12 shows a typical nucleotide. Group 1 is a phosphate or phosphoric acid group, H_3PO_4, and group 2 represents a five-carbon sugar. Depending upon the nucleotide, the sugar could be either a ribose or a deoxyribose sugar. Finally, group 3 represents a nitrogenous base. There are two groups of nitrogenous bases—purines and pyrimidines. The purines are either adenine (A) or guanine (G), and the pyrimidines are cytosine (C), thymine (T), or uracil (U).

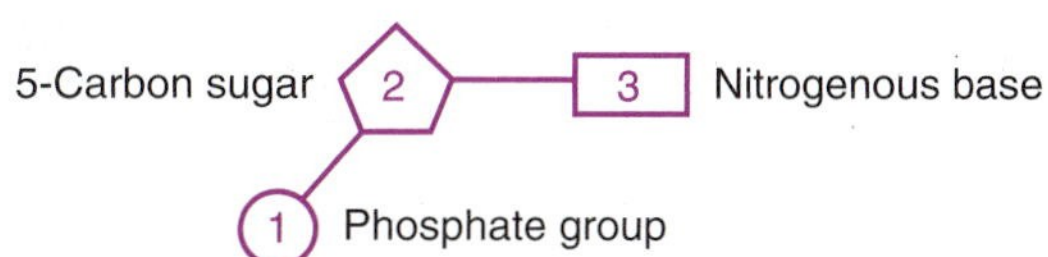

Figure 3–12 Structure of a Typical Nucleotide

Table 3–11 Differences between DNA and RNA Molecules

Type of Nucleic Acid	Type of Sugar Present	Type of Bases Present	Phosphate Group	Location	Number of Strands Present
DNA	Deoxyribose	A, T, G, C	Same as RNA	Plasma membrane, mitochondria, chromosomes, chloroplasts	2
RNA	Ribose	A, U, G, C	Same as DNA	Cytoplasm, nucleoli, ribosomes	1

DNA Structure. The nucleotide structure of a DNA molecule consists of a phosphate group, the deoxyribose sugar,* and any one of the four nitrogenous bases: adenine, thymine, cytosine, and guanine.

RNA Structure. The RNA nucleotide consists of a phosphate group, the **ribose** sugar, and any one of the following nitrogenous bases: adenine, cytosine, guanine, and uracil instead of thymine. The RNA molecule is a single-stranded molecule, whereas the DNA molecule is double stranded.

The two different types of RNA in a cell are the *messenger RNA* (mRNA) and the *transfer RNA* (tRNA). Messenger RNA carries the instructions for protein synthesis from the DNA molecule located in the nucleus of a cell into the cytoplasm. The mRNA molecule carries the code for protein synthesis from the DNA in the nucleus to the ribosomes in the cytoplasm. The tRNA molecule picks up amino acid molecules in the cytoplasm and transfers them to the ribosomes, where they are put together to form proteins. Table 3–11 shows the basic differences between the DNA molecule and the RNA molecule.

The RNA molecule is a single strand or chain of repeating phosphate, ribose, and nitrogenous base groups (Figure 3–13). The DNA molecule, on the other hand, is a double-stranded chain of repeating phosphate, deoxyribose, and nitrogenous base groups shaped as a double helix, with each strand linked by the nitrogenous base groups (Figure 3–14).

Acids, Bases, and Salts

Before ending the discussion of basic chemistry and biochemistry, a brief discussion of acids, bases, salts, and pH is essential.

Acids. Many inorganic and organic compounds that are found in living organisms and microbes and ones that we use in our daily lives can be classified into one of three groups—acids, bases, and salts. We are familiar with the sour taste of citrus fruits (grape-

*A deoxyribose sugar is a sugar that has one less oxygen atom than the ribose sugar.

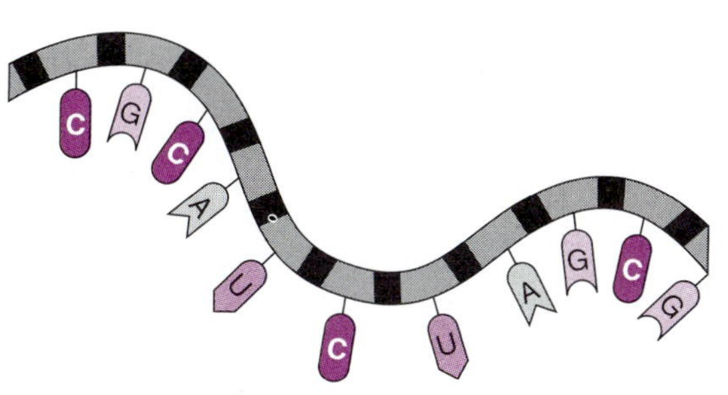

Figure 3–13 RNA Molecule

■ = phosphate; □ = sugar (ribose)
Nitrogen bases: C = cytosine; G = guanine;
U = uracil; A = adenine

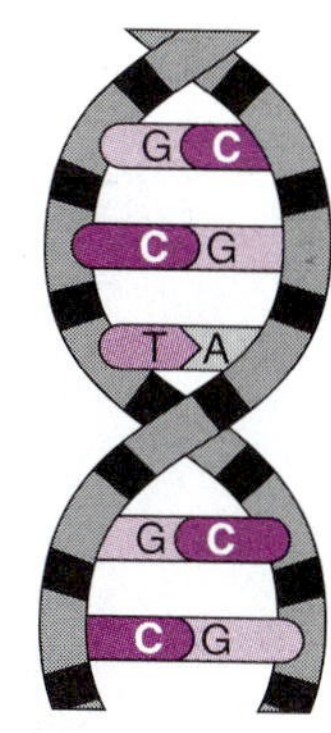

Figure 3–14 DNA Molecule

■ = phosphate; □ = sugar (deoxyribose). Nitrogen bases:
C = cytosine; G = guanine;
T = thymine; A = adenine

fruits, lemons, and limes) and vinegar. The sour taste is due to the presence of compounds called acids. What characteristics do acids have to set them apart from the bases and salts? An **acid** is a substance that, when dissolved in water, will **ionize*** into positively charged **hydronium ions** (H_3O^+) and negatively charged ions of some other element. [Basically, an acid is a substance that yields hydronium ions (H_3O^+) in solution.] For example, hydrogen chloride (HCl) in pure form is a gas, but when bubbled into water, it becomes hydrochloric acid. How does this happen? Simply, in a water solution hydrogen chloride ionizes into one hydronium ion and one negatively charged chloride ion.

$$HCl + H_2O \longrightarrow H_3O^+ + Cl^-$$

Hydrogen chloride in solution ⟶ Hydronium ion + Chloride ion

Table 3–12 gives the names of some common acids, their formulas, and where they are found.

Bases. A **base** or **alkali** is a substance that, when dissolved in water, ionizes into negatively charged **hydroxide** (OH^-) ions and positively charged ions of a metal. Bases have a bitter taste. For example, sodium hydroxide (NaOH) ionizes into one sodium ion (Na^+) and one hydroxide ion (OH^-). The reaction can be shown as follows:

$$NaOH \longrightarrow Na^+ + OH^-$$

Sodium hydrozide in solution ⟶ Sodium ion + Hydroxide ion

**Ionize* means the ability of a substance to separate into either positively or negatively charged particles when in solution.

Table 3–12 Names, Formulas, and Location or Use of Some Common Acids

Name of Acid	Formula	Where Found or Usage
Acetic acid	$HC_2H_3O_2$	Found in vinegar
Boric acid	H_3BO_3	Weak eyewash
Carbonic acid	H_2CO_3	Found in carbonated beverages
Hydrochloric acid	HCl	Found in stomach
Nitric acid	HNO_3	Industrial oxidizing acid
Sulfuric acid	H_2SO_4	Found in batteries and industrial mineral acid

Table 3–13 gives the names of some common bases, their formulas, and location or use.

Neutralization and salts. When an acid and a base are combined, they form a salt and water. This type of reaction is called a **neutralization.** In a neutralization reaction, hydrogen ions (H^+) from the acid and hydroxide ions (OH^-) from the base join to form water. At the same time, the negative ions of the acid combine with the positive ions of the base to form a compound called a **salt.** For example, hydrochloric acid and sodium hydroxide combine to form sodium chloride and water. The hydrogen ions from the acid unite with the hydroxide ions from the base to form water. The sodium ions (Na^+) combine with the chloride ions (Cl^-) to form sodium chloride ($NaCl$). When the water evaporates, solid salt remains. The neutralization reaction may be written as shown in Figure 3–15.

Indicators

Indicators are special chemicals used to test the hydrogen ion concentration present in a particular solution. They are able to do this by changing color according to the hydrogen ion concentration present in a solution. Some of these indicators are litmus paper,

Table 3–13 Names, Formulas, and Location or Use of Some Common Bases

Name of Base	Formula	Where Found or Usage
Ammonium hydroxide	NH_4OH	Household liquid cleaners
Magnesium hydroxide	$Mg(OH)_2$	Milk of magnesia
Potassium hydroxide	KOH	Caustic potash
Sodium hydroxide	$NaOH$	Lye

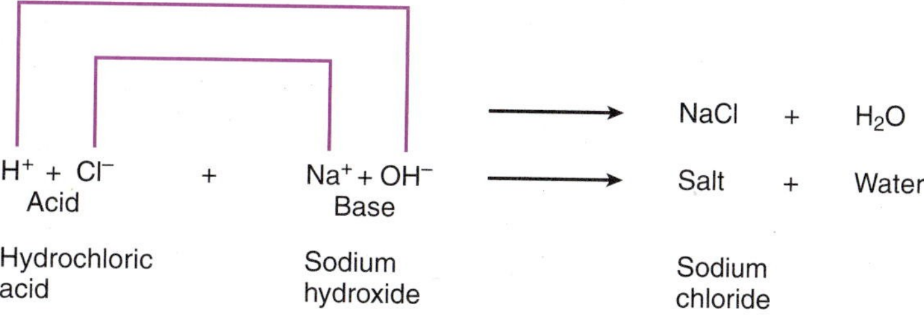

Figure 3–15 Neutralization Reaction of an Acid and a Base. Blue litmus paper turns red in the presence of an acid and stays blue in an alkali

bromthymol blue, and phenolphthalein. Bromthymol blue turns yellow in the presence of an acid but remains blue in the presence of a base. Phenolphthalein is colorless in an acid solution, but changes to pink in a basic solution.

pH

Often it is necessary to determine the pH of a solution. pH is a measure of the acidity or alkalinity (basicity) of a solution. The **pH** scale is a simplified way of stating the hydrogen ion concentration. It is derived from a logarithmic scale and expresses the degree of acidity or alkalinity of a solution. The pH range is from 0 to 14, with pH values 0 to 6.9 being acidic and pH values 7.1 to 14 being alkaline or basic. A pH of 7 indicates that a particular solution has the same number of hydrogen ions as hydroxide ions. This is a neutral pH, and pure water is neutral with a pH value of 7.0. The lower the pH number, the stronger the acid or higher the ion concentration. Thus, the greater the number above 7.0, the stronger the base or greater hydroxide ion concentration. Figure 3–16 shows the pH values of some common acids, bases, and human body fluids.

pH of Living Things

As shown in Figure 3–16, living cells and the fluids they produce are usually neither strongly acidic nor strongly alkaline. (The one notable exception is gastric juice, containing hydrochloric acid, which is found in the human stomach.) These fluids, in fact, are nearly neutral. For instance, human tears have a pH of 7.3, human blood has a pH of 7.4, and the pH of urine ranges from 5.0 to 7.5.

For living cells and microbes to function optimally, their biochemical reactions must occur at a given pH. Any marked deviation in the pH causes disruption in the sensitive biochemical processes, illness, or even death of the organism. In humans and other living organisms, the maintenance of a balanced pH, at which the fluids are neither too acidic nor too basic, is achieved through a compound called a **buffer.** Buffers are substances that, when released, maintain the required pH even in the face of contaminants or adversity. Sodium bicarbonate ($NaHCO_3$) acts as a buffer in many living organisms and microbes. Thus, buffers help a living organism to maintain a constant pH value, which contributes to the homeostasis or balanced state within all living things.

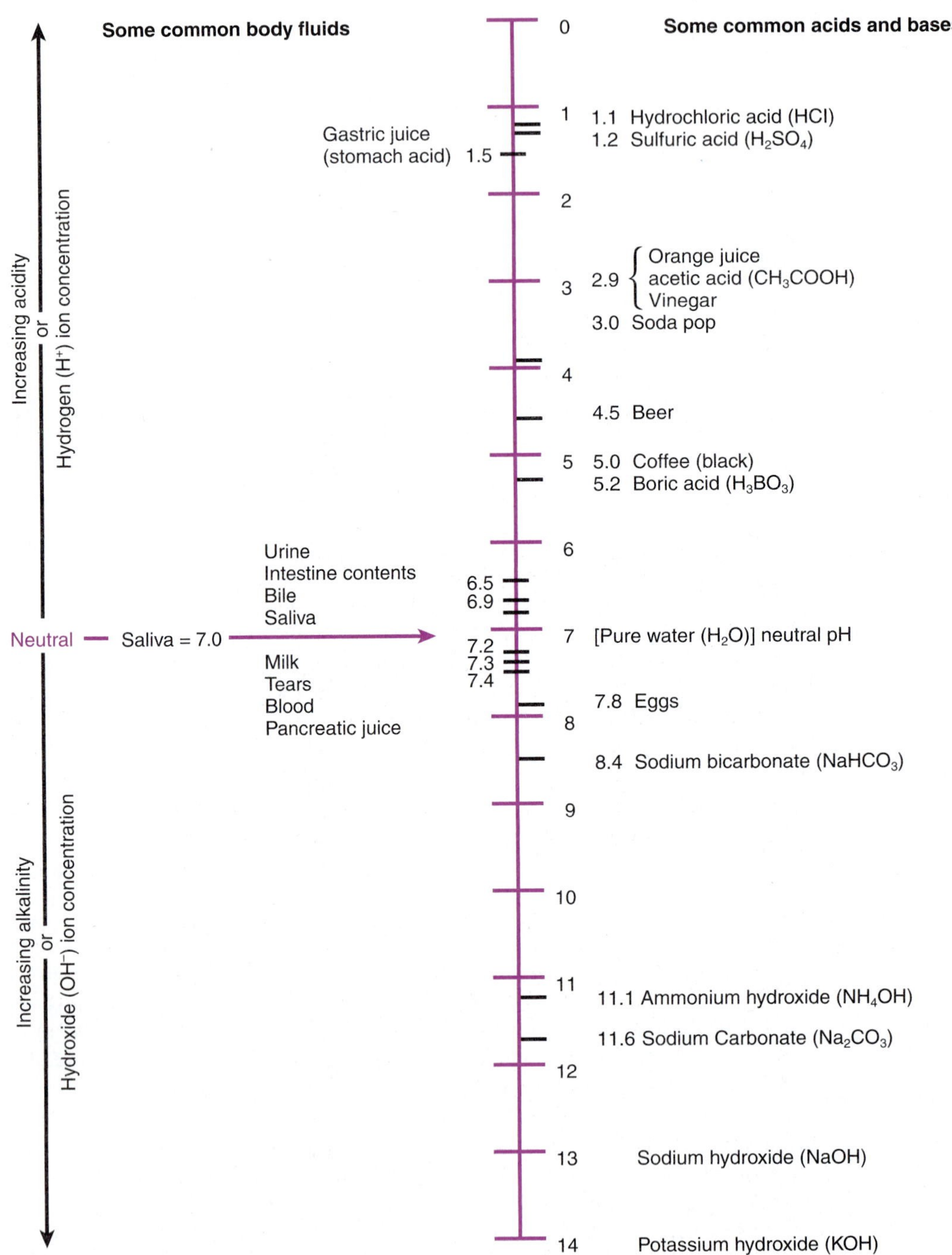

Figure 3–16 pH Values of Some Common Acids, Bases, Human Body Fluids, and Foods

SUMMARY

In this chapter we discuss some basic chemistry concepts, how substances are formed, and classifications of such particles as the atom, molecules, elements, and compounds. A periodic table of elements depicts how the elements are arranged by mass such that metals are located on the left side of the table and nonmetals are located on the right side. Living matter contains only some of the elements—with carbon, hydrogen, oxygen, and nitrogen being the abundant nonmetals—and traces of some metals as described in Table 3–1. Most reactions in living cells occur in some sort of solution or liquid in which the solute, or solid, dissolves the solid to be used for metabolic processes. Compounds are divided into two categories: organic, those containing carbon and found in nature or living things; and inorganic, those that do not usually contain carbon, but rather contain mostly metal. Organic compounds include sugars, starches, fats or lipids, proteins, alcohols, and fatty acids. Carbohydrates, important sugars for metabolizing and producing energy, are compared in discussions of monosaccharides, disaccharides, and polysaccharides.

Lipids contain long hydrogen chains and fewer carbon atoms in relation to each other than sugars. Nitrogen and phosphorus are common inclusions in lipids. Saturated and unsaturated fats are compared to show their effects on the body as well as risks for coronary artery disease. Saturated fats are clearly a higher risk because of the difficulty to break up their long, tightly packed molecular chains.

Proteins, known as building blocks, are also complex molecules. They add nitrogen and usually phosphorus to their molecular structures and comprise the outer coats of viruses and nails, hair, cartilage, tendons, ligaments, and muscle. Smaller units, called amino acids, join together to form the large protein chains. Amino acids play an important role in protein synthesis and are the base units for the composition of RNA and DNA.

Enzymes known as organic catalysts assist in the rate of chemical reactions, but do not change themselves. Enzyme rates of reaction are measured to determine muscle activity, as quantity of enzyme is not measurable. This fact is particularly important in determining whether a person with severe chest pain has suffered a coronary. When enzymes form a complex with their specific substrates, enzyme activity can then be measured. This process is called an enzyme–substrate complex.

Nucleic acids are organic compounds containing carbon, hydrogen, oxygen, nitrogen, and phosphorus. These compounds are of two types—RNA and DNA—which are found in nuclear chromosomes and genes. DNA passes genetic information while RNA helps synthesize proteins. Proteins are needed for building and repair. Nucleic acids consist of three parts: a sugar group, a nitrogen base, and a phosphate group. DNA is a double helix consisting of four nitrogenous bases (adenine, thymine, cytosine, and guanine), a deoxyribose sugar, and phosphate groups linking the two helices. RNA is a single-stranded molecule containing the nitrogenous bases of adenine, cytosine, guanine, and uracil, a ribose sugar, and repeating phosphate groups. Acids and bases, when reacted together, neutralize to form a salt and water. The human body for the most part prefers a neutral atmosphere, but many bacteria may thrive in an optimal pH of an acid or alkali environment.

STUDY AND DISCUSSION

- Individually, prepare a brief report on at least 30 of the 105 elements; discuss the origin of the name of each element.
- Lipids and oils play an important role in our daily lives. Make a list of the various lipids and oils you use every day. Divide the list into the following categories:

Foods	Cooking Oils	Cosmetics and Drugs	Household Use

- Investigate the roles of lipids, fatty acids, and cholesterols in the digestion of fats.
- There is much news and controversy over a substance called cholesterol. Prepare a report using library references and contribute your information via a class discussion, which should include the following items on cholesterol:
  1. What is cholesterol?
  2. In what part of the human body can cholesterol build up?
  3. How can cholesterol be a health hazard to humans?
  4. What foods that are very rich in cholesterol should be eliminated or minimized?
  5. What type of activity and diet would you recommend to an individual who has a cholesterol problem?

  Discuss why an athletic bodybuilder would include protein supplements in his or her daily diet.
- Vitamins are essential in our daily diet. Discuss why this is so. Make a list of at least six vitamins, and include the following information:

Vitamin	Foods Found In	Uses in the Human Body

REVIEW QUESTIONS

A. Multiple-Choice Questions: Select the letter of the choice that best completes the sentence.

1. Organic catalysts are called _____ .
   a. enzymes
   b. indicators
   c. acids
   d. ions
2. Although carbon dioxide contains carbon, it is considered to be an inorganic compound because it lacks the element _____ .
   a. sulfur
   b. hydrogen
   c. phosphorus
   d. nitrogen
3. When an acid and a base are combined, the reaction between the hydrogen ions (H^+) and the hydroxide ions (OH^-) is called _____ .
   a. neutralization
   b. ionization
   c. dehydration synthesis
   d. hydrolysis
4. Compounds that have the same molecular formula but different structural formulas are known as _____ .
   a. radioactive
   b. bases
   c. salts
   d. isomers
5. If blue litmus paper is dipped into gastric juice, it will turn _____ .
   a. blue
   b. colorless
   c. red
   d. yellow
6. Of the following acids, the weakest is _____ acid.
   a. sulfuric
   b. acetic
   c. hydrochloric
   d. nitric
7. Salt that dissolves in water is called a _____ .
   a. solute
   b. solvent
   c. mixture
   d. gas
8. When proper amounts of an acid and a base are combined, the products formed are a salt and _____ .
   a. gas
   b. water
   c. another base
   d. another acid
9. An example of an element is _____ .
   a. sugar
   b. starch
   c. water
   d. sodium
10. A solution with a pH of 12 is _____ .
    a. neutral
    b. a base
    c. organic
    d. an acid
11. A pH of 5 compared with a pH of 1 represents a hydrogen ion concentration that is _____ .
    a. half as large
    b. four times as large
    c. more acidic
    d. acidic
12. Compounds that are added to a solution to prevent sudden deviations in pH are known as _____ .
    a. ionic
    b. precipitate
    c. indicators
    d. buffers

13. Common table sugar or sucrose is an isomer of _____ .
    a. glucose
    b. deoxyribose
    c. dextrose
    d. maltose
14. Another name for glucose is _____ .
    a. grape sugar
    b. table sugar
    c. cane sugar
    d. milk sugar
15. A sugar that is used by most cells as a primary source of energy is _____ .
    a. deoxyribose
    b. glucose
    c. lactose
    d. maltose
16. Compounds that are carried to a cell's ribosomes via the tRNA molecules are _____ .
    a. amino acids
    b. fatty acids
    c. sugars
    d. lipids
17. The formula that represents a carbohydrate compound is _____ .
    a. $C_3H_4O_3$
    b. $CaHPO_4$
    c. $C_{12}H_{22}O_{11}$
    d. C_2H_5OH
18. The formation of peptide bonds between amino acids is accompanied by the _____ .
    a. addition of hydrogen
    b. release of water
    c. release of oxygen
    d. addition of water
19. A vitamin essential for the normal growth of most bacteria is _____ .
    a. uracil
    b. sulfanilamide
    c. folic acid
    d. nucleic acid
20. In cells, the molecule that can release the most energy is _____ .
    a. ATP
    b. ADP
    c. DNA
    d. RNA
21. Chemical processes that occur within most cells generally occur at a pH close to _____ .
    a. 9.1
    b. 1.1
    c. 12.8
    d. 7.1
22. Vitamins are necessary for the maintenance of living things because vitamins function as _____ .
    a. nucleotides
    b. coenzymes
    c. nucleic acids
    d. apoenzymes
23. A compound with the formula CH_2NH_2COOH is a (an) _____ .
    a. amino acid
    b. fatty acid
    c. protein
    d. complex starch
24. A nucleotide consists of a phosphate group, a sugar group, and a (an) _____ .
    a. hydroxide group
    b. nitrogenous base
    c. amino group
    d. carboxyl group
25. The pH scale ranges from _____ .
    a. 0–13
    b. 1–14
    c. 1–12
    d. 0–14

B. Completion Questions: Complete each statement with the appropriate word or words to make the statement correct. Choose from the list provided.

glycerol	amino acids
glycogen	glycerol
glucose	7.0
water	monosaccharides
base	amino
molecule	trace
carboxyl	bitter
ribose	sour
atom	enzyme
hydrolysis	oxygen

1. The sugars glucose, galactose, and fructose are examples of compounds called __________ .

2. The smallest part of an element that still possesses the original properties of the element is called a (an) __________ .

3. Elements that are present in very minute quantities in living things are called __________ elements.

4. The smallest part of a compound that still has the original properties of the compound is called a (an)__________ .

5. The reaction of dehydration synthesis is to the formation of starch as the reaction of __________ is to the digestion of starch.

6. Most inorganic compounds separate into ions when the compounds are dissolved in __________ .

7. Compounds that are basic have a (an) __________ taste.

8. A water solution of a substance containing an excess of hydroxide ions is called a (an) __________ .

9. Pure water has a pH of __________ .

10. Compounds that are acidic have a (an) __________ taste.

11. When a lipid is formed, three fatty acid molecules are joined to one __________ molecule.

12. Starch and cellulose molecules are the same in that both consist of many linked molecules of ___________ .

13. When an enzyme–substrate complex is broken down, the result is a new product and a (an) ___________ that can react again.

14. All organic compounds contain the elements carbon, hydrogen, and ___________ .

15. In liver and muscle cells, glucose molecules may be united into large storage molecules called ___________ .

16. The building blocks of large protein molecules are called ___________ .

17. The type of sugar present in an RNA molecule is called ___________ .

18. The formula NH_2 is used to designate the ___________ group.

19. The formula COOH is used to represent the ___________ group.

20. Guanine and adenine are ___________ .

C. Matching Questions: Match the terms in Column I with their corresponding terms in Column II.

Column I		Column II
_______	1. Amino group	a. O_2
_______	2. Smallest particle	b. $C_6H_{12}O_6$
_______	3. Hydrogen ion concentration	c. Glycogen
_______	4. Alkali	d. Lactose
_______	5. Oxygen	e. Enzyme
_______	6. Carbohydrate	f. NH_2
_______	7. Glucose	g. C–N
_______	8. Animal starch	h. DNA
_______	9. Milk sugar	i. Atom
_______	10. Organic catalyst	j. CH_2O
_______	11. Uracil	k. OH^-
_______	12. Hydroxide	l. Apoenzyme
_______	13. Double helix	m. pH
_______	14. Cholesterol	n. Base
_______	15. Electron loss	o. ATP
_______	16. Energy	p. Oxidation
_______	17. Peptide bond	q. Lipid
_______	18. Coenzyme	r. RNA

CHAPTER

4

Favorable Environment for Bacterial Growth

OBJECTIVES

After completing this chapter, you will be able to:

- list the conditions required by bacteria in order to grow.
- explain the difference between aerobic and anaerobic bacteria.
- describe how bacteria grow and multiply.
- explain the necessity for, and methods of, controlling the growth of bacteria.

KEY WORDS

aerobic bacteria
anaerobic bacteria
Clostridium botulinum
facultative anaerobe
microaerophilic
nitrites
obligate anaerobe
optimal temperature
pH
toxins
transverse binary fission

Like all living things, bacteria need certain conditions to survive. These basic conditions include food, moisture, and a favorable temperature for bacteria to build protoplasm and give energy to carry on their life functions. Other growth conditions include proper gaseous atmosphere and appropriate **pH** and salt concentration. When these conditions are not favorable, some bacteria form spores to await the return of favorable growth conditions.

To grow bacteria without oxygen, it is necessary to remove it by incubating the cultures in a walk-in anaerobic incubator, or use an oxygen gas replacement system, such as the Gas Pak® System, in which to grow the cultures. This system is popular for most smaller laboratories and is easy to set up. See Figure 4–1 for an example of the Gas Pak® System.

Unlike other living things, some bacteria can live and grow without the presence of atmospheric oxygen. These organisms are referred to as **anaerobic bacteria.** A bacteria that can grow only in the absence of oxygen is called an **obligate anaerobe;** organisms of the *Clostridium* genus are obligate anaerobes. Most bacteria are **facultative anaerobes** and can therefore grow with or without atmospheric oxygen. **Microaerophilic** organisms prefer to grow in a reduced oxygen environment. A reduced oxygen atmosphere can be

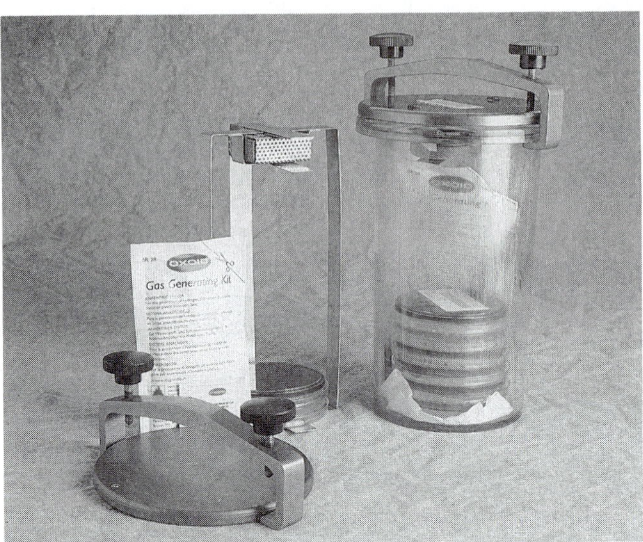

Figure 4–1 Gas Pack anaerobic system

obtained by setting the culture plates in a candle jar, lighting the candle, and sealing it before the candle is out. The candle uses up just enough oxygen before it goes out to lower the oxygen content and replace it with a 3% to 5% carbon dioxide atmosphere (see Figure 4–2). Such organisms include the *Neisseria* members that cause gonorrhea and meningitis.

Bacteria that grow in the presence of oxygen are called **aerobic bacteria.** When oxygen is an absolute requirement for growth, the organism is a strict aerobe. Examples include the *Pseudomonas* group and some species of the *Bacillus* group.

It is important for health care professionals to understand the difference between the two types of bacteria. Where free oxygen is unavailable, certain diseases caused by anaerobic bacteria, such as tetanus and lockjaw, can develop in the case of a deep wound. Such a wound, therefore, is kept open so that air may kill the anaerobic bacteria.

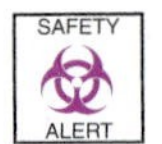

One of the most dangerous diseases known to humans is botulism, caused by ***Clostridium botulinum,*** which is anaerobic. It multiplies in the absence of oxygen. In 1971, a man died of botulism because he ate cold vichyssoise soup that was improperly canned. Proper canning requires heating to 240°F (116°C), for at least 30 minutes, to kill the spores. Because this soup was not heated enough, the spores multiplied after canning and produced the botulin. Botulin is one of the most deadly poisons known. Three quarters of an ounce of purified botulinum toxin could kill every human being on earth.

Botulinum can be killed by heating, because heat breaks down its protein molecules, making it harmless. Boiling the can of contaminated soup for 15 minutes would have killed and neutralized the deadly poison.

Nitrites, widely used as a meat preservative, have been effective for many years in preventing botulism. Unfortunately, they have also been found to induce cancer. Government restrictions have limited the use of nitrites to a degree, but they are still present in some bacon, hot dogs, and luncheon meats.

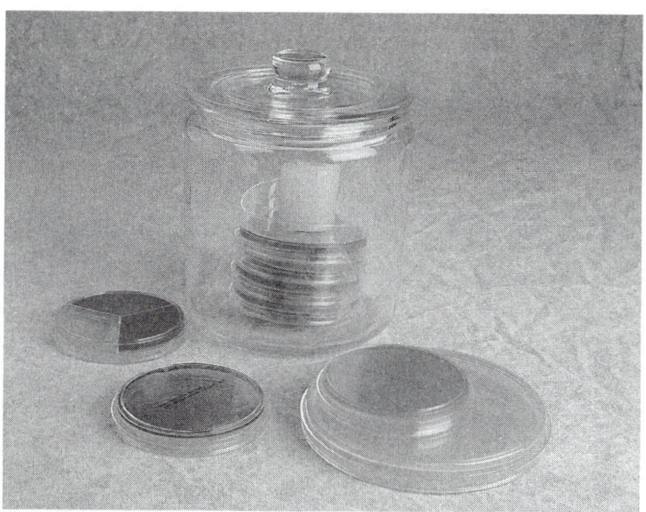

Figure 4–2 Candle jar system

Bacteria will grow wherever water, proper food, oxygen, proper temperature, and a suitable medium are present. The best medium is one that is not too acid or too alkaline, that is, at a neutral pH.

Most bacteria grow best in a nutritive fluid that is approximately neutral or equal to pH 7. Our blood is slightly alkaline (pH 7.35 to pH 7.45). When bacteria produce too much acid from fermentation, they will finally die when they reach a certain point of intolerance. This situation is good for us, as we would soon be killed if bacteria were not curbed in their rapid rate of reproduction.

Most bacteria grow best in moderate temperatures, although some grow only at body temperature. Each species has a minimum, a maximum, and a best temperature at which it will grow. The best temperature is called the **optimal temperature.** Bacteria capable of infecting humans usually have an optimal temperature close to that of human body temperature (37°C). A health professional working with cultures of certain bacteria must know the best bacteria for that culture in order to carry on the experiment.

Most microorganisms dislike light and may be killed by direct rays of sunshine. Molds, for example, prefer darkness for their growth.

ENVIRONMENTAL CONTROL

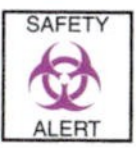

Bacterial growth can be encouraged in nature and in the laboratory by supplying the conditions that allow them to grow. This may be done without knowing, such as when food is left out of the refrigerator.

Bacteriologists grow bacteria in the laboratory by using nutrient agar, nutrient broth, gelatin, litmus milk, and other media.

Table 4–1 Common Methods of Food Preservation

Method	Action
Salting Drying Preserving in a heavy syrup	Removal of water
Pickling	Addition of excessive amounts of acid
Freezing	Introduction of an unfavorable temperature
Canning	Heating and excluding of organisms

It is possible to limit or inhibit the growth of bacteria by producing conditions that either slow the process or make growth impossible. Such conditions include:

- Lack of food
- Dryness—kills most bacteria but not spore-forming bacteria
- Too acid or too alkaline a medium—antiseptics retard the growth of bacteria; disinfectants kill bacteria
- Unfavorable temperature—cold (below freezing) retards the growth; heat (boiling point) kills most non-spore-forming bacteria
- Light—direct rays of the sun and ultraviolet light are harmful to bacteria

Methods of preserving food depend upon producing unfavorable conditions for the growth of bacteria. Table 4–1 presents some common ways of preserving foods.

GROWTH AND REPRODUCTION

Bacteria, under the favorable conditions discussed, reproduce by a method called **transverse binary fission.** In this method, a cell divides in half after developing a transverse cell wall around the bacteria, as shown in Figure 4–3a.

Bacteria may reproduce at the rate of two cells from every one cell every half hour. In a period of 12 hours, one single bacterium may reproduce over 16 million descendants to form bacterial colonies (Figure 4–3b). The rapid rate of increase is illustrated in Table 4–2. Unless bacteria are checked in their growth, they would soon overwhelm all other forms of life.

As bacteria grow, they give off poisonous wastes and enzymes. These are called **toxins** and may cause disease or result in food spoilage. Fortunately for us, a bacterial culture reaches its maximum population and stops growing when its food supply is exhausted. Thus, overpopulation and the accumulation of waste kill off more of the bacteria.

One can readily see how important it is to check the growth of bacteria once they have gained entrance into the human body. Disease spreads so rapidly that sometimes a few hours may mean the difference between life and death.

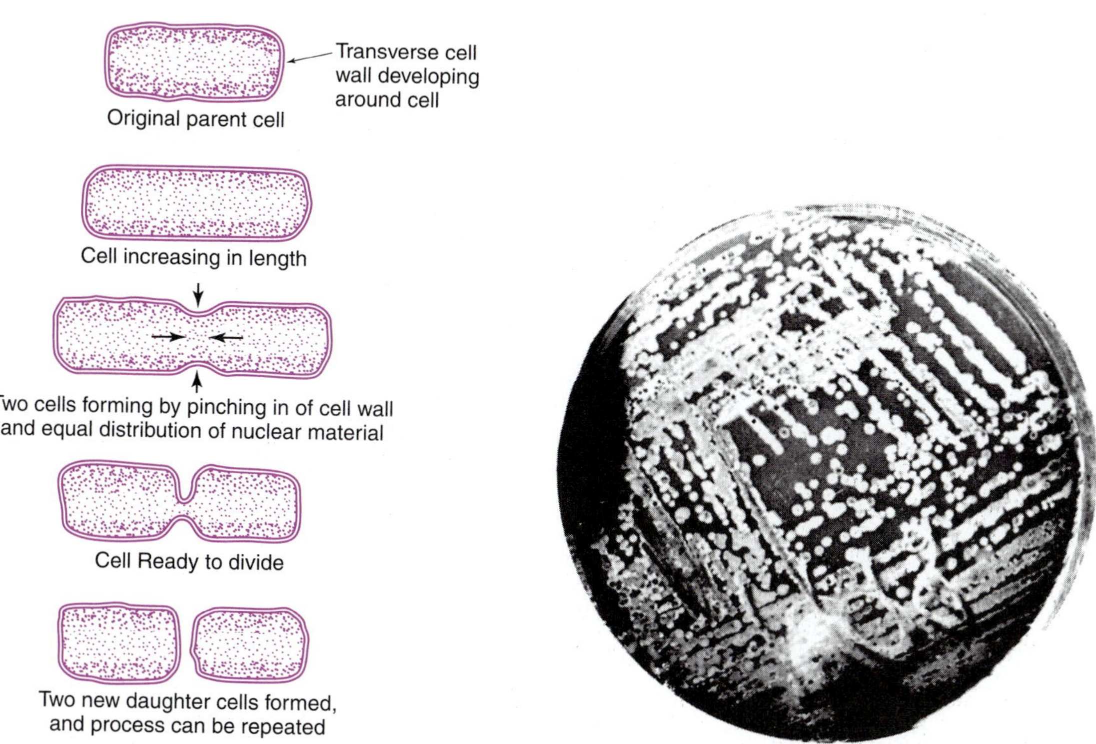

Figure 4–3 (Left) Bacillus; (right) petri dish with colonies of bacteria (*Courtesy National Committee for Careers in Medical Technology*)

Table 4–2 Reproduction of Bacteria

Time in Hours	Bacterial Cells	Time In Hours	Bacterial Cells
0	1	6½	8192
½	2	7	16,384
1	4	7½	32,768
1½	8	8	65,536
2	16	8½	131,072
2½	32	9	262,144
3	64	9½	524,288
3½	128	10	1,048,576
4	256	10½	2,097,152
4½	512	11	4,194,304
5	1024	11½	8,388,608
5½	2048	12	16,777,216*
6	4096		

*Assuming all bacteria are living after 12 hours

SUMMARY

This chapter discusses optimal temperatures, food, and atmospheric conditions that bacteria prefer for growth and multiplication. Some bacteria are strict aerobes, meaning they can grow only in the presence of oxygen. *Pseudomonas* species are cited as the prime example. Others are obligate anaerobes, meaning that they can only grow in the absence of oxygen. Facultative anaerobes, also referred to as aerobes, can grow with or without oxygen, whereas microaerophilic bacteria prefer a reduced oxygen environment for growth. Most bacteria prefer a rather neutral pH for optimal growth, approximately pH 7.0. The pH of the human body hovers around pH 7.2 to 7.4. Similarly, the best temperature for the growth of most bacteria is body temperature (37°C); a few yeast grow well at 25°C or room temperature. Bacteria prefer to grow in darkness. Sunlight usually kills bacteria. Food needs include a moist environment and a source of protein, which nutrient agar provides quite nicely. Some bacteria have special growth needs, such as the enteric organism needing bile salts to grow, which closely duplicates the bowel environment.

Numerous methods slow or inhibit the growth of bacteria, but do not kill bacteria. Disinfectants, ultraviolet light, and most antibiotics actually kill bacteria.

Bacteria reproduce by binary fission, and double their numbers approximately once every 20 minutes when growth conditions are favorable. Toxins or poisons produced by bacteria may cause disease, but they also destroy the food upon which they are growing. Fortunately when a culture of bacteria overpopulate they usually die out due to lack of food supply.

STUDY AND DISCUSSION

- Discuss the importance of refrigeration in keeping food safe and edible.
- Describe how the human body meets requirements for supplying a favorable environment for some bacteria.
- Explain how the health care professional can help provide an environment unfavorable to bacteria for the patient, both at home and in the hospital.
- Define aerobic and anaerobic bacteria. Describe the difference in health care procedures in the treatment and prevention of diseases caused by each type.
- Examine under the microscope various prepared slides of bacteria that show transverse binary fission.
- Explain why bacteria do not reproduce indefinitely.
- Explain how the health care professional can help to inhibit the growth of bacteria in the home, in the hospital, and in patients.
- Using library references, prepare a simple chart showing the various methods by which microorganisms reproduce. Include a brief explanation of each method, a list of the organisms that use that method, and a simple sketch showing each method of reproduction.
- Perform the following experiment.

Procedure 4–1 Determination of Conditions Favorable for Bacterial Growth

Equipment and Materials Needed

Agar	Incubator
9 Petri dishes	Refrigerator
Sterilizer	Oven

Method

1. Prepare eight petri dishes with sterilized, moist agar as described in earlier experiments.
2. Place some dry agar in another petri dish and sterilize it.
3. Keep one petri dish closed for a control. Label it.
4. Expose all the other sterilized agar plates to the air of the room for 5 minutes.
5. Cover. Put them in the following places for a few days:
   a. In a dark closet at moderate temperature
   b. In direct sunlight
   c. In a hot oven for a few hours
   d. At room temperature
   e. In a refrigerator for the entire experiment
   f. Another at room temperature, apart from (d) above
   g. One petri dish with dry agar in a dark closet at room temperature
   h. A regular petri dish with regularly prepared agar in the same place
6. Label and examine each dish every 24 hours.

Observations and Conclusions

Examine all petri dishes every day and record your observations on this chart:

Condition	First Day	Second Day	Third Day	Fourth Day
Darkness Sunlight				
Hot oven Room temperature				
Refrigerator Room temperature				
Dry agar Moist agar				

Questions

1. What conclusions do you draw from this experiment?

2. Why was one petri dish kept unopened?

REVIEW QUESTIONS

A. General Questions: Provide complete answers to each of the following.

1. List five conditions that bacteria need to grow.

2. Define the terms *aerobic bacteria* and *anaerobic bacteria.*

3. Indicate why nondisposable diapers should be sterilized and, if possible, hung outdoors in direct sunlight to dry.

4. Explain why thermometers must be disinfected after each usage.

5. Explain why frequent bathing is important to preventing infections.

6. Explain what causes the odor of perspiration.

7. Name four ways to inhibit the growth of bacteria in food, and explain how it is done.

8. Suggest why the test tubes and flasks in this picture are covered with cotton.

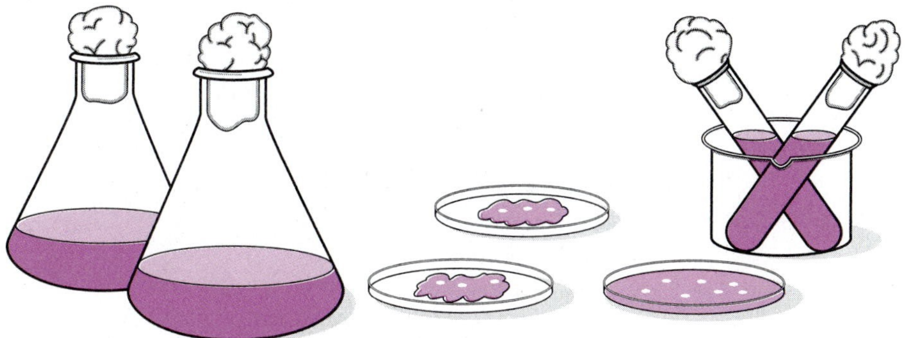

9. What are toxins?

10. What are some effects of toxins?

11. How often do bacteria reproduce, and by what method?

12. Why is it important to discover the presence of bacteria soon after they have entered the body?

13. Explain how colonies of bacteria will be visible on a petri dish after 24 hours.

B. Multiple Choice Questions: Select the letter of the choice that best answers the question.

1. The presence of carbon dioxide in the atmosphere enhances the growth of _____.
   a. *Staphylococcus*
   b. Micrococcus
   c. *Neisseria*
   d. *Pseudomonas*
2. The ideal temperature for growing most bacteria is
   a. 22°C
   b. 37°C
   c. 56°C
   d. 98.6°C
3. Bacteria require _____ for growth.
   a. food, moisture, warmth, neutral pH
   b. food, moisture, water
   c. food, neutral pH, water
   d. food, optimum temperature, neutral pH
4. Facultative anaerobes grow _____.
   a. best in oxygen
   b. best with added carbon dioxide
   c. with and without the presence of oxygen
   d. best without any oxygen
5. Toxins are _____.
   a. chemicals required for growth of bacteria
   b. poisons given off by bacteria
   c. by-products of fermentation of bacteria
   d. needed nutrients for bacterial growth

C. Completion Questions: From the following list of terms fill in the blanks with the correct choice.

obligate aerobes	pickling	transverse binary fission
facultative anaerobes	freezing	budding
obligate anaerobes	canning	nitrites
microaerophilic	salting	nitrates

1. Bacteria that can grow only in the absence of oxygen are called
   ________________.
2. The addition of excessive amounts of acid to preserve food is called
   ________________ .
3. Bacteria that prefer reduced oxygen are called ________________.

4. Bacteria are reproduced by ________________.

5. ________________ are used as a meat preservative to prevent botulism.

D. Matching Questions: Match the terms in Column I with their corresponding terms in Column II.

Column I		Column II
_______	1. Transverse binary fission	a. Needs oxygen
_______	2. Nitrites	b. Food
_______	3. Aerobic	c. 116°C
_______	4. Anaerobic	d. Preservative
_______	5. Agar	e. No oxygen
_______	6. pH for bacterial growth	f. Reproduction
_______	7. Canning temperature	g. 7.35
_______	8. Growth temperature	h. Removes water
_______	9. Salting	i. 37°C
_______	10. Blood pH	j. 7.0

SECTION 1

ACHIEVEMENT REVIEW

A. Insert the word or phrase that best completes the following statements.

1. Tiny organisms so small they can only be seen with the aid of a microscope are called ____________________.

2. These organisms were first discovered over 250 years ago by ____________________.

3. It was not until the late 1800s that scientists proved that ____________________ cause disease.

4. One-celled animals are called ____________________.

5. Simple plants are called ____________________.

6. The study of microbiology includes the study of:

   a. __________ c. __________ e. __________

   b. __________ d. __________ f. __________

B. Choose the word or expression that best completes the following statements from the list provided.

sunshine	spores	optimal
sterilization	reproduce	shape
flagella	absorb water	toxins
size	disinfection	cocci
structure	pH change	unfavorable temperature

1. Bacterial cells often differ from one another in ____________________, ____________________, and ____________________.

2. Tiny structures that project from the cell wall of motile bacteria are called ____________________.

3. The type of bacteria that lacks motility is the ____________________.

4. Some bacteria form resistant bodies called ____________________.

5. During the inactive period as described in (4) above, the bacterium is unable to ____________________ or ____________________.

6. Two methods of retarding the growth of bacteria are ___________________ and ___________________.

7. Two methods of killing bacteria are ___________________ and ___________________.

8. In general, ___________________ temperatures favor the growth of bacteria.

9. Most bacteria dislike ___________________ of any kind.

10. Poisonous excretions produced by bacteria are called ___________________ .

C. **Identify the parts of the microscope** (**see photo below**).

1. __________	5. __________	9. __________	12. __________
2. __________	6. __________	10. __________	13. __________
3. __________	7. __________	11. __________	14. __________
4. __________	8. __________		

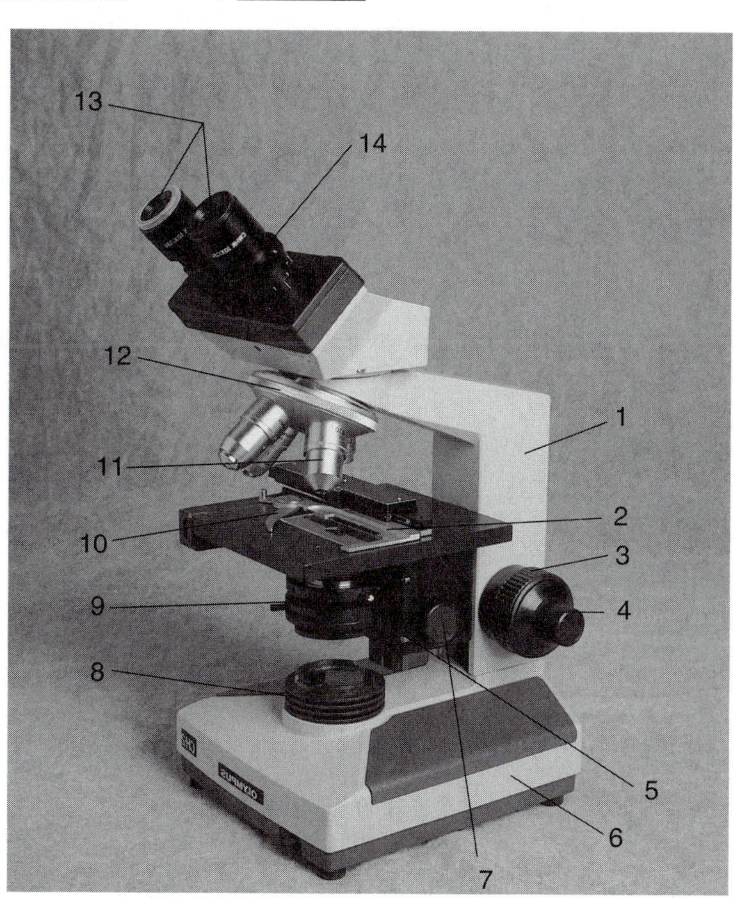

D. Insert the word or expression that best completes each statement.

30	Spallanzani	250,000	anesthetized
45	neutral	food	coldness
Streptococcus	acidic	water	kill
60 minutes	disinfectant	contamination	temperature
sterile	25,000	moisture	Lister
16×10^6	fumigated	darkness	Koch
Redi	sterilized	pasteurized	

1. It is possible for a bacterium to divide after __________________ minutes.
2. Most bacteria prefer a __________________ medium.
3. An electron microscope may magnify __________________ times.
4. All methods of preserving foods depend on producing __________________ conditions for the growth of bacteria.
5. The effect of direct sunlight on bacteria is to __________________ them.
6. Under favorable conditions, a single bacterial cell may produce __________________ of bacteria in 12 hours.
7. Four conditions needed by bacteria for growth are __________________, __________________, __________________, and __________________.
8. The medium agar provides bacteria with both __________________ and __________________.
9. Refrigeration retards the growth of bacteria because it produces the unfavorable environmental condition of __________________.
10. Something free from bacteria is referred to as __________________.
11. All health care professionals should wash their hands thoroughly with disinfectant soap and water after tending patients to prevent __________________.
12. The man who deserves the greatest credit for introducing the control of germs in operations is __________________.
13. To prevent infection, surgical instruments are __________________.

SECTION 2

STRUCTURE AND BEHAVIOR OF MICROORGANISMS

CHAPTER 5

The Cellular Structure and Characteristics of Eukaryotic Cells

OBJECTIVES

After completing this chapter, you will be able to:

- identify the structure of a typical cell.
- define the function of each part of the eukaryotic animal cell.
- describe the processes that transport materials in and out of a cell.

KEY WORDS

absolute zero
active transport
Adenosine triphosphate (ATP)
ameboid
autolysis
cell
cell membrane
cellular respiration
cell wall
centrioles
centrosome
chitin
chromatin
chromosome
cilia
cristae
cyclosis
cytologist
cytoplasm
diffusion
diploid
ectoplasm
endoplasm
endoplasmic reticulum (smooth and rough)
enzyme
equilibrium
eukaryote
filtration
flagella
glucan
Golgi apparatus
haploid
hemolyze
hypertonic solution
hypotonic solution
isotonic solution
lipid

EY WORDS (cont.)

oprotein
osome
ozyme
meiosis
microfilament
microtubule
mitosis
mitochondria
nuclear membrane
nucleolus
nucleus
organelle
osmolality
osmosis
osmotic pressure
phagocytosis
phospholipid bilayer
pinocytic vesicle
pinocytosis
polyribosome
prokaryote
refractive
ribosome
selective permeable membrane
sheath
silica
solutes
solvent
spindle-fiber apparatus
vacuole

THE CELL

When a field of grass is seen from a distance, it looks like a solid green carpet. Closer observation, however, shows that it is not a solid mass but is made up of countless separate blades of grass. So it is with the body of a plant or animal; it seems to be a single entity, but when any portion is examined under a microscope, it is found to be made up of many small, discrete parts. These tiny parts, or units, are called **cells.** All living things—plant or animal, unicellular or multicellular, large or small—consist of cells. A cell is microscopic in size. The cell is the basic unit of structure and function of all living things.

Cells are grouped into two major categories. The more complex cells of plants, animals, protozoa, fungi, and most algae are the **eukaryotes** (Figure 5–1). The less complex cells of bacteria and cyanobacteria (blue-green algae) are the **prokaryotes.** *Eukaryote* means "true nucleus," and *prokaryote* means "before nucleus." **Cytologists** specialize in the pathology of the cell, whose changes in internal structures give important clues as to the cause or source of diseases.

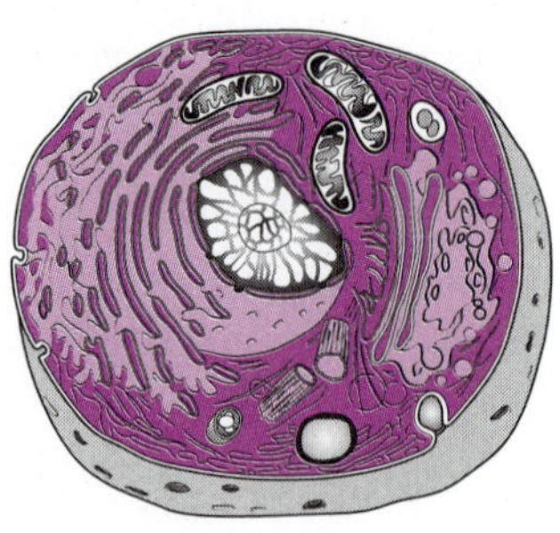

Figure 5–1 Eukaryotic cell

Because cells are microscopic, a special unit of measurement is used to determine their size—the micrometer (μm), or micron (μ). This measure is used to describe both the size of cells and their cellular parts (refer to Table 2–1).

To better understand the structure of a cell, let us compare a living entity—such as a human being—to a house. The many individual cells of this living organism are comparable to the many rooms of a house. Just as each room is bounded by four walls, a floor, and a ceiling, a cell is bounded by a cell membrane. Cells, like rooms, come in a variety of shapes and sizes. Every kind of room or cell has its own unique function. A house can be made up of a single room or many rooms. In much the same fashion, a living thing can be made up of only one cell (unicellular), or many cells (multicellular). A cell is made up of certain basic parts. Just as rooms have walls, are filled with air, and usually have a central piece of furniture, cells consist of a cell membrane, cytoplasm, and, in the case of eukaryotic cells, a nucleus. Additional furnishings in the eukaryotic cell are referred to as **organelles.** The name *organelle* means "little organ." Some organelles are easily seen under the light microscope, but others can be seen only with an electron microscope.

"Basic" and "typical" are terms used to identify structures common to most living cells. For an example of an animal cell, see Figure 5–2.

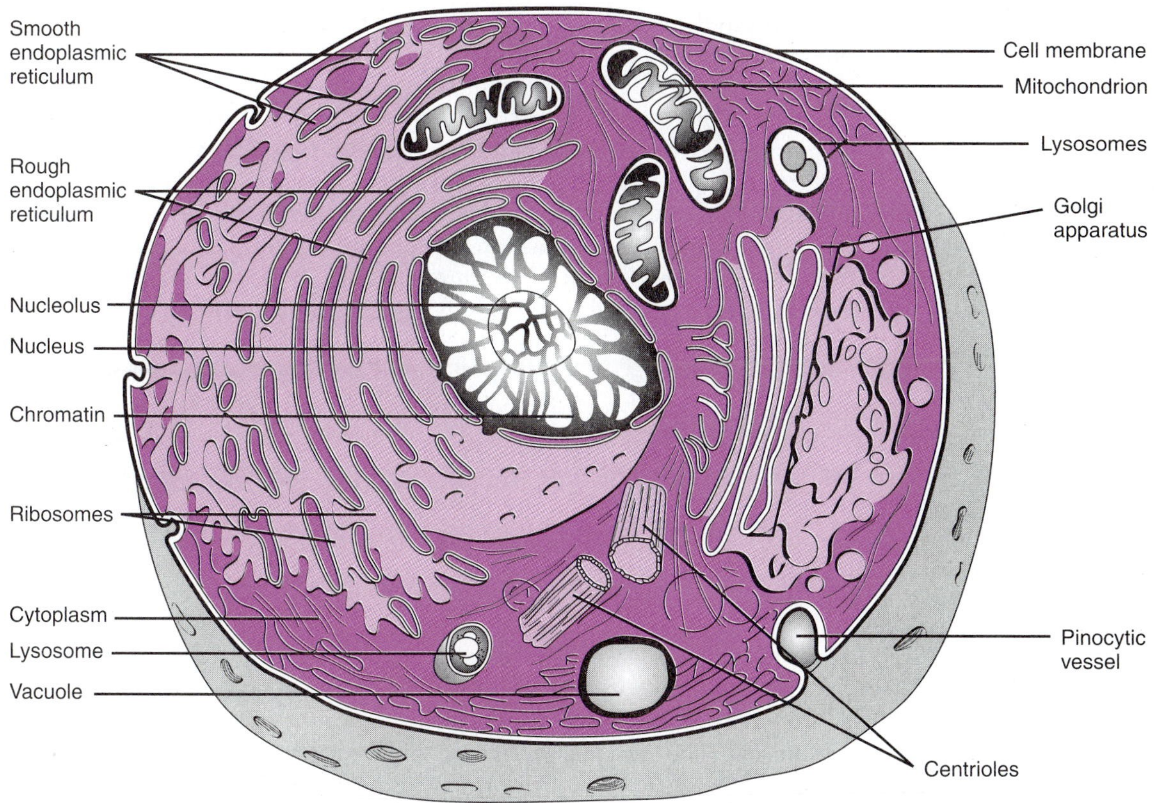

Figure 5–2 Fine structure of a typical animal cell

EUKARYOTIC CELL STRUCTURE

The Nucleus

The **nucleus** is the most important structure within the cell. Usually located near the center of the cell, it is the control center for all cell activity, and it is from within the nucleus that cell division is initiated. Various dyes or stains, such as iodine, can be used to make the nucleus stand out. The nucleus stains vividly because it contains DNA (deoxyribonucleic acid) and protein. Both readily absorb stains. Surrounding the nucleus is a membrane called the **nuclear membrane.**

The DNA and protein are arranged in a loose and diffuse state called **chromatin.** When the cell is ready to divide, the chromatin condenses to form short, rodlike structures called **chromosomes.** There is a specific number of chromosomes in the nucleus for each species. The number of chromosomes for humans is forty-six, or twenty-three pairs.

When a cell reaches a certain size, it may divide to form two new cells. When this occurs, the nucleus divides first by a process called **mitosis.** During this process, the nuclear material is distributed to each of the two new nuclei. This step is followed by division of the **cytoplasm** into two approximately equal parts through the formation of a new membrane between the two nuclei. It is only during the process of nuclear division that the chromosomes can be seen (Figure 5–3).

In mitosis the total number of chromosomes in the daughter cells is the same as in the parent cell. This number is referred to as a **diploid** or 2N number. In humans the diploid number is 46 and the haploid number is 23. Cells that are involved in sexual reproduction, such as the human egg and sperm, must undergo another cell division process to reduce their number from 2N to N or **haploid** number. This division ensures that, upon union, the fertilized cell will be able to begin its growth process of mitosis with the full complement of 2N chromosomes. This second type of cell division, whose purpose it is to reduce the number of chromosomes to a haploid number, is called **meiosis.** Mitosis involves all but the sex cells, and two daughter cells with a diploid number of chromosomes are produced. Meiosis, on the other hand, involves only sex cells and ultimately results in four offspring, each with a haploid number of chromosomes (Figure 5–4).

Chromosomes are important because they store the hereditary material—DNA—passed on from one generation of cells to the next.

The Cell Membrane

Every eukaryotic cell is surrounded by a **cell membrane,** sometimes called a plasma membrane. The cell membrane separates the cell's cytoplasm from its external environment and from the neighboring cells. It also regulates the passage or transport of certain molecules into and out of the cell, while preventing the passage of others. This is why the cell membrane is often called a "selective semipermeable membrane." The cell membrane is made up of a double layer of phospholipid molecules (**phospholipid bilayer**) with protein molecules embedded in the **lipid** layers. It is these molecules that regulate the passage of nutrients and waste into and out of the cell.

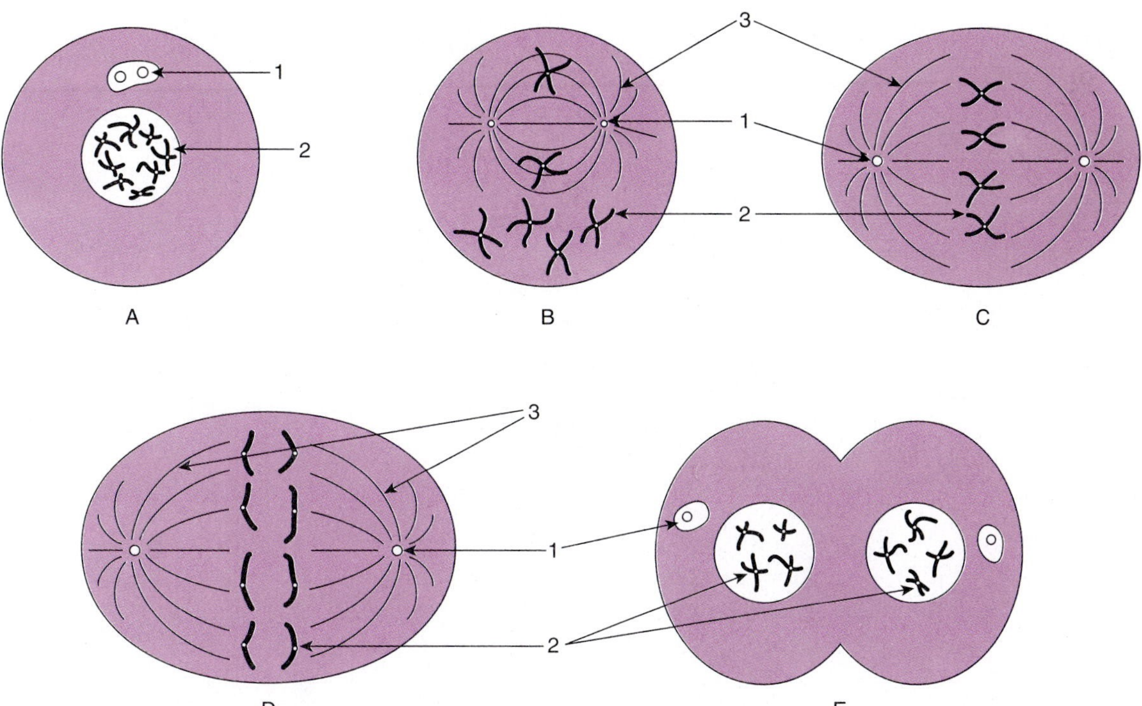

Figure 5–3 Process of mitosis: (A) resting or interphase; (B) prophase; (C) metaphase; (D) telophase; (E) anaphase. 1 = centrioles; 2 = chromatin chromosomes; 3 = spindle fibers

The Cytoplasm

The cytoplasm, often thought of as the body of the cell, is a sticky semifluid material found between the nucleus and the cell membrane. It may be divided into two layers: an outer layer known as the **ectoplasm** and an inner layer called the **endoplasm.** Chemical analysis of the cytoplasm shows that it is made of proteins, lipids, carbohydrates, minerals, salts, and a great deal of water (70% to 90%). Each of these substances varies greatly from one cell to the next and from one organism to the next. The cytoplasm is the background for all the chemical reactions that take place in a cell, such as protein synthesis and cellular respiration. Molecules are transported about the cell by the circular motion of the cytoplasm (**cyclosis**). Embedded in the cytoplasm are organelles, or cell structures, that help a cell to function. These include the nucleus, mitochondria, ribosomes, Golgi apparatus, endoplasmic reticulum, lysosomes, and the centriole.

The Nucleolus and the Ribosomes

Within the nucleus are one (nucleolus) or more **nucleoli.** Each nucleolus is a small round dense body (see Figure 5–2). The nucleolus takes part in protein synthesis and manufactures the **ribosomes** that are made up of ribonucleic acid (RNA) and protein.

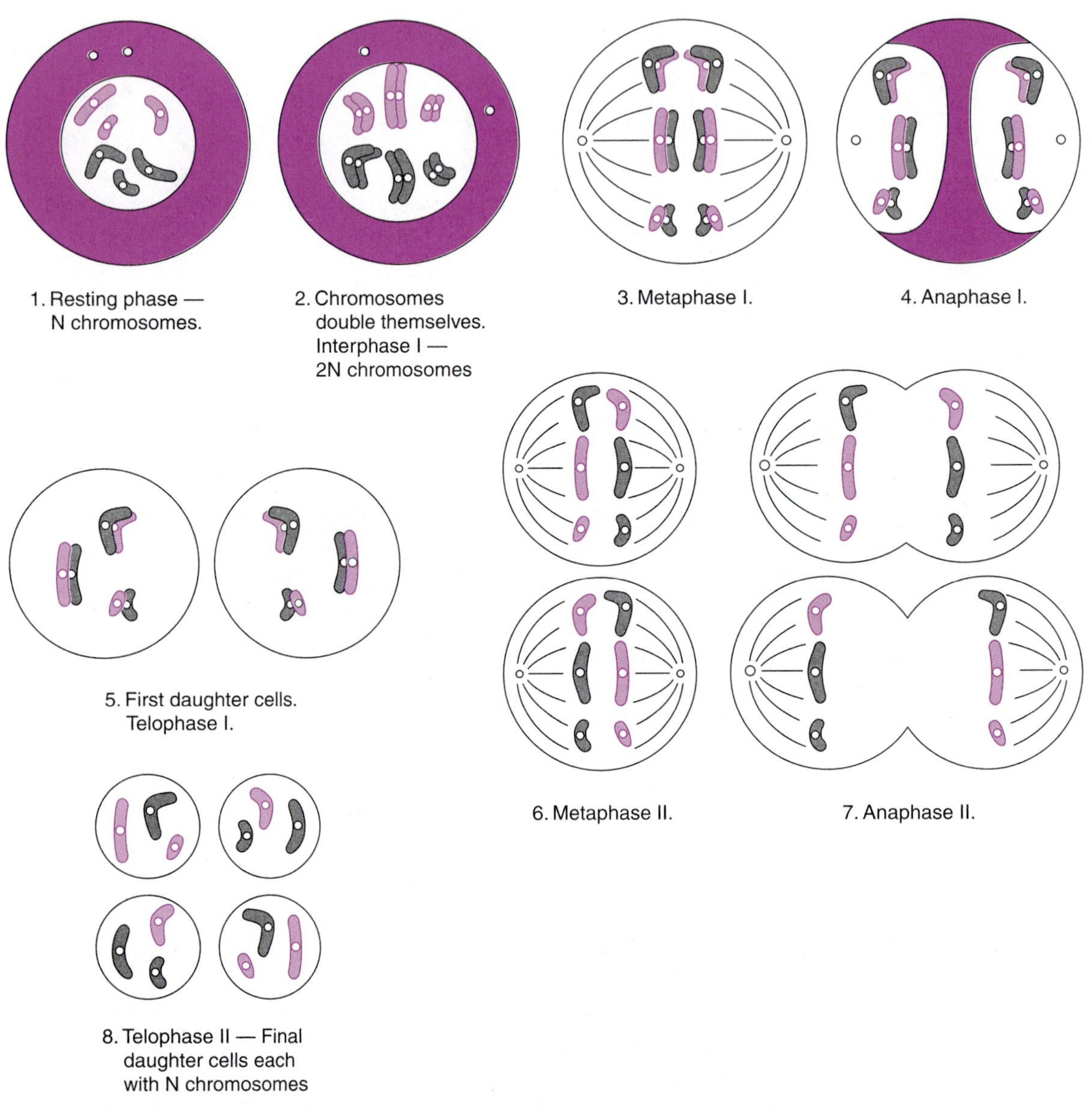

Figure 5–4 Process of meiosis

The ribosomes move out to the cytoplasmic area, where they can be found attached to the walls of the endoplasmic reticulum, floating freely in the cytoplasm, or formed into clusters called **polyribosomes.** Ribosomes, among the smallest of cell structures, are commonly referred to as the protein factories of the cell because their function is one of the most important.

The Endoplasmic Reticulum

Crisscrossing the cellular cytoplasm is a fine network of tubular structures called the **endoplasmic reticulum** (*reticulum* means "network"). Some of this endoplasmic reticulum connects the nuclear membrane to the cell membrane. Thus, it serves as a channel for the transport of proteins and other materials in and out of the nucleus and provides some structural support for the cell. Sometimes the endoplasmic reticulum will accumulate large masses of proteins and act as a storage area.

There are two types of endoplasmic reticulum—rough and smooth. Rough endoplasmic reticulum has the ribosomes studding the outer membrane, which gives it a coarse appearance. Smooth endoplasmic reticulum has no ribosomes on the outer membrane and it synthesizes the lipids.

The Mitochondria

All of a cell's energy comes from spherical or rod-shaped organelles called **mitochondria** (singular, mitochondrion; *mito* means "thread," *chondrion* means "granule"). These mitochondria vary in shape and number. There can be as few as a single one in each cell or as many as a thousand or more. Cells that need the most energy have the greatest number of mitochondria. Energy, in the form of **adenosine triphosphate (ATP),** is organized in the mitochondria and released to all parts of the cell as needed. Because they supply the cell's energy, mitochondria are also known as the "powerhouse" of the cell.

The electron microscope identifies the mitochondria as a double-membraned structure: It has an outer and an inner membrane. The inner membrane is folded inward to form shelflike ridges called **cristae. Enzymes** are chemicals found in the cristae. These enzymes help the mitochondria undergo **cellular respiration,** which is a chemical reaction that breaks down carbohydrate, lipid, and protein molecules to release energy, carbon dioxide, and water. ATP is the product of cellular respiration and of the oxidation of glucose and oxygen.

The Golgi Apparatus

The **Golgi apparatus** was discovered in 1898 by the Italian scientist, Camillo Golgi. It is also called Golgi bodies or the Golgi complex. It is an arrangement of layers of membranes resembling a "stack of pancakes." Scientists believe that this organelle synthesizes carbohydrates and combines them with protein molecules as they pass through the Golgi apparatus. In this way the Golgi apparatus stores and packages secretions for discharge from the cell. It follows logically that these organelles are abundant in the cells of gastric glands, salivary glands, and pancreatic glands.

Lysosomes

Lysosomes are oval or spherical bodies that originated in the Golgi apparatus and are found in the cellular cytoplasm. They contain powerful digestive enzymes that digest protein molecules. Their enzyme, **lysozyme,** is capable of breaking down foreign materials. The lysosome thus helps to digest old, worn-out cells, bacteria, and foreign matter. Lysozyme can also digest old, broken down parts of the cell as well as destroy the whole cell by a process known as **autolysis.** If a lysosome should rupture, as sometimes happens, the lysosome will start digesting the cell's proteins, causing it to die. For this reason lysosomes are also known as "suicide bags."

Pinocytic Vesicles

Large molecules such as proteins and lipids, which cannot pass through the cell membrane, will enter a cell by way of the pinocytic vesicles. The **pinocytic vesicles** form by having the cell membrane fold inward to form a pocket. Some of the fluid surrounding the cell flows into this pocket. The fluid contains large molecules in solution. The edges of the pocket then close and pinch away from the cell membrane, forming a bubble or **vacuole** in the cytoplasm. The contents of the vacuole are separated from the cytoplasm by a cell membrane. This process by which a cell forms pinocytic vesicles to take in large molecules is called **pinocytosis** or "cell drinking."

MOVEMENT OF MATERIALS ACROSS CELL MEMBRANES

The cell membrane, aside from housing the cellular organelles, also controls passage of substances into and out of the cell. This process is important because a cell must be able to acquire materials from its surrounding medium, after which it either secretes synthesized substances or excretes wastes. The physical processes that control the passage of materials through the cell membrane are diffusion, osmosis, filtration, active transport, phagocytosis, and pinocytosis. Diffusion, osmosis, and filtration are passive processes, which means they do not need energy to function. Active transport, phagocytosis, and pinocytosis are active processes that require an energy source.

Diffusion

Diffusion is a physical process whereby molecules of gases, liquids, or solid particles spread or scatter themselves evenly through a medium. When solid particles are dissolved within a fluid, they are known as **solutes.** Diffusion also applies to a slightly different process, in which solutes and water pass across a membrane to distribute themselves evenly throughout the two fluids, which remain separated by the membrane. Generally, molecules move from an area in which they are greatly concentrated to an area in which they are less concentrated. The molecules will, finally, distribute themselves evenly within the space available; when this happens, the molecules are said to be in a state of **equilibrium** (Figure 5–5).

The three common states of matter are gases, liquids, and solids. Molecules will diffuse more quickly in gases and more slowly in solids. Diffusion occurs due to the heat energy of molecules. As a result, molecules are always in constant motion, except at

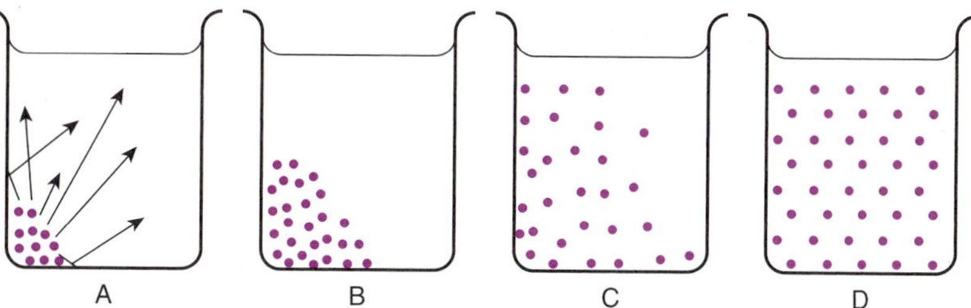

Figure 5–5 The process of diffusion

(A) A small lump of sugar is placed into a beaker of water. Its molecules dissolve and begin to diffuse outward; (B) and (C) The sugar molecules continue to diffuse through the water from an area of greater concentration to an area of lesser concentration; (D) Over a long period, the sugar molecules are evenly distributed throughout the water, reaching a state of equilibrium.

absolute zero (−273°C). In all cases, the movement of molecules increases with an increase in temperature.

A few familiar examples of the rates of diffusion may be helpful. For instance, if one thoroughly saturates a wad of cotton with ammonia and places it in a far corner of a room, as the ammonia diffuses throughout the room one can soon smell it everywhere. Another test for diffusion is to place a pair of dye crystals on the bottom of a water-filled beaker. Later, they will uniformly permeate and color the water. This diffusion process will take quite a while, especially if no one stirs, shakes, or heats the beaker. In still another test, a dye crystal placed on an ice cube moves even more slowly through the ice. Diffusion of the dye can be done faster by melting the ice.

The diffusion rate of molecules in the various media (gas, liquid, and solid) depends upon the distances between each molecule and how freely they can move. In a gas, molecules can move more freely and quickly; within a liquid, molecules are more tightly held together. In a solid substance, molecular movement is highly restricted and thus very slow. Regardless of the material being in a solid, liquid, or gas, the solute (the material being dissolved or diffused) will move from the region of a higher concentration to a lower concentration at a rate determined by distance to travel and the density of the **solvent.**

Diffusion plays a vital role in permitting molecules to enter and leave a cell. Oxygen diffuses from the bloodstream, where it dwells in greater concentration. From the bloodstream, the oxygen enters the fluid surrounding a cell, then into the cell itself, where it is far less concentrated. In this manner, the flow of blood through the lungs and bloodstream provides a continuous supply of oxygen to the cells. Once oxygen has entered a cell, it is utilized in metabolic activities.

Osmosis

Osmosis is the diffusion of water through a selective permeable membrane (such as the cell membrane) from an area of greater concentration of water to an area of lesser concentration. A **selective permeable membrane** is any membrane through which some solutes can diffuse, but others cannot. For example, sausage casing is a selective permeable

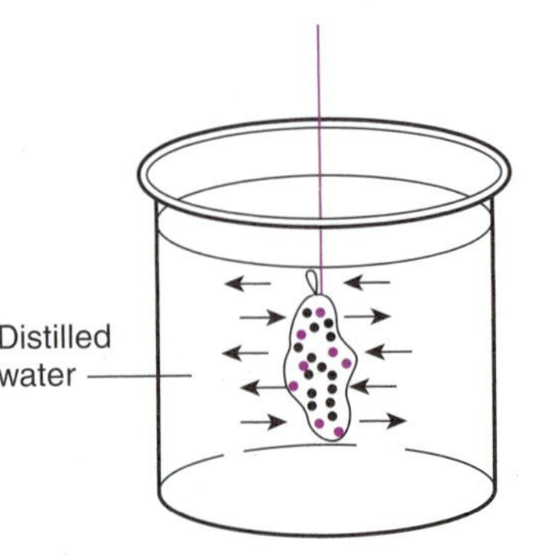

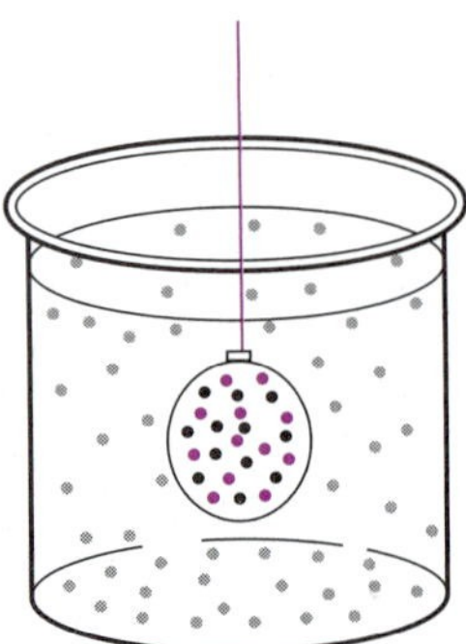

- Gelatin
- Salt
- Sucrose

Figure 5–6 Osmosis is the diffusion of water through a selective permeable membrane. A sausage casing is an example of a selective permeable membrane (Left) In the initial stage, the sausage casing contains a solution of gelatin, salt, and sucrose. The casing is permeable to water and salt molecules only. Since the concentration of water molecules is greater outside the casing, water molecules will diffuse into the casing. The opposite situation exists for the salt. (Right) Ten to 12 hours later, the sausage casing swells because of the net movement of water molecules inward. However, the volume of distilled water in the beaker remains constant.

membrane that can be used to substitute for a cell membrane. A solution of salt, sucrose (table sugar), and gelatin is placed into the sausage casing. This mixture is then suspended into a beaker filled with distilled water (Figure 5–6). The sausage casing is permeable to water and salt, but not to gelatin and sucrose. Thus, only the water and salt molecules can pass through the casing. Eventually, more salt molecules will move out because we began with a greater concentration of these molecules inside. At the same time, more water molecules move into the casing, since there were more outside when we began.

This is yet another example of diffusion whereby molecules move from a region of higher concentration to a region of lower concentration. The volume of water increases inside the casing, causing it to expand because of the entry of water molecules. When the number of water molecules entering the casing is equal to the number exiting, an equilibrium has been achieved; the casing will expand no further.

The pressure exerted by the water molecules within the casing at equilibrium is called the **osmotic pressure,** which is expressed as millimeters of mercury (mm Hg). It is important to remember that every solution has a potential osmotic pressure.

The osmotic pressure of a solution is dependent upon the number of molecules of solute dissolved in a solution. The higher the osmotic pressure (**osmolality**) of a solution, the greater the number of molecules in that solution; and the greater the concentration of molecules, the stronger the "pull" or attraction for water molecules. Simply stated, water molecules move toward the area of greater osmolality.

In physiology, the osmotic characteristics of various solutions are determined by the manner in which they affect red blood cells. In other words, the osmolality of a given solution is compared with that of blood plasma. For instance, if a human red blood cell is placed into a solution with the same osmotic pressure as human blood plasma, the red blood cell will remain unchanged. This type of solution is known as an **isotonic solution.**

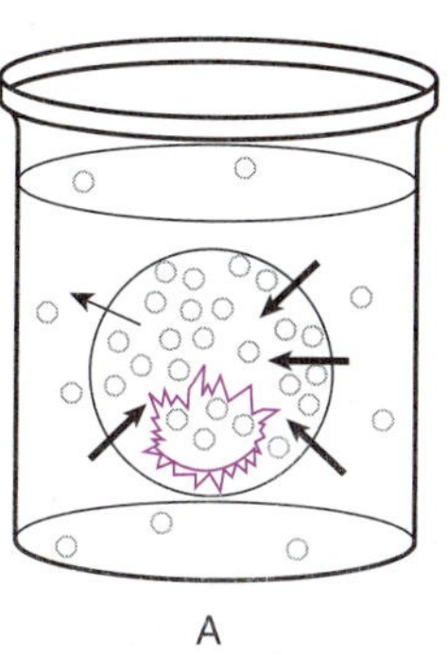

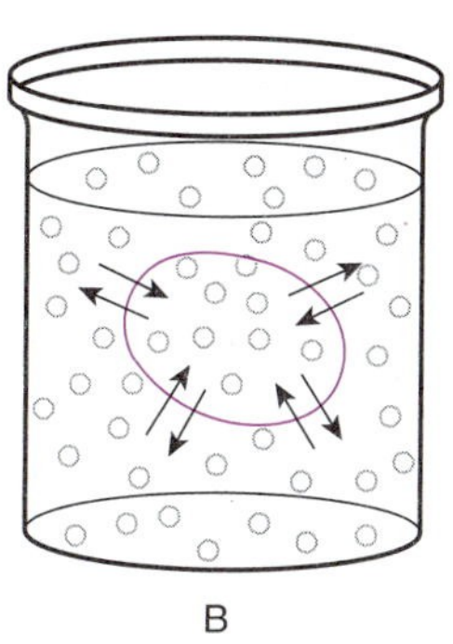

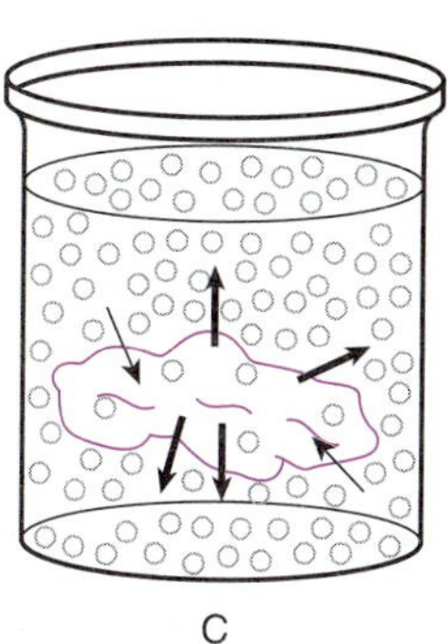

Figure 5–7 Movement of water molecules in solutions of different osmolalities
(A) Hypotonic solution (fresh water)—a red blood cell will swell and burst because water molecules are moving into the cell. (B) Isotonic solution (human blood serum)—a red blood cell remains unchanged, because the movement of water molecules into and out of the cell are the same. (C) Hypertonic solution (seawater)—a red blood cell will shrink and wrinkle up because water molecules are moving out of the cell.

Another way to appreciate the concept of osmotic pressure in an isotonic solution is to add a few red blood cells to a 0.1% saline solution (**hypotonic**), a 0.85% (or 0.9%) saline solution (**isotonic**), and a 1.0% saline solution (**hypertonic**). Since an isotonic solution has the same concentration of salt and water on both sides of the red cell, there is equal pressure applied to both sides of the red-cell membrane. Thus, the movement of water entering or leaving the cells is about the same. The cells in the hypotonic solution have a greater concentration of saline inside the red cells, thus water moves into the red cell to try to equalize the salt concentrations on both sides of the red-cell membrane. The red cell swells with the added water, and eventually it will burst, releasing the contents of the cell into the water. When a red cell breaks open and releases its hemoglobin content, the cell is said to have **hemolyzed.** Red blood cells in the hypertonic solution react differently. Because the salt concentration is greater in the saline solution, water rushes out of the red cell, causing it to shrivel up and become crenated. In summary, in a hypotonic solution, the osmolality is lower than that of blood plasma, and the red blood cell will swell and burst. This is caused by the water molecules moving into the cell. However, a red blood cell placed inside a hypertonic solution, such as seawater (with a higher osmolality than that of blood plasma), will shrink and wrinkle up because of the water moving out of the cell (Figure 5–7).

Filtration

Filtration is the movement of solutes and water across a semipermeable membrane, resulting from some mechanical force such as blood pressure or gravity. The solutes and water move from an area of higher pressure to an area of lower pressure. The size of the membrane pores determines which molecules are to be filtered. Thus, filtration allows for the separation of large and small molecules. Such filtration takes place in the kidneys. The process allows larger protein molecules to remain within the body and smaller ones to be excreted as waste (Figure 5–8).

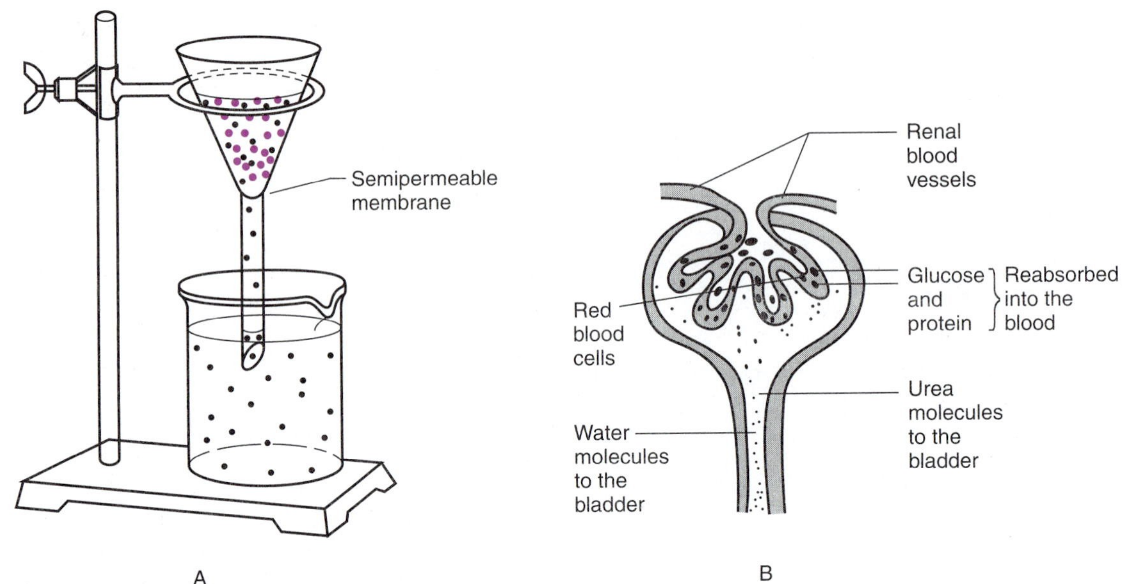

Figure 5–8 Filtration is a passive transport process
(A) Filtration—small molecules are filtered through the semipermeable membrane, while the large molecules remain in the funnel. (B) Example of filtration in the human body—glomerulus of kidney. Large particles such as red blood cells and proteins remain in the blood, and small molecules such as urea and water are excreted as a metabolic excretory product—urine.

Active Transport

Active transport is a process in which molecules move across the cell membrane from an area of lower concentration, against a concentration gradient, to an area of higher concentration. This process requires the high-energy chemical compound ATP. The ATP is supplied by the cell membrane.

How does active transport work? One theory suggests that a molecule is picked up from the outside of the cell membrane and brought inside by a carrier molecule. Both molecule and carrier are bound together, forming a temporary carrier–molecule complex. This carrier–molecule complex shuttles across the cell membrane; the molecule is released at the inner surface of the membrane. From here it enters the cytoplasm. At this point, the carrier acquires energy at the inner surface of the cell membrane. Then it returns to the outer surface of the cell membrane to pick up another molecule for transport. Accordingly, the carrier can also convey molecules in the opposite direction from the inside to the outside (Figure 5–9).

Phagocytosis

Phagocytosis, or "cell eating," is quite similar to pinocytosis, with an important difference: In pinocytosis, the substances engulfed by the cell membrane are in solution; in

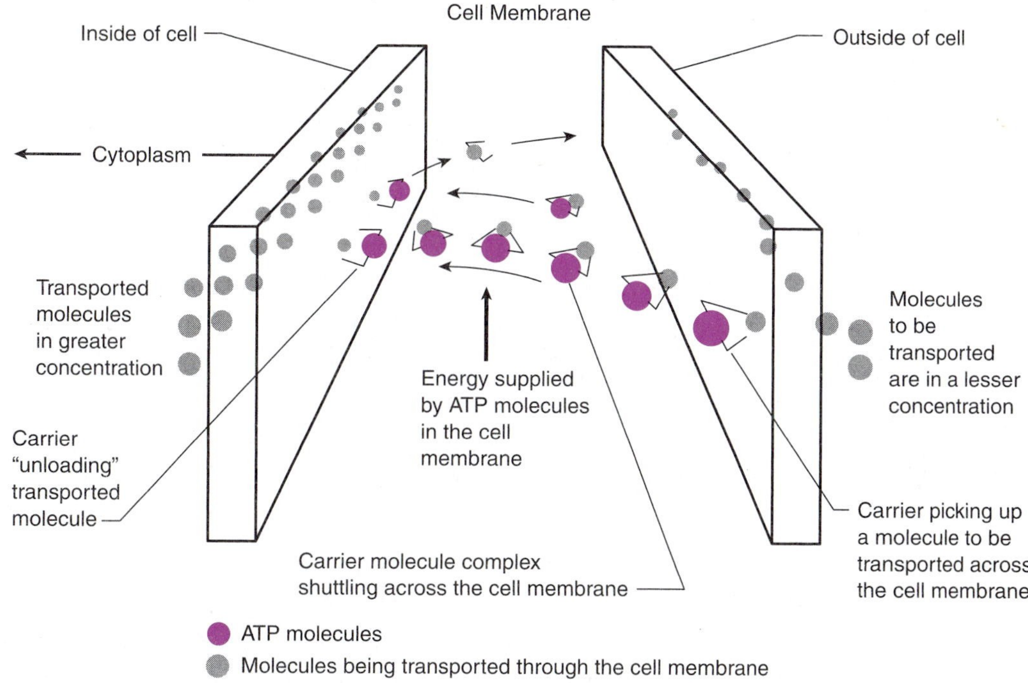

Figure 5–9 Active transport of molecules from an area of lesser concentration to an area of greater concentration, according to one theoretical model, with the help of ATP energy molecules as carriers

phagocytosis, the substances engulfed are within particles. Human white blood cells are capable of phagocytosis. They will phagocytize bacteria, cell fragments, or even a damaged cell. The particulate substance will be engulfed by an enfolding of the cell membrane to form a vacuole enclosing the material. When the material is completely enclosed within the vacuole, digestive enzymes pour into the vacuole from the cytoplasm to destroy the entrapped substance.

Pinocytosis

As stated earlier, pinocytosis or "cell drinking" involves the formation of pinocytic vesicles that engulf large molecules in solution. The cell then ingests the nutrient for its own use.

OTHER CYTOPLASMIC INCLUSIONS

Other microscopic structures found in the cytoplasm help a eukaryotic cell to function. These include the centrioles, microtubules, microfilaments, cilia, and flagella.

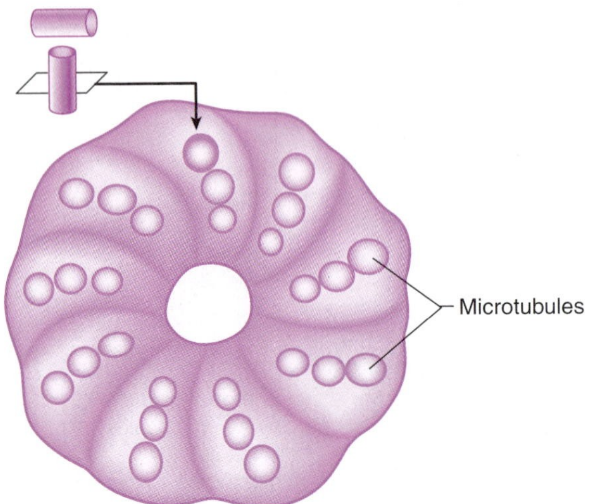

Figure 5–10 Larger view of the centrioles

Centrioles

The **centrioles** are two-cylindrical organelles found near the nucleus in a tiny round body called the **centrosome.** The centrioles are placed perpendicular to each other. Figure 5–2 shows two centrioles near the nucleus, while Figure 5–10 shows a larger view of the centrioles. The illustration in Figure 5–10 is based on an electron microscope picture. It shows that each centriole is made up of nine groups of three microtubules. During eukaryotic mitosis or cell division, the two centrioles separate from each other. In the process of separation, thin cytoplasmic spindle fibers form between the two centrioles. This structure is called a **spindle-fiber apparatus.** The spindle fibers attach themselves to individual chromosomes to help in the even and equal distribution of these chromosomes to two daughter cells. See Figure 5–3 showing the spindle fibers attracting the chromosomes to the centriole, now placed at opposite ends of the cell.

Microtubules and Microfilaments

Microtubules are made of protein, and as the name implies, are an array of long, thin microscopic tubules. They play a role in cytoplasmic membrane function and cell shape as well as forming the mitotic spindle-fiber apparatus.

Microfilaments are arrays of thin microscopic fibers or filaments containing two contractile proteins—actin and myosin. Microfilaments provide for the mechanism of **ameboid*** movement. There are also intermediate filaments, but their function is not yet known.

*Ameboid means "like an amoeba" (a unicellular bloblike organism) in form or in movement.

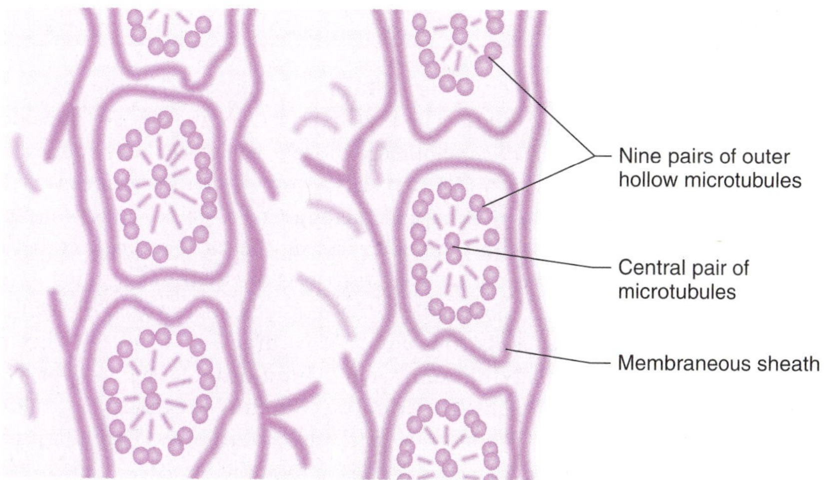

Figure 5–11 Cross section of eukaryotic flagella from *Trichonympha*

Cilia and Flagella

Many motile eukaryotic microorganisms propel themselves through water by the use of protein extensions called **cilia** or **flagella.** Eukaryotic flagella are far more complex than prokaryotic flagella. Both organelles consist of a bundle of nine pairs of hollow protein fibers on microtubules surrounding a central pair. This entire arrangement is enclosed in a membranous **sheath,** or covering. See Figure 5–11 for a cross section of eukaryotic flagella from protozoa *Trichonympha.*

The microtubules that make up the cilia and flagella started from a basal body within the cytoplasm. Cilia can be likened to short flagella.

Surface Layers

As mentioned, a eukaryotic cell is surrounded by a **lipoprotein** (lipid and protein) cell membrane. Most animal cells do not have any other surface layer surrounding the cell membrane. However, some cells do have this structure, called a **cell wall.** The chemical composition of most eukaryotic cell walls tends to vary, but in general they are much simpler than bacterial cell walls. The cell walls of most algae and fungi are made from a polysaccharide called cellulose, which makes the cell wall very rigid. Other fungi also have cell walls made from repeating subunits of glucose; however, the bonding between these glucose subunits is different from that found in cellulose. The resulting polymer is called **glucan.** There is another type of polymer, made up of subunits of *N*-acetylglucosamine forming **chitin,** which is found in some fungal cell walls. Other cell walls can be made from inorganic minerals such as **silica,** which is a very fine, sandlike material used in making glass.

SUMMARY

This chapter examines cellular structure and characteristics of eukaryotic cells. Any cell including human cells that have a true nucleus are considered to be eukaryotic cells. Eukaryotes also include the more complex cells of plants, animals, protozoa, fungi, and algae. Cells, as in animal cells, come in various shapes (no single shape), whereas plant cells tend to be square or rectangular in shape. Functioning parts of the cells are called organelles, with the nucleus being the most important, because it houses the chromosomes and genetic DNA. Mitosis is the method by which cells divide and multiply, producing exact look-alike daughter cells, each with a diploid or 2N numbers of chromosomes. Sex cells (ova and sperm) divide and multiply in numbers, but each daughter cell has half the number of chromosomes, haploid or N numbers. This process is known as meiosis. The most common organelles in cells include the nucleus, cytoplasm, cell membrane, nucleolus, ribosomes, endoplasmic reticulum, mitochondria, Golgi apparatus, lysosomes, pinocytic vesicles, centrioles, microtubules, microfilaments, cilia, and flagella.

For nutrients to pass across a cell membrane, a process of diffusion occurs. This process equalizes the molecules on both sides of the cell membrane. Osmosis is the diffusion of water across a selective (semi) permeable membrane.

The concentrations of solutions are compared with their action on red blood cells. If the solution in which the red cells bathe remain unchanged, then the osmotic pressure is the same on both sides of the cell and the solution is said to be isotonic, which is comparable to a 0.85% saline (salt) solution. Conversely, if the saline concentration is greater inside the cells than outside the cells, water moves into the red cells to equalize the saline concentration. The cell then swells and eventually bursts or hemolyzes, releasing its hemoglobin into the water or solution of a lesser saline concentration. This solution is a hypotonic solution. If the reverse were to occur, whereby the saline concentration was greater outside the cell, fluids from within the cell would rush out to equalize the osmotic pressure on the exterior of the cell. The cell then shrinks or crenates, and the solution is then said to be hypertonic. Fluids containing nutrients also move across cell membranes by filtration and active transport.

Some cells such as bacteria are able to engulf foreign materials to rid the body of their effects. This process is called phagocytosis and the polynuclear white blood cells (granulocytes) are the first to react. Phagocytosis is somewhat similar to pinocytosis, or cell drinking, a process that engulfs large molecules in solution.

STUDY AND DISCUSSION

- Study a prepared slide of a typical animal cell and one of a typical plant cell. From your close observations, write at least two differences between these two types of cells.
- If possible, visit a laboratory where different types of cells are studied under microscopes. A blood analysis laboratory or hospital laboratory would be interesting.

REVIEW QUESTIONS

A. Multiple-Choice Questions: Select the letter of the choice that best completes the sentence.

1. The organelle that most resembles the endoplasmic reticulum in basic structure is the _____ .
   a. plasma membrane
   b. Golgi apparatus
   c. nuclear membrane
   d. vacuole
2. All eukaryotic cells contain nuclear material, cytoplasm, and a _____ .
   a. plasma membrane
   b. chloroplast
   c. cell wall
   d. centrosome
3. Cristae or inner folds are characteristic of _____ .
   a. pinocytic vessels
   b. mitochondria
   c. chloroplasts
   d. ribosomes
4. Chemical analysis of the plasma or cell membrane indicates the presence of _____ .
   a. protein and cellulose
   b. lipid and starch
   c. protein and lipid
   d. protein and starch
5. The organelles that are the site for protein synthesis are the _____ .
   a. ribosomes
   b. mitochondria
   c. Golgi bodies
   d. lysosomes
6. Chromatin material is generally found in a structure called the _____ .
   a. pinocytic vesicle
   b. Golgi apparatus
   c. lysosome
   d. nucleus
7. The chemical compound most plentiful in the cytoplasm is _____ .
   a. ribonucleic acid
   b. oxygen
   c. glucose
   d. water
8. The term that is most closely related to chromatin is _____ .
   a. astral ray
   b. nucleolus
   c. DNA
   d. ribosome
9. RNA is most plentiful in the part of the nucleus called the _____ .
   a. Golgi apparatus
   b. nucleolus
   c. vacuole
   d. plasma membrane
10. A cell obtains energy during the process of _____ .
    a. secretion
    b. ingestion
    c. respiration
    d. excretion
11. Dissolved gases pass in and out of a cell through the _____ .
    a. cell membrane
    b. nuclear membrane
    c. nucleus
    d. ribosomes
12. ATP is a chemical that is produced by _____ .
    a. assimilation
    b. oxidation
    c. digestion
    d. absorption
13. All of the following are organelles except _____ .
    a. Golgi bodies
    b. ribosome
    c. phase-contrast microscope
    d. lysosome

14. Diffusion is the process by which _____ .
    a. ions or molecules do not move
    b. the same number of molecules or ions move in opposite directions
    c. molecules or ions move from an area of high concentration to an area of lower concentration
    d. molecules or ions migrate from an area of low concentration to an area of high concentration
15. A major feature of the cell or plasma membrane is that _____ .
    a. it is permeable only to water
    b. it selectively controls the passage of materials
    c. it is nonliving
    d. it is present only in animal cells
16. The following can readily pass through the cell membrane:
    a. starch
    b. glucose
    c. proteins
    d. fats
17. Molecules pass through a membrane from an area of lower concentration to an area of higher concentration by a process called _____ .
    a. diffusion
    b. digestion
    c. dehydration synthesis
    d. active transport

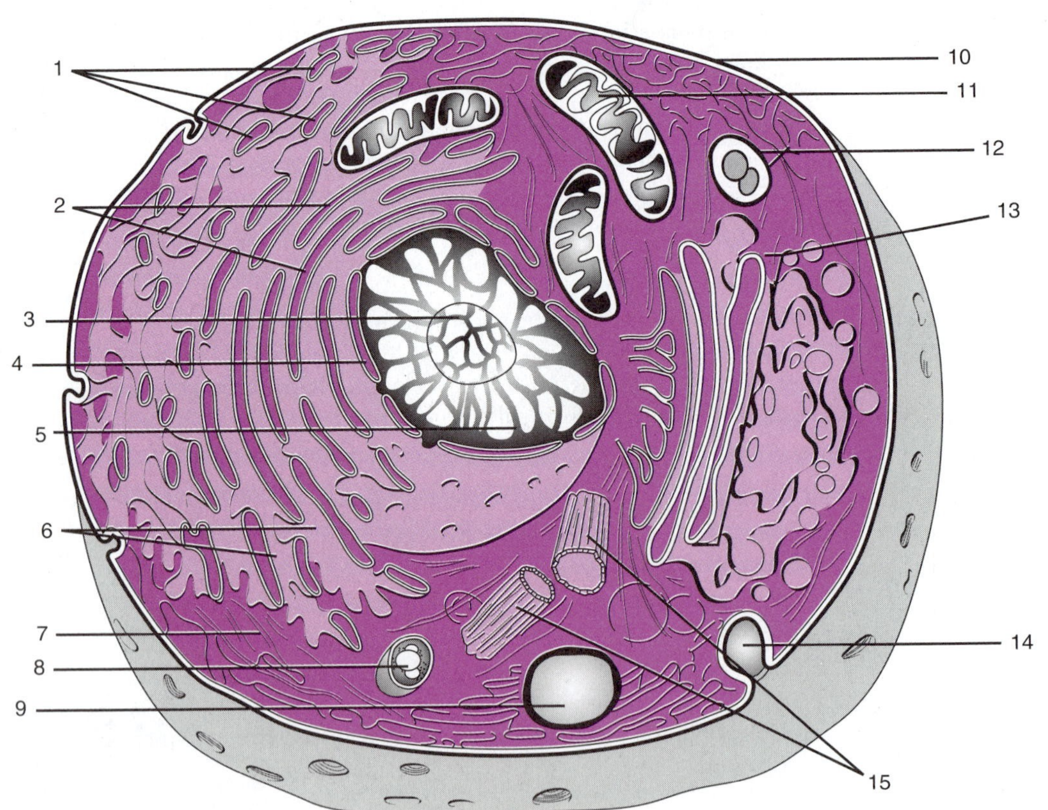

B. Identification Questions: Study the diagram of a typical cell (left). Identify the structures labeled with the numbered callouts.

1. ____________________
2. ____________________
3. ____________________
4. ____________________
5. ____________________
6. ____________________
7. ____________________
8. ____________________
9. ____________________
10. ____________________
11. ____________________
12. ____________________
13. ____________________
14. ____________________
15. ____________________

C. Matching Questions: Match each of the terms in Column I with its correct description in Column II.

Column I

_______ 1. Nucleus
_______ 2. Ribosome
_______ 3. DNA
_______ 4. Cytoplasm
_______ 5. Nerve
_______ 6. Reproduction
_______ 7. Cells
_______ 8. Mitosis
_______ 9. Mitochondria
_______ 10. Cell membrane

Column II

a. Small units of which all plants and animals are made
b. Exposed outer edge of the cell
c. Process by which cells divide
d. Example of a specialized cell
e. Dense inner portion of the cell
f. Cell powerhouse from which energy is released
g. Portion of the cell between the nucleus and cell membrane
h. Ability lost by some specialized cells
i. Hereditary material within the chromosome
j. Cell structure where chromosomes are located
k. Organelle involved in protein synthesis

CHAPTER 6

The Cellular Structure and Characteristics of Prokaryotic Cells

OBJECTIVES

After completing this chapter, you will be able to:

- state a function for each part of a typical bacterial cell.
- state the difference between an encapsulated bacterium and a nonencapsulated bacterium.
- differentiate between the cell walls of a gram-negative bacterium and a gram-positive bacterium.
- describe the four different groups of flagellated bacteria.
- describe the value of sporogenesis.

KEY WORDS

animalia
autolysis
basal body
binary fission
capsule
caries
cell envelope
cell wall
conjugation
cytochrome
dehydrogenase
dormant
encapsulated
endospore
exoenzyme
flagella
flagellin
fimbriae
germinate
glycocalyx
mesosome
nonencapsulated
nucleoid
pili
pilus bridge
plaque
plasmid
polyribosome
prokaryote
refractive
spore
sporogenesis
unit membrane
virulence

PROKARYOTIC CELL STRUCTURE

The structure of a prokaryotic cell is much simpler than the structure of a eukaryotic cell. Prokaryotic cells do not have as many internal membrane-bound organelles as do eukaryotic cells. However, there is one notable exception—the prokaryotic cell envelope is very complex.

The cytoplasm of bacteria is surrounded by the cytoplasmic membrane and the cell wall, and others may have a third layer called the **capsule.** These two or three layers together are called the **cell envelope.** The description of the typical structure of a **prokaryote** will proceed from the capsule (the outermost layer) to the structures found within the cytoplasm (Figure 6–1).

Capsule or Slime Layer

As discussed, the outermost layer found on most prokaryotic algae and bacteria is the capsule or "slime" layer. The capsule is a thick, sticky layer of gelatinous material synthesized by enzymes found at the surface of the bacterial plasma membrane. The surrounding

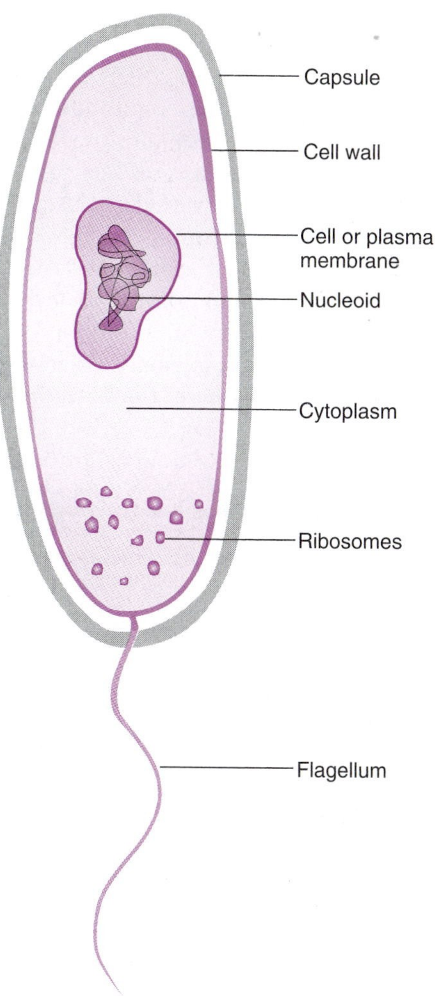

Figure 6–1 Basic prokaryotic bacterial cell with a flagellum

capsule, when negatively stained (that is, when the background is stained instead of the material being examined), is quite visible under the microscope. (For more information on negative stains and other stains, see Chapter 13). Most of the bacterial capsule is made from polysaccharides such as dextran, dextrin, levan, and cellulose, which may unite with lipids and proteins. The chemical composition of the capsule varies according to the species of microbe. Other capsules may be made up of polypeptides made from one or two amino acids. For example, the bacterium *Bacillus anthracis* makes a polypeptide capsule from the amino acid D-glutamic acid. Knowledge of the chemical composition of a bacterial capsule was and still is important. For instance, before the development of sulfa drugs and antibiotics, it was important to know the specific type of bacterium causing an infection. The treatment was quite species-specific because of the slight differences in the capsular chemical makeup.

Not all prokaryotic bacterial species have capsules around them. The ones that have capsules are **encapsulated** bacterium and those that do not are **nonencapsulated** bacterium. When grown on nutrient agar, encapsulated bacterium are smooth (S), glistening, and mucoid. The nonencapsulated ones form dry and rough (R) colonies.

A bacterial capsule is a multifunctional structure. It gives a protective covering and can also function as a reservoir for stored food or as a place for waste disposal. A capsule is found around some disease-causing bacteria. It is believed that the capsule enhances its infective ability. Nonencapsulated bacteria are quickly engulfed and destroyed by white blood cells in the human body. If a disease-causing bacterium lost its capsule, it would also lose its infective or invasive ability **(virulence).**

There is a variation on the bacterial capsule called a **glycocalyx.** The glycocalyx is made of a loose meshwork of fibrils coming outward from the bacteria. This structure helps bacteria to stick to environmental surfaces, including the cells of their animal and plant hosts. For instance, the bacterium *Streptococcus mutans* sticks tightly to tooth enamel via the glycocalyx. Bacteria of the same or different species get trapped in the fibril meshwork of the glycocalyx, forming a filmy layer on the tooth's surface, commonly called dental **plaque.** The acidic substances produced by plaque bacteria erode the tooth enamel, causing dental **caries.** Glycocalyx needs sucrose for its synthesis. Thus, there is a direct link between the development of dental caries and sucrose consumption by human beings.

Cell Wall

The bacterial **cell wall** is found between the outermost capsule or slime layer and the inner cytoplasmic membrane. The chemical composition of the cell wall is responsible for its rigid nature, which gives shape to the bacterial cell. The strength and rigidity of the bacterial cell wall has been demonstrated in the laboratory: Bacteria of different sizes and shapes were subjected to extremes of different physical conditions. These conditions were very low and high osmotic pressures and subfreezing temperatures followed by rapid thawing. The cell walls of these bacteria were not broken, and they still retained their shape. Besides contributing to the shape of the bacteria, the cell walls seem to be needed for proper bacterial growth and division. Bacteria whose cell walls have been removed cannot undergo normal growth or cell division.

The study of the special characteristics of the cell wall is of importance to the health care provider. It is through the use of different stains on the various types of cell walls that bacteria can be easily detected. Certain bacteria, because of their staining ability, can be divided into two groups—gram-negative and gram-positive. Each has special characteristics unique to its cell wall.

It is vital for the health care provider to have some knowledge and understanding of the different cell types and their structure. This is essential in helping us to classify microbes and to understand the differences in their structure, chemical composition, and chemical activities. This knowledge will help the health care professional select the proper chemicals or drugs to combat disease-causing microbes that affect our daily lives and health.

Characteristics of gram-positive cell walls. The cell walls of gram-positive bacterium are much thicker than gram-negative cell walls. This dense cell wall is due to layer upon layer of the peptidoglycan molecule. Each layer is firmly connected to the other layers by amino acid bridges. This entire interconnected meshlike molecule gives the cell wall its rigidity and strength. The gram-positive peptidoglycan cell wall has an added part to its structure—the teichoic acids.

Characteristics of gram-negative cell walls. The cell wall of a gram-negative bacterium is also made from a peptidoglycan layer. However, its cell wall is not as thick as that of a gram-positive bacterium. A gram-negative cell wall can be broken down by mechanical forces more easily than the gram-positive cell wall. The gram-negative cell wall has other compounds joined to the peptidoglycan layer, including lipoprotein, liposaccharide, and phospholipid that envelop the peptidoglycan layer. Of these three organic compounds, the liposaccharide is of most interest. This layer allows a gram-negative bacterium to secrete toxins that are either deadly or harmful to the host organism. Purified liposaccharides have been isolated and extracted from various gram-negative strains in the laboratory. Upon injection into a susceptible host, liposaccharides cause symptoms characteristic of diseases caused by the entire bacterium. When stained, the acetone-alcohol easily dissolves the cell wall allowing the red counterstain to remain. As a result, when stained using the Gram stain method, this cell wall is insoluble in acetone-alcohol, and the primary color purple remains. When the decolorization agent is left on the slide longer than the prescribed time, the purple will be washed away.

Cytoplasmic Membrane

Located beneath the cell wall is a very thin membrane covering called the "cytoplasmic membrane" (also called the "plasma membrane" or the "protoplasmic membrane"). It is found between the cell wall proper and the cytoplasm.

Chemically, it is made up of about 60% protein and 40% lipid. The chemical and physical structures of prokaryotic and eukaryotic plasma membranes are quite similar. As viewed through the electron microscope, they appear as two dark bands with a light band in the middle. These two very similar looking plasma membranes are also called **unit membranes.**

The cytoplasmic membrane is a selective, semipermeable membrane with a host of functions. Because it is a selective semipermeable membrane, it will control the passage of nutrients and waste products into and out of the cell.

A second function of the cytoplasmic membrane resides in special respiratory enzymes called **cytochromes** and **dehydrogenases.** These enzymes take part in a chemical reaction called aerobic cellular respiration or, technically speaking, electron transport and oxidative phosphorylation. This reaction, essentially, breaks down nutrients to yield energy in the form of ATP molecules. These molecules are used to help power the bacterial cell's many chemical activities. These respiratory enzymes are located in inward foldings of the cytoplasmic membrane called **mesosomes.** These mesosomes can be compared with the mitochondrial cristae of eukaryotic cells.

A third function involves the excretion of hydrolytic **exoenzymes** or extracellular enzymes. All organisms, including microbes, rely on larger organic molecules such as lipids, polysaccharides, and proteins as a source of nutrients and energy. However, these very large organic molecules cannot penetrate the cytoplasmic membrane. So, they are digested or hydrolyzed outside the bacterial cell by exoenzymes. Depending on the species of microbe, these enzymes are located either on the outside of the cell or in the periplasmic space between the cell wall and the cytoplasmic membrane of the bacterium. Thus, large organic molecules passing through the cell wall will encounter these enzymes. Digestion occurs, and the resultant smaller molecules can then be transported through the cytoplasmic membrane via the permeases. (A permease is any number of enzymes designed to help transport a soluble nutrient molecule across the cell membrane into a cell.)

The enzymes needed for the manufacture of the cell wall, cytoplasmic membrane lipids, and DNA are located in the cytoplasmic membrane.

Mesosomes

Mesosomes are inward foldings of the bacterial cytoplasmic membrane. Apparently, these mesosomes help to increase the surface area of the cytoplasmic membrane. Several functions are attributed to the mesosomes. As mentioned, special respiratory enzymes called "cytochromes," which are part of the electron transport system producing high-energy ATP molecules, are found in the mesosomes. There are mesosomes located near the center of the bacterial cell that can help form a new cell wall or septum as the cell divides. The DNA of the bacterial nucleoid seems to be continuous with the mesosome. Therefore, it is possible that the mesosome helps to synthesize and divide the DNA during bacterial cell division, or replication. The mesosomes seem to be found in gram-positive bacteria but not in gram-negative bacteria.

Nucleoid

Prokaryotic cells, like eukaryotic cells, contain DNA in some localized area. However, prokaryotic DNA is *not* bounded by a discrete nuclear membrane. Thus, prokaryons do not have a distinct, discrete nucleus. This DNA area in the bacterial cell is called by one of several terms: *bacterial chromosome, chromatin body, nuclear equivalent,* or *nucleoid.*

For our purposes, the term **nucleoid** will be used. The nucleoid and its DNA can be seen through the light microscope when stained with a Feulgen stain, which is specific for DNA. Each bacterial chromosome is made from a single DNA strand, which is 1 millimeter (mm) long when unfolded. The bacterial DNA is acidic, and it is surrounded by basic proteins. All this seems to be coiled around an RNA core, which helps to hold the DNA in a coiled, compact form. This highly coiled DNA is packed into a volume approximately 10% of the volume of the bacterial cell. When the prokaryotic DNA starts duplicating and dividing, it does not form a mitotic spindle-fiber apparatus as eukaryotic DNA does. Bacterial DNA also carries genetic information to help it manufacture thousands of enzymes and proteins, as well as to help control the chemical activities of the bacterium.

Plasmids

Besides the genetic information contained in the regular bacterial chromosome, additional genetic information is carried in a structure called a **plasmid.** A plasmid is found in some bacteria, and because it contains genetic information that is not part of the regular chromosome, it is also called an "extrachromosomal DNA." The genetic information carried in the plasmid provides for additional characteristics and is not needed for bacterial life. The plasmid has two functions: It can transfer genetic information between bacterium in a reproductive process called "conjugation," and the information the plasmid transfers can determine whether a bacterium becomes resistant to one or several antibiotics.

Ribosomes

Found within the bacterial cytoplasm are thousands of submicroscopic particles. The majority of these particles are clustered ribosomes, called **polyribosomes** (*poly* meaning "many"), found throughout the cytoplasm. As in eukaryotic cells, these bacterial ribosomes will help in the synthesis of proteins. Up to 15,000 of these ribosomes are found in the cytoplasm, depending on how quickly the bacterial cell is making proteins. Thus, the faster the rate of protein synthesis, the greater the number of ribosomes present in the bacterial cell. The ribosomes serve as a physical site for the attachment of amino acids to form long polypeptide protein chains.

Flagella

Flagella are long, threadlike extensions composed entirely of protein. They function as organs of locomotion on the bacteria that possess them. These motile bacteria are called "flagellated bacteria." The flagellated bacteria are grouped according to the number and arrangement of their flagella. These characteristics are unique for each flagellated species. Thus, the presence of flagella on a bacterium can be used for classification purposes. The four groups are the monotrichous, the amphitrichous, the lophotrichous, and the peritrichous. Monotrichous bacteria possess a single polar flagellum, whereas amphitrichous bacteria have flagella at both ends. Lophotrichous bacteria contain a tuft of flagella at one end, and peritrichous bacteria have flagella all over their surface area. The four different groups of flagellated bacteria are illustrated in Figure 6–2.

The bacterial flagellum is made from a single protein subunit called **flagellin.** The flagellin subunits combine to form the flagellum, which is a hollow cylindrical structure. It has been demonstrated in the laboratory that the flagella are directly responsible for bacterial motility. When flagella are mechanically removed from bacteria by gentle whirling in a blender, they remain alive but immobile. However, if these immobile bacteria are incubated in a medium containing flagellin, new flagella are quickly made. The process is quite fast; within 3 to 6 minutes, motility is restored along with the growth of a new flagellum.

The flagellum is attached to the bacterium by a structure made up of a hook and a **basal body.** This structure in turn is firmly anchored into the cell wall and the cytoplasmic membrane.

For flagella to propel a bacterium through a liquid medium, the flagellum spins around its long axis. The bacterium itself will spin in the opposite direction. Figure 6–3 shows how a flagellum propels a bacterial cell through a liquid medium.

The surfaces of many cells and microbes have fine, short threadlike extensions. These extensions are called **pili.** They may be of the same or different lengths depending on their location. They may help to move fluid across the surface of a microbe. They are of medical importance in that they are responsible for the attachment of bacteria to the surfaces of human cells, and their attachment may be the source of the exchange of genetic information that is related to antibody production as a result of the protein-rich pilin present in pili.

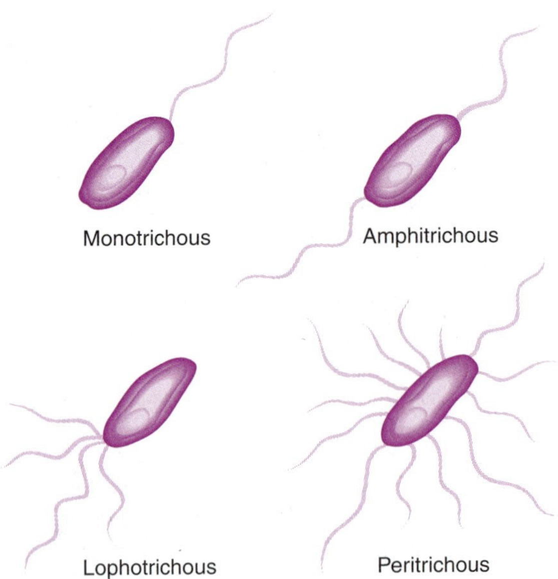

Figure 6–2 The four different groups of flagellated bacteria—monotrichous, amphitrichous, lophotrichous, and peritrichous

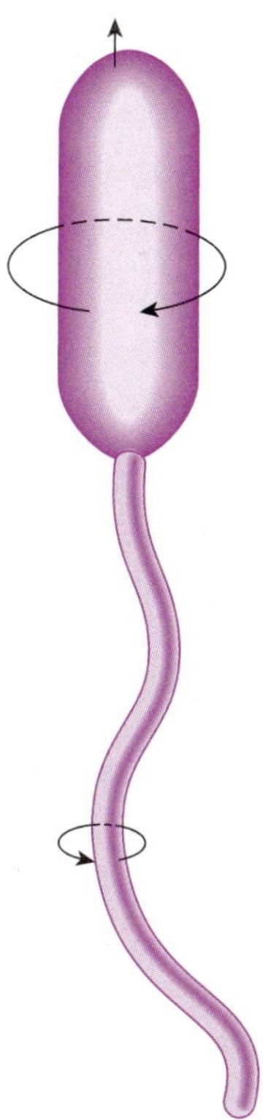

Figure 6–3 Movement of a flagellum as it propels a bacterium through a liquid medium

Pili (Fimbriae)

Many gram-negative bacteria (and, so far, only one gram-positive bacterium) have hundreds of rigid, hairlike appendages extending from their surfaces. As stated, these extensions are called pili (Latin, "hairs") or **fimbriae** (Latin, "fringes"). They are shorter and thinner than flagella, and they consist of protein subunits wound around one another to form a hollow cylindrical structure.

The two different types of pili are the ordinary pili and the F or sex pili. The ordinary pili allow a bacterium to stick to another or to other membrane surfaces, such as the intestinal lining and red blood cells. They also help to keep bacteria near the surface of a liquid or to absorb more oxygen and nutrients when the supply is low. It is believed that disease-causing bacteria tend to be piliated. For example, the strains of *Neisseria gonorrhoeae* that cause gonorrhea all have pili. Strains that have pili attach more readily to many kinds of eukaryotic cells. Nonpiliated bacterial strains fail to cause gonorrhea. The F or sex pilus allows a bacterium to transfer genetic information from one bacterium to another via an attachment called the **pilus bridge.** This process is called **conjugation.**

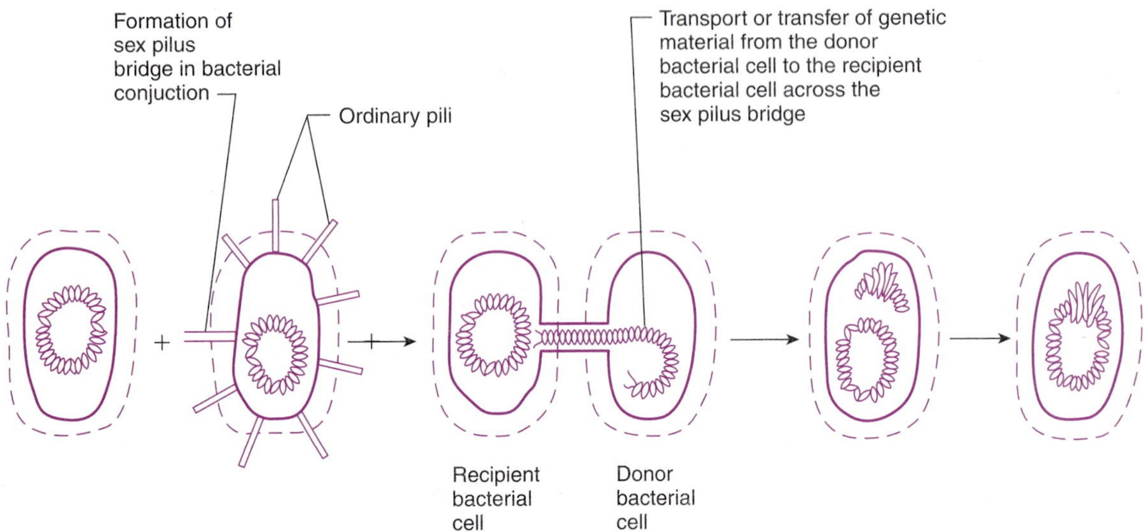

Figure 6–4 Bacterial conjugation

Conjugation is a form of sexual reproduction in which a donor bacterium (male) contributes some or all of its DNA to a recipient (female), which then incorporates differing genetic information into its own chromosome by recombination and passes the recombined set on to its progeny by replication. **Binary fission,** on the other hand, involves the division of a cell into two daughter cells after DNA replication and nuclear division. This division is a form of asexual reproduction. Figure 6–4 shows the process of conjugation between two bacterium.

Endospores or Spores

Some bacterial types are able to form a highly specialized protective covering called an **endospore** or **spore.** These spore-forming bacteria include two common rod-shaped bacteria: the aerobic genus *Bacillus* and the anaerobic genus *Clostridium.* Other bacteria that are spore formers are the coccus *Sporosarcina* and the rickettsial agent of Q fever, *Coxiella burnetii.* (More information on bacteria and rickettsias is found in Chapters 7 to 11.) A spore is formed when a normally growing vegetative bacterium is subjected to less than the best growing conditions, for instance, lack of food, moisture, oxygen, and the proper temperature. This process of spore formation is called "sporulation" or **sporogenesis.** During sporogenesis, the DNA is surrounded by several protein coats. The spore thus formed is resistant to most chemicals, drying, freezing, heating, and radiation.

Spores can survive for many years on dust particles. It has been estimated that spores can live up to 150,000 years. The most notable characteristic of a spore is that it has virtually no metabolic activities. However, when the dried, **dormant** spore lands on a moist, nutrient surface, it will **germinate** (develop into a new vegetative bacterial cell).

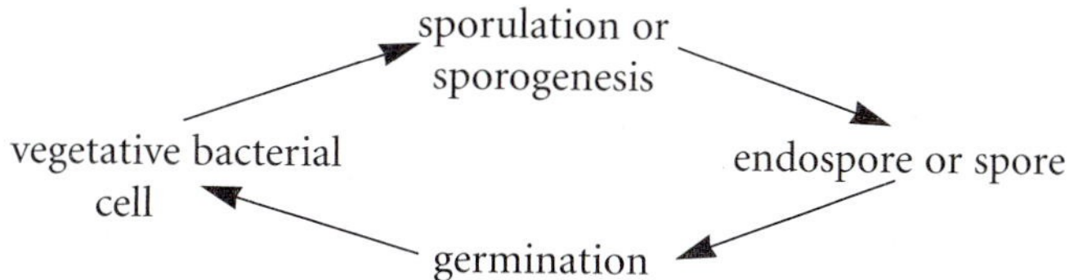

However, germination is not reproduction, as only one vegetative bacterial cell develops from one spore. A spore only helps a vegetative bacterial cell to live in less than the best conditions.

Not only are spores resistant, but some bacteria produce deadly toxins from spores. It is important that foods that might contain these spores be properly processed. Thus, knowledge of the structure and behavior of spores is vital to the health care professional.

Spores are easily detected under a good compound light microscope. They are highly **refractive,** having the ability to bend light from a straight line as it passes through the spore. Spores also do not absorb most stains through their very thick, protein spore coat, as do the remainder of the bacterium.

SUMMARY

This chapter examines the structure and characteristics of the simpler prokaryotic cells. Although these kinds of cells do not have many complex organelles, they do have a complex cell envelope, which consists of the cytoplasm surrounded by a cytoplasmic membrane and the cell wall. Some even have a third layer called a capsule. Simple organelles also include ribosomes, granular inclusions, a basal body, nucleoid, mesosome, and sometimes (if motile) a flagellum. Capsules may be difficult to see by ordinary staining methods; however the "negative" staining results are quite visible. The chemical composition of the capsule is important to the identification of the bacterium. Capsular bacteria are shiny and mucoid on culture, while on similar culture media, non-capsular bacteria are dry and rough. Capsular bacteria are also more virulent because they make it harder to shed the capsule when engulfed as a foreign body. When the capsule is shed, though, they lose their virulence and infectability.

Cell walls have distinct gram staining traits, so it is important to know into which group the bacterium falls, especially for antibiotic therapy determination. The two types are gram positive and gram negative, named for a researcher who developed the staining technique. Gram positive bacteria have cell walls that cannot be dissolved by a solution of acetone-alcohol, thus they retain their purple primary stains. Gram negative bacteria, on the other hand, have cell walls that are soluble in acetone-alcohol. This causes the cell wall and purple color to dissolve when washed in acetone-alcohol, leaving the bare cell covered in its cytoplasmic membrane to accept the red counterstain. This membrane consists of 60% protein and 40% lipid and functions the same as the eukaryotic cell membrane in breathing and metabolizing energy for the cell. The difference is the type of organelle assistance to accomplish these functions. Cytochrome and dehydrogenase enzymes aid in cell respiration and extracellular hydrolytic coenzymes situated in space between the cell wall and cytoplasmic membrane and are taken into the cell when digestion occurs.

Mesosomes, generally found only in gram positive bacteria, may have a function in helping synthesize and divide DNA during cell division or replication. They also are part of the active transport system, producing high energy ATP molecules to assist in cell division.

Nucleoids (e.g. the nucleolus) house DNA which carries genetic information to help manufacture enzymes and proteins. Each bacterial chromosome is made of one strand of DNA that is one millimeter long when unfolded. The DNA is coiled around an RNA core. Additional genetic information is carried in the plasmids, which are also known as extra-chromosomal DNA. The plasmid has two functions: to transfer genetic information between bacterium and to determine whether a bacterium is resistant or sensitive to one or several antibiotics through the information it carries. Thousands of ribosomes aid in the synthesis of proteins.

Flagella are responsible for the locomotive capabilities of bacteria, and depending on the location of flagella, bacteria can be classified into one of four groups: monotrichous, amphitrichous, lophotrichous, and peritrichous. Pili, hairlike extensions found on many gram negative bacteria, consist of protein subunits. These pili may be F or sex pili that allow bacteria to stick to another's chromosomal DNA during replication, or they may help keep bacteria near the surface of a liquid to be able to absorb more oxygen and nutrients. It is believed that disease-causing bacteria including *Neisseria gonorrhoeae* all have pili. Binary fission is an asexual reproductive method involving the splitting of a cell into two daughter cells, each with the same genetic information as the parent cell.

Some bacteria can form spores as protection from unfavorable environmental conditions for many years. In the spore form, bacteria are virtually dormant, but when moisturized in nutrients, they germinate and produce new bacterial cells unharmed by the long dormancy.

STUDY AND DISCUSSION

- Perform a Gram stain on several different kinds of bacteria. Record their staining properties. What color are gram-positive organisms? Gram-negative organisms? What color do yeasts stain?
- Study stained prepared slides of gram-positive and gram-negative cocci and rods from groups representing the following: 1. Staphylococci and Streptococci 2. Enterobacteriacae and Heamophilis 2. Bacillus and Clostridium and 4. Neisseria and Morexella. Describe similarities and differences within each of the four group pairs.
- If possible visit a clinical microbiology laboratory and tour the specialty areas in the Department of Microbiology. Make written observations of the methods used to identify the different microorganisms.

REVIEW QUESTIONS

A. Multiple-Choice Questions: Select the letter of the choice that best completes the sentence.

1. Bacteria may survive unfavorable conditions by _____ .
   a. forming spores
   b. splitting in half
   c. forming flagella
   d. forming pili

2. A type of glassware *most commonly* used for growing bacteria is a _____ .
   a. cup
   b. glass plate
   c. petri dish
   d. beaker
3. Poisons produced by bacteria are known as _____ .
   a. enzymes
   b. proteins
   c. drugs
   d. toxins
4. All of the following are types of "infectious agents," except _____ .
   a. worms
   b. proteins
   c. viruses
   d. bacteria
5. Viruses can be seen with the aid of the _____ .
   a. compound light microscope
   b. electron microscope
   c. phase-contrast microscope
   d. oil-immersion objective
6. Simple organelles of a prokaryotic cell include _____ .
   a. ribosomes, nucleoid, chloroplast, and mitochondria
   b. ribosomes, lysosomes, granular inclusions, and mesosomes
   c. ribosomes, mesosomes, nucleoid, and a basal body
   d. nucleus, cell wall, mitochondria, and ribosomes
7. Capsular bacteria are _____ .
   a. more virulent
   b. easy to stain
   c. always a gram-positive rod
   d. dry and dull on culture media
8. Organelles of locomotion are _____ .
   a. pilli
   b. flagella
   c. chromosomal DNA
   d. mesosomes
9. All prokaryotic cells are enveloped by a cell membrane and a _____ .
   a. capsule
   b. chitlin layer
   c. basal bodies
   d. cell wall
10. It was important to know which bacteria was causing the infection since antibiotic treatments were specific for certain bacteria because of the chemical makeup of the _____ .
    a. cell wall
    b. capsule layer
    c. cell membrane
    d. gram staining characteristics
11. Linnaeus developed the classification system that used
    a. dissimilar characteristics.
    b. one English name.
    c. conservation of energy.
    d. binomial nomenclature.
12. The branch of biology that deals with classification is
    a. microbiology.
    b. taxonomy.
    c. cytology.
    d. botany.
13. Of the following, the most closely related group of organisms is called a(n)
    a. kingdom
    b. genus.
    c. species
    d. order
14. Protists include
    a. algae and protozoa.
    b. algae and mosses.
    c. protozoa and mammals.
    d. birds and reptiles.
15. The number of protista kingdom is
    a. 2.
    b. 3.
    c. 4.
    d. 5.

16. The Latin classification for humans is *Homo sapiens,* which is the
    a. kingdom and phylum.
    b. phylum and class.
    c. genus and species.
    d. genus and family.
17. The correct arrangement of the following groups from the highest to the lowest. 1 = class; 2 = family; 3 = phylum; 4 = orders; 5 = genus; 6 = species is
    a. 3-2-4-1-5-6.
    b. 3-4-1-6-5-2.
    c. 3-4-1-5-6-2.
    d. 3-1-4-2-5-6
18. The kingdom containing organisms that are neither plants nor animals is
    a. fungi.
    b. protists.
    c. slime molds.
    d. mosses.
19. Two organisms are in the same species if they
    a. can mate and produce fertile offspring.
    b. can live together in a similar environment.
    c. can eat the same foods.
    d. are dissimilar.

B. Complete the statements below using terms from the list below. Not all terms will be used.

negative	mucoid and shiny	Plasmid
gram staining characteristics	conjugation	positive
capsule	mesosomes	dry and rough.
ribosomes	flagella	cellulose
pili	basal body	binary fission

1. Thick gelatinous layer __________ .
2. __________ contains respiratory enzymes.
3. Capsular bacteria are __________ .
4. Bacteria are characterized by their __________ .
5. Bacteria with thicker cell walls are gram __________ .
6. Thread-like extensions on bacteria made of protein __________ .
7. Contains bacterial DNA __________ .
8. A form of sexual reproduction __________ .
9. Fine hairlike structures found protruding from the cytoplasmic membrane of bacterial cells are __________ .
10. Aids in the synthesis of proteins __________ .

CHAPTER

7

The Structure and Behavior of Bacteria

OBJECTIVES

After completing this chapter, you will be able to:

- describe the size, shape, and structure of bacterial cells.
- detail the potential dangers of bacteria to human beings.

KEY WORDS

bacillus (bacilli)
bacterial chromosome
capsule
cell membrane
cell wall
coccus (cocci)
diplobacilli
diplococci
flagellum (flagella)
Micrococcus tetragenus
micrometer
nucleoid
ocular micrometer
saprophyte
sarcina
Sarcina lutea
slime layer
spirilla
spores
staphylococci
Staphylococcus aureus
streptobacilli
streptococci
Streptococcus pyogenes
tetrad
virulence

Bacterial organisms are so minuscule (tiny) that they cannot be measured by the usual methods. It is necessary to use a special unit of measurement, the **micrometer** (μm), or micron. The micrometer is equal to 1/1000 of a millimeter, or 1/25,400 of an inch. The meter (1000 millimeters) is the standard unit of measurement in the metric system.

Common bacteria average from 0.5 μm to 1.0 μm in length. They are studied by examining living and dead organisms under the high-power lens or under the oil-immersion lens of a microscope. To calibrate (measure) the dimensions of bacterial cells as seen on the microscopic field, an ocular micrometer scale may be fitted into the ocular lens. The **ocular micrometer** is a disk etched with tiny equidistant lines, not unlike a small ruler. When studying bacteria through an ocular microscope equipped with such a disk, the tiny lines are superimposed upon the bacteria, making calibration possible. Bacteria are more easily seen when they are stained. Only when millions of bacteria are massed together to form a colony can they be seen with the naked eye.

Studies with the electron microscope, using magnifications of from 80,000× to 200,000×, show that bacterial cells have a definite cell wall and a cell membrane. Surrounding some bacterial cells is the **capsule** or **slime layer,** which is the sticky covering secreted by the bacteria. This capsule is made up of various starchlike substances and cellulose, which protect the bacteria against the host's defenses. Encapsulated bacteria have a much greater infective capacity (**virulence**) than nonencapsulated bacteria; the loss of the capsule can mean the loss of this virulence. For instance, the streptococcus that causes streptococcal pneumonia has a distinct capsule. These **streptococci** are an example of diplococci, which remain in pairs after cell division.

The **cell wall** is a structure found between the capsule and the cell membrane; the wall's rigidity helps it to maintain the shape of the bacterial cell. It is believed that a bacterial cell needs the cell wall for normal growth and division. Beneath the cell wall is the **cell** (cytoplasmic) **membrane,** which helps to regulate the passage of nutrients and wastes in and out of the bacterial cell.

The nucleus in a bacterial cell is not a well-defined structure as it is in higher plant and animal cells. Instead, the nucleus is diffused throughout the cell. Other names, such as **bacterial chromosome** and **nucleoid,** have been suggested for this structure, due to the difference between bacterial nuclei and other nuclei. The cytoplasm, a gel-like fluid that contains the nucleus, is colorless and transparent.

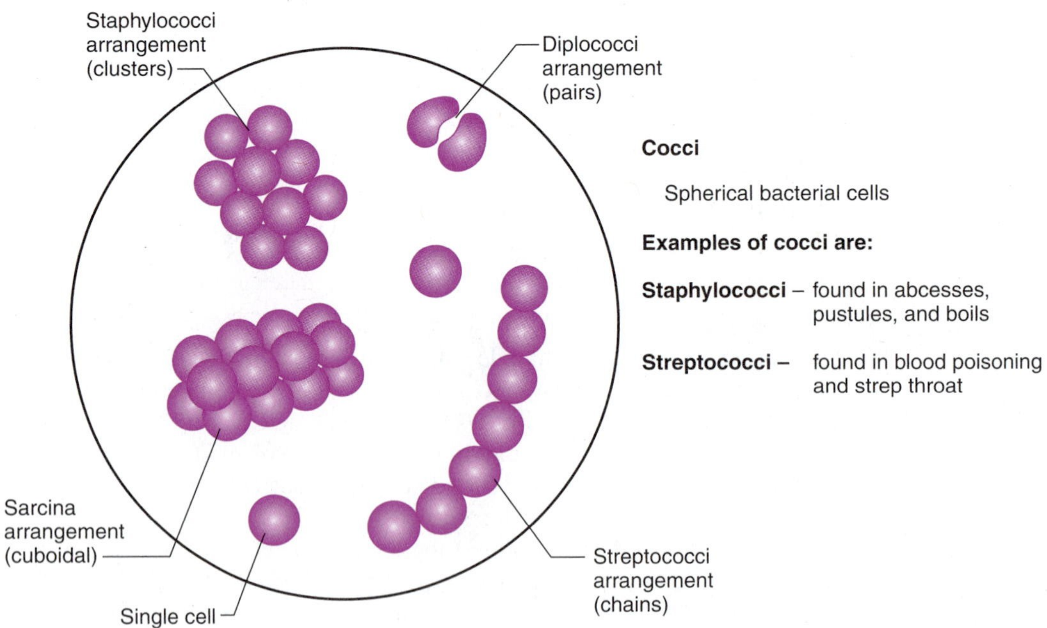

Figure 7–1 Cocci

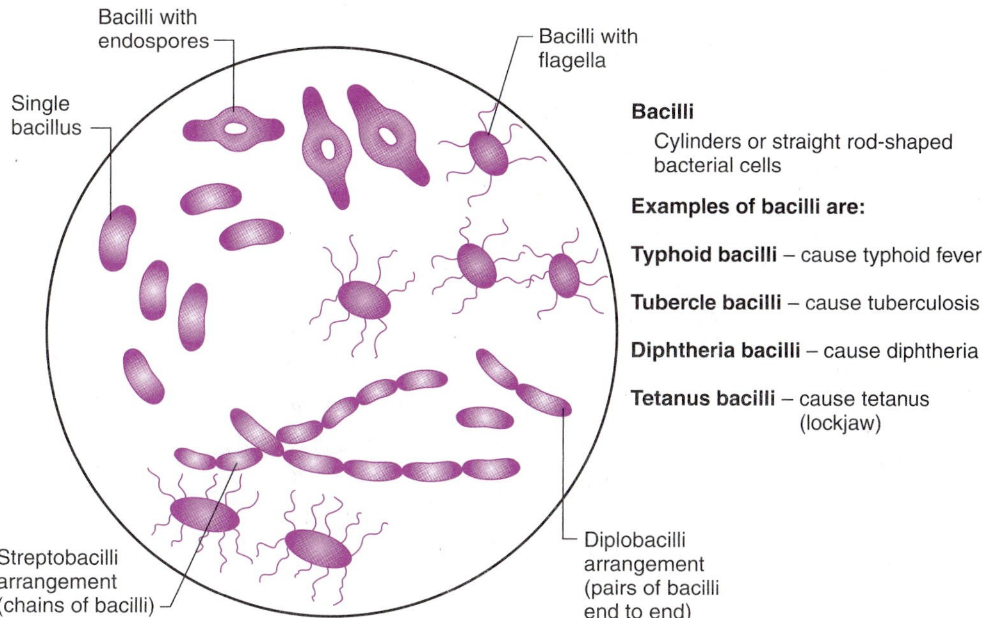

Figure 7–2 Bacilli

Cell shape, which is definite and fairly constant, is used to classify bacteria into three main groups: spherical-shaped or **cocci** (sing., **coccus**) (from the Greek *coccus,* meaning "berry"); rod-shaped or **bacilli** (sing., **bacillus**) (Latin for "little stick or rod"); and spiral-shaped or **spirilla** (from the Latin *spira,* meaning "coil") (see Figures 7–1 through 7–3).

Bacterial cells often are arranged into particular patterns, because their cell walls remain attached to each other after cell division. When cocci are grouped into pairs they are called **diplococci** (Figure 7–4). Diplococci-type bacteria cause such diseases as gonorrhea, meningitis, and pneumonia. Some diplococci are encapsulated as shown in Figure 7–4. For example, *Diplococcus pneumoniae* may be shiny and mucoid on culture media, or dry and pitted like a target. The mucoid strain is encapsulated, whereas the dry, pitted strain is nonencapsulated.

Streptococci are cocci arranged into long chains, like beads on a string. One example is ***Streptococcus pyogenes,*** which causes sore throats. Cocci arranged in clusters like bunches of grapes are known as **staphylococci,** such as ***Staphylococcus aureus,*** which is responsible for abscesses and boils. A group of four cocci surrounded by a capsule is known as a **tetrad.** ***Micrococcus tetragenus*** is such a tetrad; it is often found in the sputum of tuberculosis patients.

The cocci arranged in a cuboidal structure is the **sarcina.** ***Sarcina lutea*** is a **saprophyte** or nonpathogenic species of this type, commonly present in dust.

Some species of bacilli may appear singly, or, more often, in pairs called **diplobacilli.** Other species forming long chains are the **streptobacilli.**

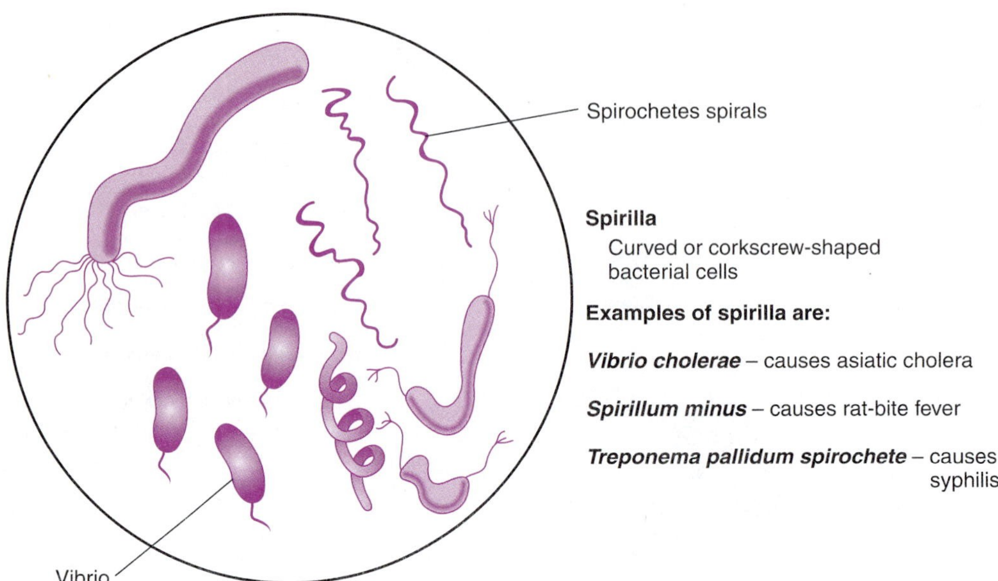

Figure 7–3 Spirilla

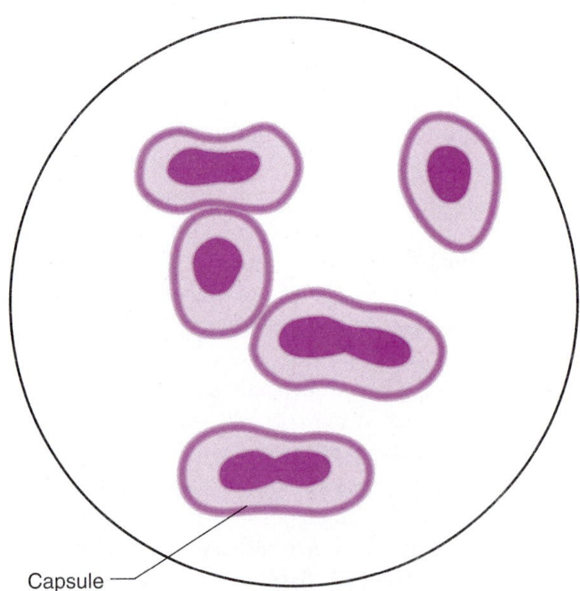

Figure 7–4 *Streptococcus pneumoniae* diplococci

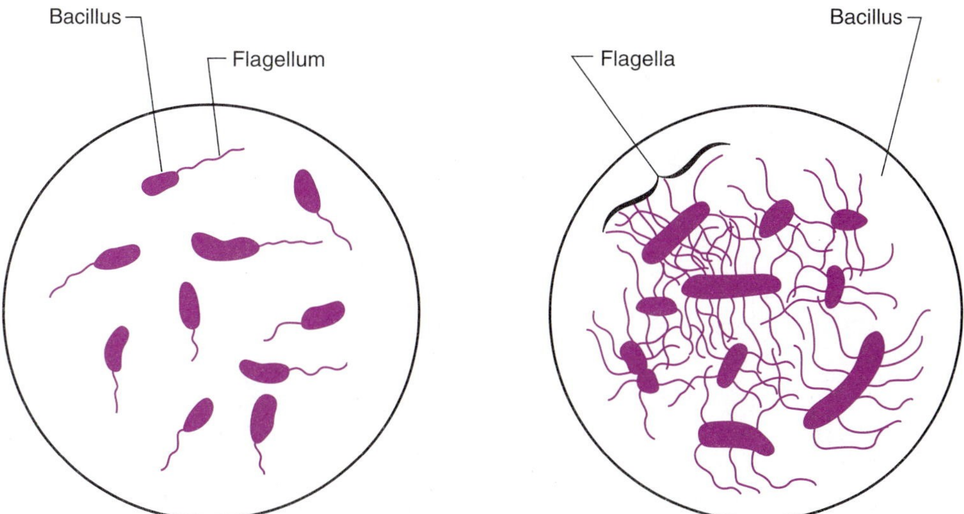

Figure 7–5 Some bacilli have only one flagellum; some have many flagella

Many bacteria have one or more long threadlike projections from the cell membrane or capsule. These filaments are called **flagella** (sing., **flagellum**) (Figure 7–5). They propel the bacterium by a rotary movement similar to that of a propeller on a boat. Flagella can be demonstrated only by special staining methods or by the use of an electron microscope. Most spiral-shaped bacteria are motile (able to move); sphere-shaped cocci are nonmotile. Many of the rod-shaped bacteria are motile. One example is the bacillus that causes typhoid fever. It is a very motile rod because of the presence of flagella. Other bacilli, such as the one that causes diphtheria, do not have flagella and therefore are not motile. Compare the three groups in Figure 7–6.

Bacilli have the ability to form resistant bodies called **spores** (Figure 7–7), or endospores. When spores develop, the protoplasm changes so that nothing can enter or leave the cell. This makes the bacteria very resistant to drying, temperature changes, and the action of stains and disinfectants. They become very hard to kill and may present a health hazard.

During the spore stage the bacterial cell is alive but inactive. As soon as favorable conditions again present themselves, the spore absorbs water and the bacteria cell becomes active again. Thus, bacteria can survive for months or even years under unfavorable conditions. Only the rod-shaped bacteria form spores; spiral-shaped and spherical bacteria do not form spores.

The health care professional must be familiar with the bacteria that form spores, as they present a special problem in sterilization techniques. The killing of spores requires strict and longer sterilization procedures than are needed for bacteria that do not form spores.

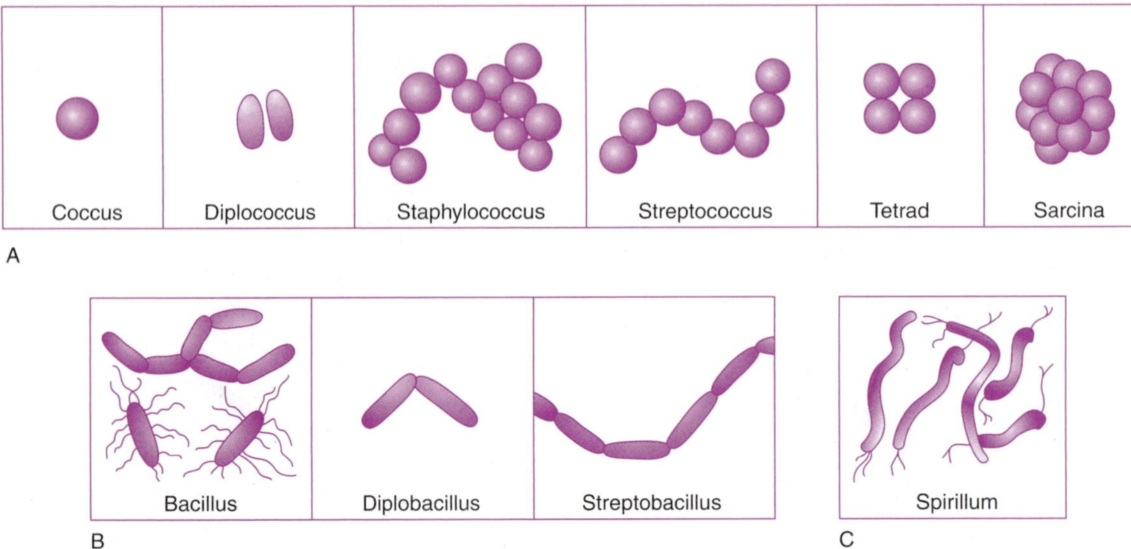

Figure 7–6 Examples of the three different types of bacteria (A) cocci, (B) bacilli, (C) spirals

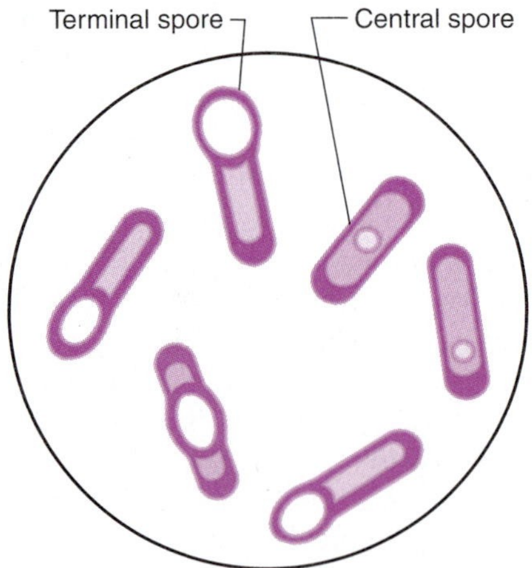

Figure 7–7 Bacilli with central and terminal spores

When environmental conditions are unfavorable some bacilli, such as the *Bacillus* and *Clostridium* species, form spores as a survival against adverse conditions. Techniques used to kill normal bacteria may just be sufficient to bring spore-forming bacteria out of their spore stage to become active bacteria again. Therefore, sterilization techniques must be sufficient to kill not only bacteria but their spores as well.

SUMMARY

In this chapter we see that bacteria come in three basic shapes: the round, actually spherical cocci (coccus, sing.), the rod or bacilli (bacillus, sing.), and the spirals or spirilla which are curled rods. All forms of bacteria can only be seen with the aid of a microscope, because they measure only a thousandth of a millimeter or less. The particular arrangement of cocci, especially seen from a liquid culture, is an excellent indicator of the family to which the bacteria might belong. For example, among the cocci, streptococci are found in chains, staphylococci in clusters, diplococci in pairs, and some are even arranged in tetrads (micrococci) or cuboids (sarcina). Capsulated bacteria are usually in pairs or tetrads, and are more virulent than their nonencapsulated relatives.

Bacilli, too, have variable rod shapes and many are even motile because of flagella attached to the sides or ends. Some bacilli are cigar shaped, some form spores (e.g., the *Clostridium* species), and some are barely identifiable as bacilli. A trademark of corynebacteria is that they resemble "chicken scratch" when stained samples are viewed under the microscope. Some arrange themselves end to end in long chains; some are very small, yet easily recognized as bacilli. Bacilli size and shape can also be slight indicators as to the species' family. Lactobacilli often arrange themselves end to end. Enteric organisms are generally small- to medium-size rods. Haemophilus organisms are usually very tiny. Many enteric organisms have flagella for motility. Some proteus species are so motile that they spread all over the culture plate instead of forming discrete colonies. Cocci and spirilla are not motile.

STUDY AND DISCUSSION

Procedure 7–1 Examination and Identification of Bacteria Using the Compound Microscope

- Under the high-power lens, examine stained slides of various types of bacteria. Identify each type you examine.
- Examine under the microscope prepared slides of the following formations of spherical bacteria:
  a. Pairs, as in pneumonia (*Diplococcus*)
  b. Cuboidal packets, found in the soil (*Sarcina*)
  c. Strings of beads, such as those that cause throat infections (*Streptococcus*)
  d. Grapelike clusters, found in boils and abscesses (*Staphylococcus*)

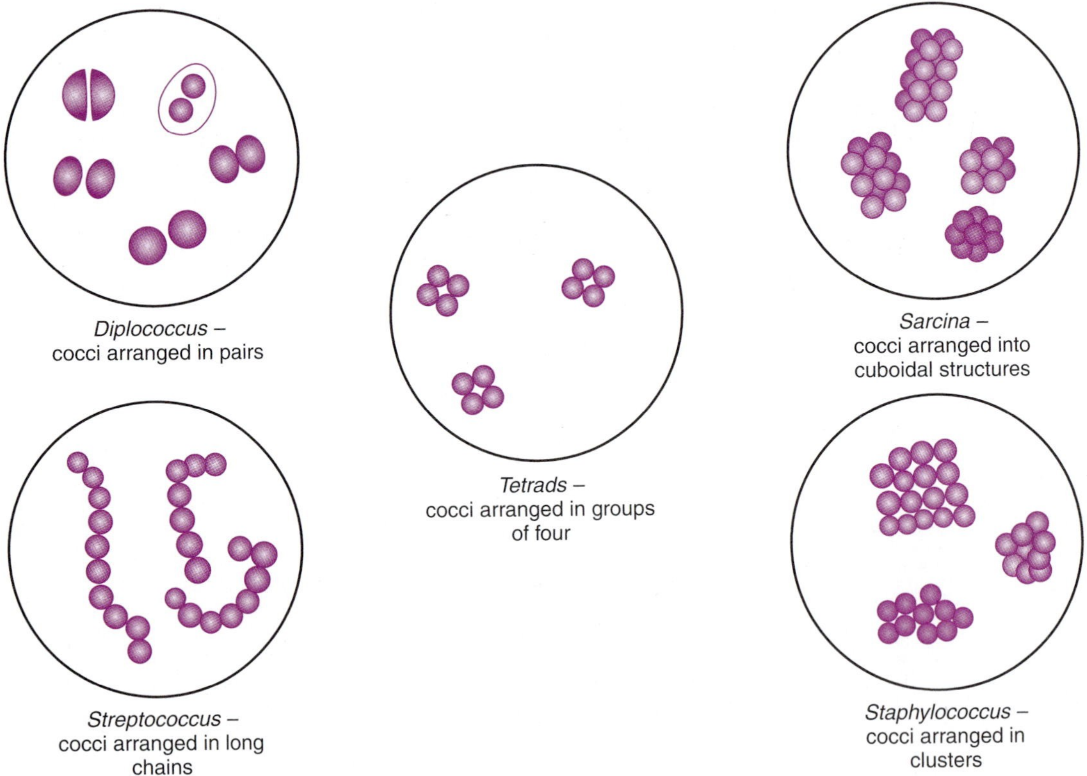

Diplococcus – cocci arranged in pairs

Tetrads – cocci arranged in groups of four

Sarcina – cocci arranged into cuboidal structures

Streptococcus – cocci arranged in long chains

Staphylococcus – cocci arranged in clusters

- Using library references, list several bacteria which form spores. What diseases do these bacteria cause?
- List several cytoplasmic inclusions or structures found in bacteria, and state their functions.

REVIEW QUESTIONS

Procedure 7–2 Recognition of Bacteria Structures

A. General Questions: Provide complete answers to each of the following.

1. In the spaces provided, identify the types of bacteria.

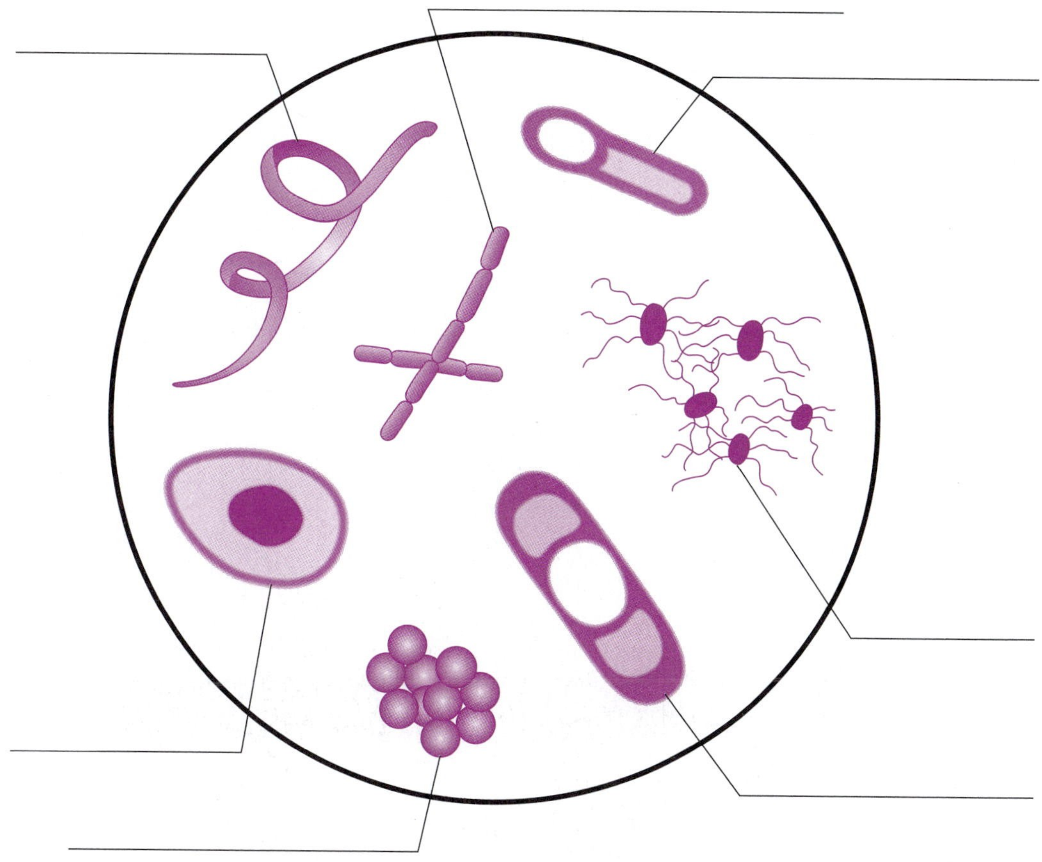

2. What is a flagellum? What is its function?

3. What is a spore? What is its function?

4. What genera of bacteria form spores? Why are they dangerous?

5. What is a capsule?

6. What characteristic of a cell wall helps a bacterial cell to maintain its shape?

7. What does a pathogenic bacterium have that a nonpathogenic bacterium usually does not have?

8. a. In terms of an inch, how large is a bacterium?

   b. What is the unit of measurement bacteriologists use to measure bacteria?

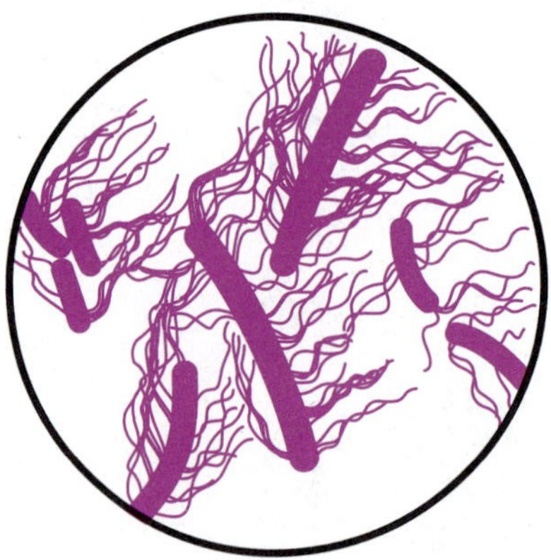

Typhoid fever – motile bacilli

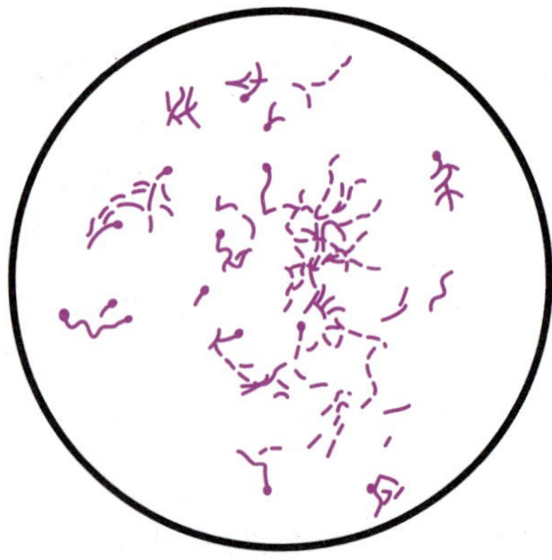

Diphtheria – diphtheroids

c. With what is the ocular lens on a microscope fitted to assist in the measurement of bacteria?

9. Name a disease caused by:
   a. Spherical bacteria in clusters

   b. Spherical bacteria in chains

   c. Spherical bacteria in pairs

   d. Rod-shaped bacteria

   e. Spiral-shaped bacteria

10. Name the type of bacteria that causes typhoid fever and diphtheria. Describe these bacteria and tell how they differ.

11. What precautions must be taken when killing bacterial cells that have spores?

B. Multiple-Choice Questions: Select the letter of the choice that best answers the question.

1. Some diplococci-type bacteria cause such diseases as _____ .
   a. pneumonia, meningitis, gonorrhea
   b. tuberculosis, pneumonia, histoplasmosis
   c. meningitis, gonorrhea, influenza
   d. diphtheria, pneumonia, gonorrhea

2. Streptococci are found in _____ arrangements.
   a. pairs
   b. chains
   c. clusters
   d. cuboidal
3. Staphylococci are found in _____ arrangements.
   a. pairs
   b. chains
   c. clusters
   d. cuboidal
4. Sarcina are found in _____ arrangements.
   a. pairs
   b. chains
   c. clusters
   d. cuboidal
5. Cholera is caused by a _____ bacteria.
   a. spirochete
   b. capsulated
   c. vibrio
   d. cuboid

C. From the following list of terms, fill in the blanks with the correct choice.

spores	hardy	100
flagella	resistant	1000
light microscope	electron microscope	darkfield microscope
spiral bodies	ruler	200,000
virulent	arrow	1,000,000

1. Motile bacteria contain ________________ .

2. Encapsulated bacteria are more ________________ than nonencapsulated bacteria.

3. Spore-forming bacteria can withstand harsh environmental conditions, therefore are more ________________ than most.

4. A micrometer is a tiny ________________ etched into the ocular lens.

5. A/an ________________ magnifies more than ________________ times while a/an ________________ magnifies up to ________________ times.

D. Matching Questions: Match the terms in Column I with their corresponding terms in Column II.

Column I		Column II
_______	1. capsule	a. rod
_______	2. cocci	b. coffee bean
_______	3. flagella	c. tetrad
_______	4. vibrio	d. groups of four
_______	5. spiral	e. slime layer
_______	6. bacilli	f. spherical
_______	7. spores	g. spirochete
_______	8. diplococcus	h. motility
_______	9. micrococcus	i. protection
_______	10. tetrads	j. curved rod

CHAPTER 8

Introduction to the Phylum, Protista

OBJECTIVES

After completing this chapter, you will be able to:

- name the microorganisms that comprise the five protist groups.
- suggest some uses for algae.
- give some examples of specific disease-causing organisms, and explain why this knowledge is necessary for proper health care.

KEY WORDS

acquired immunodeficiency syndrome (AIDS)
actinomyces
Aedes
algae
amoeba
aerobic
Animalia
anaerobic
Anopheles
arachnids
arthropods
Ascaris
Aspergillus
Bacillus
bacteria
binomial nomenclature
cestodes
carotene
carrier
Clostridium
Cryptococcus
dermatophytes
diatoms
digenea
Diphyllobothrium
Echinococcus
Entamoeba
Enterobacteriaceae
Enterobius
Euglena
Fasciola
Fasciolopsis
fungi
gametocyte
Giardia
Haemophilus
helminths
hepatitis B
Histoplasma
Hymenolepis
molds
multicellular
Mycobacteria
Necator
Neisseria
nematodes
OSHA
Paragonimus
Paramecium
parasite
pathogenicity
Pediculus
Penicillium
photosynthesis
Phthirus
Plantae
Plasmodium
primordial
Protista
protists
protozoa
rickettsias
saprophytes
Sarcoptes

KEY WORDS (cont.)

Schistosoma
silica
slough
spirochetes
staphylococci
streptococci
Strongyloides
Taenia
taxonomy
Toxoplasma
trematodes
Trichomonas
Trichuris
Trophozoite
typhoid fever
unicellular
viruses
Volvox
yeasts

PRINCIPLES OF CLASSIFICATION

Since the time of the Greek philosopher Aristotle (384 to 322 B.C.), people have studied, described, named, and tried to classify animals, plants, and microorganisms in some logical and meaningful way. In the attempt to assemble and categorize the huge amount of biological data on living organisms, many classification schemes have developed and gone by the wayside. The current classification system was developed by Carolus von Linne, usually known as Karl Linnaeus (1707–1778), a Swedish biologist.

Classification or **taxonomy** is a formal science in its own right. Taxonomy is a branch of biology that deals with the classification of living organisms. The classification scheme is based on similarities in the structure, embryonic development, and evolutionary origins among organisms. Even though the Linnaean classification system is used, there is still no universal consensus among current biologists and microbiologists on *one* system. That is one reason why some microorganisms have been named only to be renamed at some later date.

Today's five-kingdom system (see Table 8–2) was developed from the three-kingdom system—**Plantae, Animalia,** and **Protista**—into which all known organisms are classified. Protista, which means "primitive," contains all of the protists, which are unicellular or simple multicellular organisms. The lower protists contain the prokaryotic cyanobacteria—the blue-green algae and the bacteria. The higher protists include the eukaryotic microorganisms—protozoa, algae, and fungi. The viruses are not classified under this classification scheme, because they are not cellular.

Binomial nomenclature. The Linnaean system is currently used for the naming of all organisms. In Karl Linnaeus's system, two Greek or Latin names are used for each plant and animal. Hence, his system is called the **binomial** ("two") **nomenclature** ("system of names") system. The first name is the *genus* name, and the first letter of the genus is always capitalized. The second name is the *species* name, and it begins with a lowercase letter. Some genus and species names of common bacteria, fungi, yeasts, protozoa, and algae are found in Table 8–1.

Taxonomy. One of the most commonly accepted taxonomic schemes classifies all known living organisms into the three kingdoms. After "kingdom," the classification scheme continues to group related organisms into closer and smaller clusters as their similarities become more detailed and exacting. Table 8–2 shows the subdivisions of the entire classification scheme.

Table 8–1 Genus and Species Names of Some Common Bacteria, Protozoa, Algae, Fungi, and Yeasts

Bacteria	*Acetobacter aceti (A. aceti)* *Bacillus subtilis (B. subtilis)* *Clostridium butyricum (C. butyricum)* *Corynebacterium diphtheriae (C. diphtheriae)* *Enterobacter cloacae (E. cloacae)* *Escherichia coli (E. coli)* *Klebsiella pneumonia (K. pneumoniae)* *Lactobacillus delbrueckii (L. delbrueckii)* *Mycobacterium tuberculosis (M. tuberculosis)* *Neisseria gonorrhoeae (N. gonorrhoeae)* *Pseudomonas aeruginosa (P. aeruginosa)* *Rickettsia prowazekii (R. prowazekii)* *Salmonella chloerae-suis (S. chloerae-suis)* *Shigella dysenteriae (S. dysenteriae)* *Staphylococcus aureus (S. aureus)* *Streptococcus pyogenes (S. pyogenes)* *Treponema pallidium (T. pallidum)* *Vibrio cholerae (V. cholerae)*
Fungi	*Aspergillus niger (A. niger)* *Claviceps purpurea (C. purpurea)* *Neurospora sitophila (N. sitophila)* *Penicillium notatum (P. notatum)* *Rhizopus stolonifer (R. stolonifer)*
Yeasts	*Candida albicans (C. albicans)* *Cryptococcus neoformans (C. neoformans)* *Endomyces decipiens (E. decipiens)* *Saccharomyces cerevisiae (S. cerevisiae)* *Trichosporon pullulans (T. pullulans)*
Protozoa	*Balantidium coli (B. coli)* *Entamoeba histolytica (E. histolytica)* *Giardia lamblia (G. lamblia)* *Leishmania donovani (L. donovani)* *Paramecium candatum (P. candatum)* *Plasodium vivax (P. vivax)* *Trichomonas vaginalis (T. vaginalis)* *Trypanosoma cruzi (T. cruzi)*
Algae*	*Acetabularia* *Chlamydomonas* *Chlorella* *Euglena* *Sargassum* *Spirogyra* *Vaucheria* *Volvox*

*Usually referred to by their genus names only.

Table 8–2 Arrangement of the Modern Classification Scheme

1. The main division of all plant, animal, and microscopic organisms is the	*Kingdom*
2. In each kingdom similar classes make up a	*Phylum*
3. In each phylum similar orders make up a	*Class*
4. In each class similar families make up an	*Order*
5. In each order similar tribes make up a	*Family*
6. In each family similar species make up a	*Genus*
7. In each genus similar organisms make up a	*Species*

The smaller the classification or grouping, the more similar the organisms will be. For example, members of the same genus are comparable in embryonic development and structure, which implies descent from a common ancestor.

Besides the three-kingdom system, as discussed, there is now a five-kingdom system proposed by Whittaker in 1969 that is currently in use by many biologists and microbiologists.

Whittaker's five-kingdom system is based on three levels of cellular organization and the three main types of nutrition: photosynthesis, absorption, and ingestion. Whittaker's system adds the kingdoms Monera, which includes all bacteria, and Fungi, which includes all yeasts and molds. The five kingdoms and their important features and members are listed in Table 8–3.

A theory of the evolutionary relationships among the major members of the five-kingdom system is shown in Figure 8–1. On the right side are the members of the current five-kingdom system. Included in this listing are the major groups of present-day microorganisms. The horizontal line shows the time period from the **primordial** past (since the beginning of life) to the current time. The vertical scale shows relative evolutionary process. Following this evolutionary time scheme, the earliest type of cell to arise on earth was an anaerobic (not needing oxygen for its growth) prokaryote. This primitive anaerobic prokaryote branched off into three different evolutionary paths. The first path leads to photosynthetic organisms. These are organisms that use sunlight to synthesize their own food. A second branch later gives rise to organisms undergoing **aerobic** respiration: These organisms require oxygen for their growth. The third path leads to an ancestral **anaerobic** ("proto") growth (without oxygen) eukaryote that later gives rise to more advanced eukaryotes.

The modern-day eukaryotes from algae to animals arose by a sequence of further events. In subbranch A, a cyanobacteria establishes a symbiotic (mutually helpful) relationship inside an anaerobic protoeukaryote. The anaerobic protoeukaryote becomes an anaerobic photosynthetic eukaryote. The chloroplast needed for photosynthesis inside the anaerobic photosynthetic eukaryote developed from the cyanobacteria. Later, the anaerobic photosynthetic eukaryote develops into an aerobic photosynthetic eukaryote. This happens when an aerobic prokaryote establishes a symbiotic relationship inside the anaerobic photosynthetic eukaryote. Subbranch B shows this event. The mitochondria

Table 8–3 Members of the Five-Kingdom System and Their Important Features

Monera	Prokaryotic cell; heterotrophic* or photoautotrophic† nutrition; unicellular; filamentous or mycelial; others possess flagella, pili, and spores	Eubacteria (true bacteria) Cyanobacteria (blue-green bacteria) Archaebacteria
Protista or Protoctista	Eukaryotic, unicellular or multicellular microorganisms; heterotrophic or photoautotrophic; motile types have flagella or cilia	Protozoa Slime molds Red, brown, and green algae Seaweed
Fungi	Eukaryotic, unicellular or multicellular organisms; heterotrophic and nonphotosynthetic	Molds Yeasts Mushrooms Plant smuts and rusts
Plantae (Plants)	Eukaryotic, multicellular organisms; autotrophic, photosynthetic nutrition; differentiation and specialization of plant tissue	Vascular plants Conifers Ferns Mosses Worts
Animalia (Animals)	Eukaryotic, multicellular organisms; heterotrophic nutrition; differentiation and specialization of animal tissue; vertebrate or invertebrate	Mollusks Arthropods Fish Amphibians Reptiles Birds Mammals and humans

*Heterotrophic is a type of nutrition in which an organism takes in and uses preformed organic molecules.

†Photoautotrophic is a type of nutrition in which an organism synthesizes its own food from very simple substances in its environment. In this case, the process needs energy from sunlight (*photo-* = light) for the food synthesis.

needed for aerobic respiration inside the aerobic photosynthetic eukaryote developed from the aerobic prokaryote.

These two events later give rise to an aerobic photosynthetic eukaryote. In turn, it leads to the present-day higher algae. Loss of the chloroplast explains the development of the protozoa and then the fungi and slime molds.

The archaebacteria is a form that has had little or no evolution from the anaerobic prokaryote.

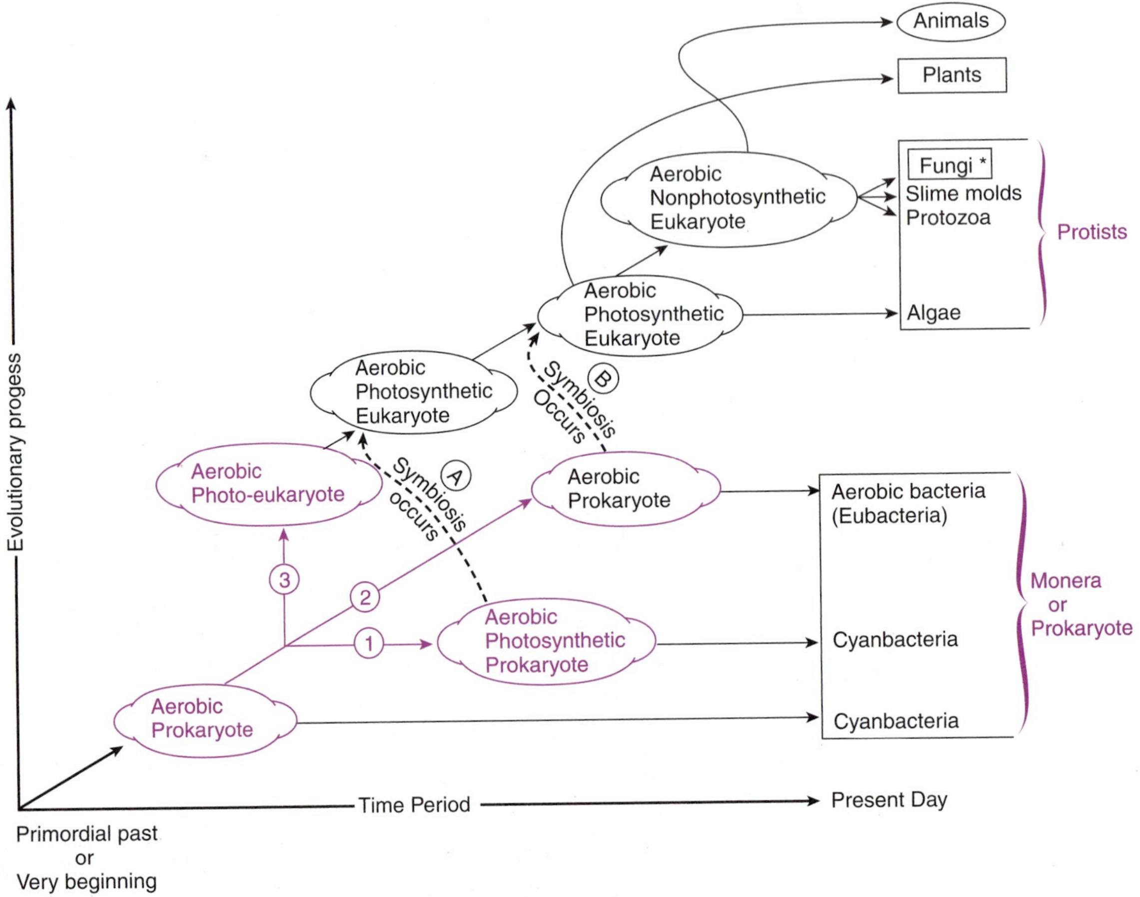

Figure 8–1 Evolutionary relationships of the major members of the five-kingdom system

THE PROTISTS

As discussed, several classification schemes have been in use, namely the two-group system including plants (Plantae) and animals (Animalia) which has been the most widely used; the three-group system including plants, animals, and the protists (Protista); and the five-group system including the aforementioned plus the Monera and Fungi. For the purposes of this textbook, we will include bacteria, fungi, and **parasites** in the Protista kingdom. **Protists** include the lower members of the plant and animal kingdoms but do not really fit into either of the plant or animal categories. These include the **algae,** fungi (yeasts and molds), parasites, and **bacteria.** Bacteria may be further subdivided into the true bacteria, **actinomyces** (moldlike bacteria), **spirochetes** (protozoalike bacteria), and **rickettsias** (viruslike bacteria). The **viruses** are sometimes included with the protists, but they are noncellular and nonliving structures in that they cannot survive outside of a living host. A virus must parasitize or live in a healthy cell to obtain its nutrition. The parasites are divided into **protozoa** (single celled), **helminths** (wormlike invertebrates), and **arthropods** (insects, spiders, ticks, and mites). Most are unicellular and some are multicellular, yet protists do not have multiple cells, specialized tissues, or organs. They have no definite cellular arrangement to their structure. Many are microscopic; thus, they are generally categorized as microorganisms. Some of the fungi, such as the mushrooms, are quite large, as are some of the parasites in the roundworm and flatworm families.

Algae

Algae are simple plant structures containing chlorophyll. They can be either **unicellular** (one celled) or **multicellular** (more than one cell). Generally, they are not pathogenic. Lacking roots, stems, or leaves, algae are independent plants. They are able to live in fresh or salt water, in moist soil, and on rocks, plants, and trees.

Algae have economic importance in soil fertility, as a food, and in commercial usage. In these days of growing environmental awareness and the development of natural resources, there are facts about algae that everyone should know. The growth of algae contributes to fertilizing soil and controlling soil erosion. In the Far East, algae have been used for the cultivation of rice because of their ability to return nitrogen to the soil.

Floating on water in either strands or colonies, algae combine with other microscopic life to provide food for marine animals. Algae may even increase the oxygen concentration when dispersed in natural waters. They do so through a chemical process called photosynthesis. **Photosynthesis** is the process whereby chlorophyll absorbs light energy from the sun; then, in the presence of water and carbon dioxide, it forms starch, water, and oxygen.

The yellow pigment found in many algae is **carotene,** a form of vitamin A. Green algae is rich in vitamins B_1, C, and K.

Some kinds of algae, **diatoms,** produce a mineral called **silica,** which has a wide variety of commercial uses. Silica is used in insulating materials, as a filter for making drinking beverages clearer, as a cosmetic base, and as a polishing material. Certain algae serve as sources of medicinal products; for example, rockweed, kelp, and Irish moss. Even agar culture material, used to grow microorganisms in the microbiology laboratory, comes from algae.

In the food industry, algae are used to gel jams, as a stabilizer for salad dressings and ice cream, and as an emulsifier for puddings.

By themselves, algae are not pathogenic. However, some types (bloom) eaten by shellfish are toxic to the humans, animals, and birds that later eat the shellfish.

Fungi

The **fungi** are very simple, plantlike structures that do not contain chlorophyll. Thus, they cannot carry on photosynthesis and produce their own food. They are **saprophytes,** organisms that obtain their nutrition from dead, decaying organic material. In a very real sense, fungi are the scavengers of the microbes.

Yeasts are the unicellular forms of fungi (Figure 8–2). **Molds** are the filamentous, multicellular fungi often found on bread, cheese, and fruit (Figure 8–3). Molds are of great importance to people, because they are the major source of antibiotics. Both yeasts and molds have some harmful and some beneficial members. They are relatively large

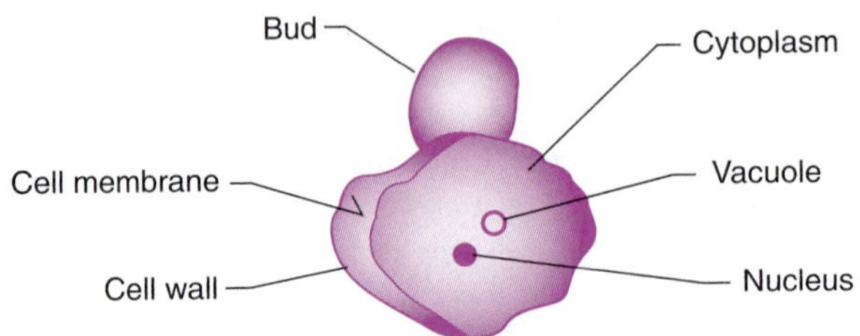

Figure 8–2 Single yeast cell

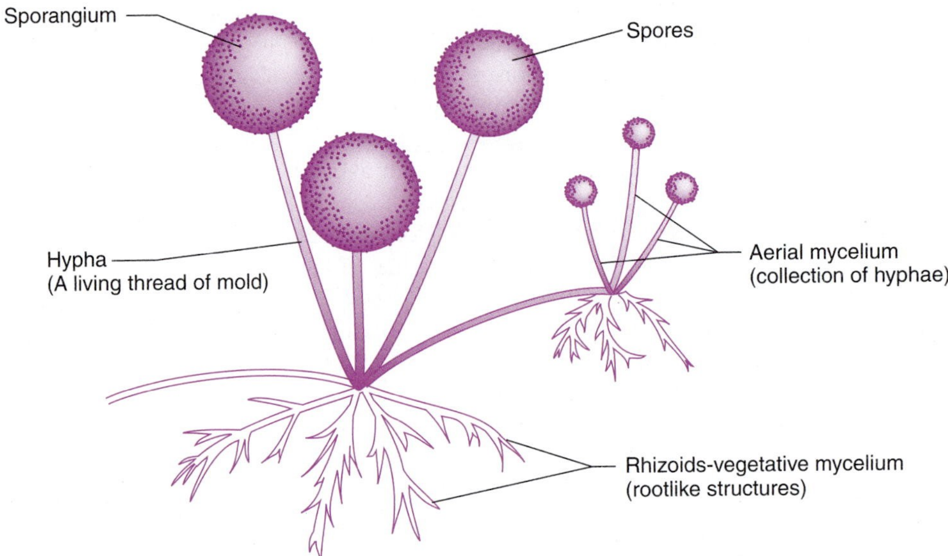

Figure 8–3 Black mold or bread mold

spherical or oval cells, visible under the low-power magnification of the microscope. Mold filaments are visible to the naked eye.

The molds are filamentous fungi known primarily for their growth on foods and their use in making antibiotics. The Rhizopus is black bread mold. ***Penicillium*** is used to make penicillin and flavor various cheeses. The ***Aspergillus*** mold as found on peanuts can be very toxic to humans. Some of the clinically significant fungi are yeasts of the ***Candida*** group; systemic fungi; the **dermatophytes,** which cause nail and skin diseases; and other deep-seated fungi, including ***Histoplasma*** and ***Cryptococcus,*** which cause pulmonary, lung, and meningococcal infections. These will all be described in Chapter 9.

Parasites

Included as parasites are the single-celled protozoa, the wormlike helminths, and the arthropods, including insects, lice, spiders, mites, and ticks.

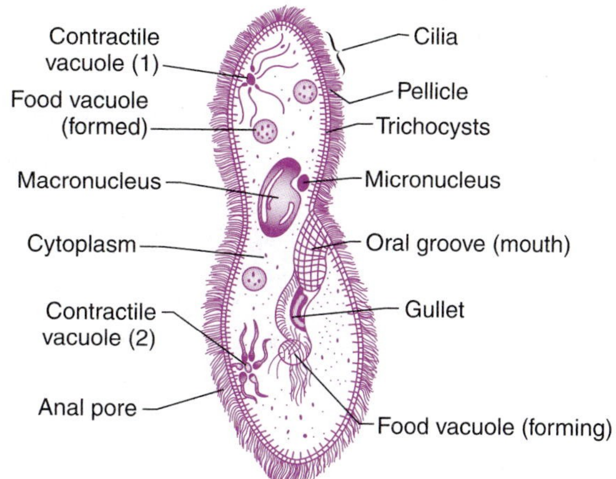

Figure 8–4 A paramecium—a ciliate

The protozoa are relatively large, single-celled organisms. One of the largest and most frequently demonstrated is the ***Paramecium*** (Figure 8–4). It can be found in pond water living off green plants and other water parasites. It is not implicated in human parasitic infections. Five paramecia would fit across the head of a pin. The paramecium and the **amoeba** (another protozoan living in pond water) (Figure 8–5), can easily be seen with the low-power objective of a microscope. Other freshwater protozoa that may be of biological interest include the ***Volvox*** (Figure 8–6) and the ***Euglena*** (Figure 8–7). These protozoa do not cause disease in humans, whereas other members of the protozoa group,

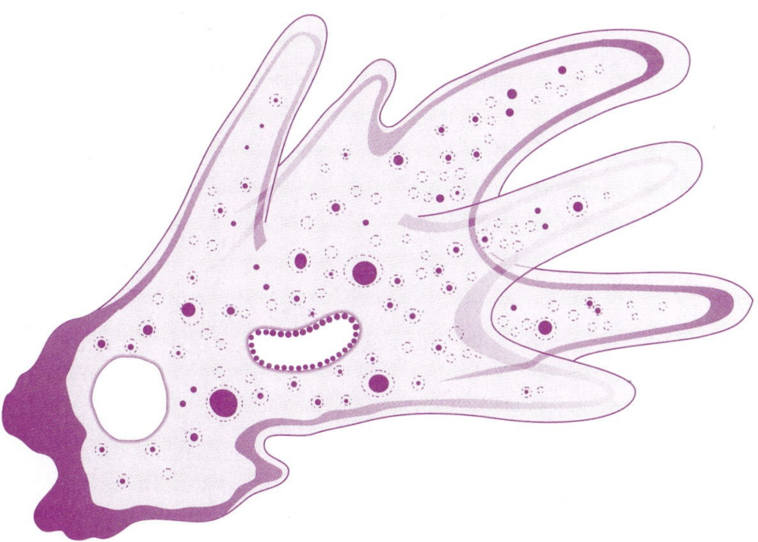

Figure 8–5 An amoeba

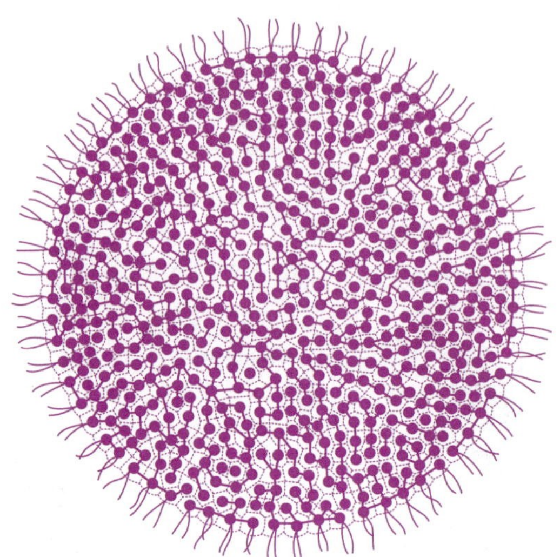

Figure 8–6 A *Volvox*

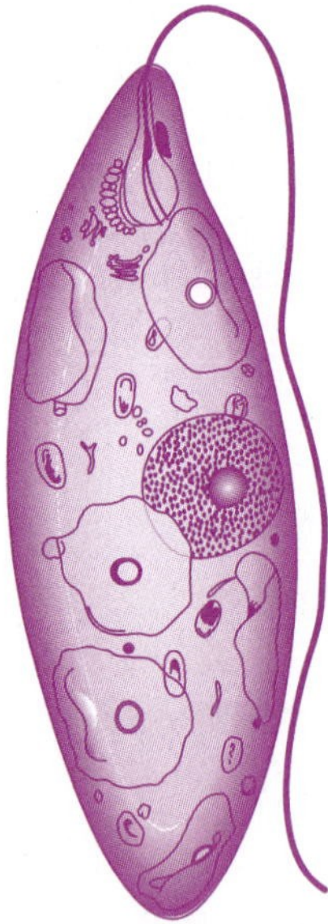

Figure 8–7 An *Euglena*

including the ***Plasmodium*** (Figure 8–8), which causes malaria; the ***Entamoeba*** (Figure 8–9) and ***Giardia*** (Figure 8–10), which cause dysentery; the ***Trichomonas*** (Figure 8–11), which causes genital infections; and the ***Toxoplasma,*** which causes toxoplasmosis, are pathogenic to humans and will be discussed in Chapter 10.

The helminths include the roundworms or **nematodes,** the flatworms (tapeworms) or **cestodes,** and the **trematodes** (subclass **digenea**), which are called flukes. Adult round-

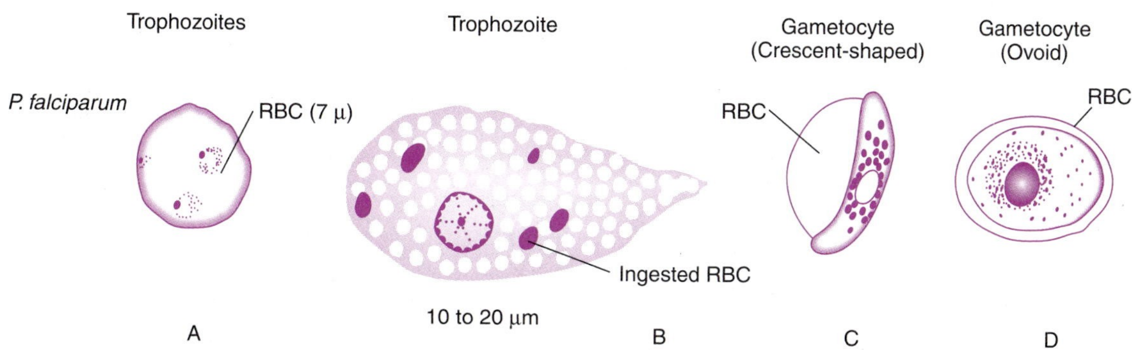

Figure 8–8 Plasmodium: A & B. **Trophozoites** C & D. **gametocytes**

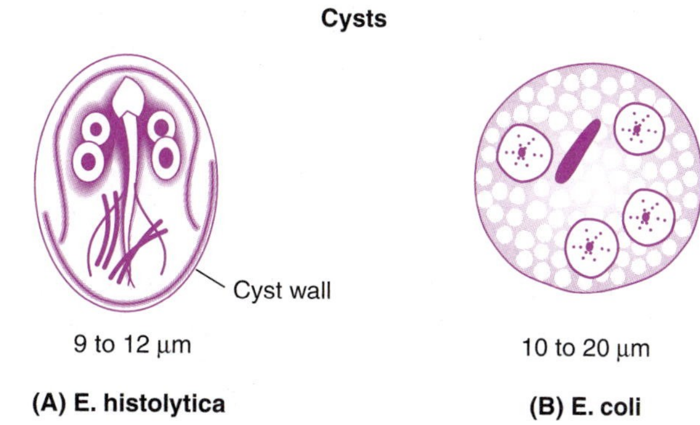

Figure 8–9 Entamoeba cysts (A) ***Entamoeba histolytica,*** (B) ***Entamoeba coli***

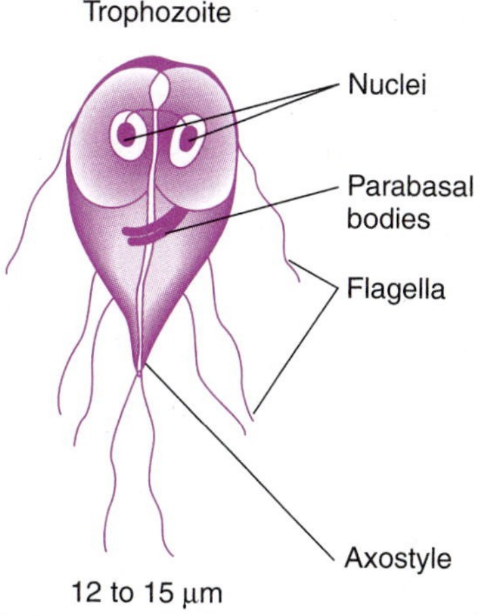

Figure 8–10 *Giardia lamblia*

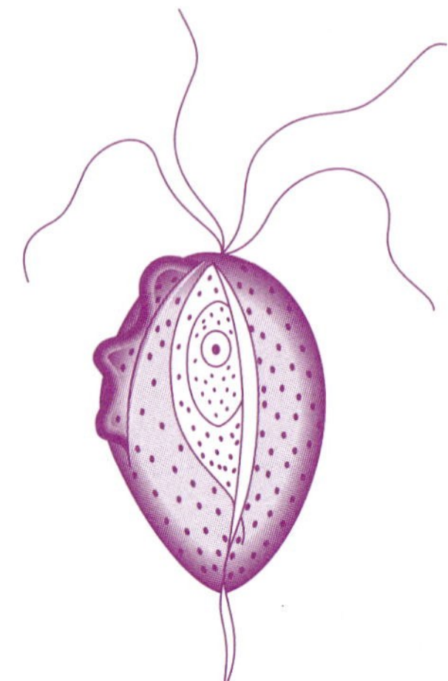

Figure 8–11 *Trichomonas vaginalis*

worms and flatworms may be examined directly or in cross section. The presence of their eggs (Figure 8–12) in stool or tissue is sufficient to make a diagnosis of the disease. Almost all helminths found in humans are infectious. One of the most common intestinal roundworm infections, the pinworm (***Enterobius***) is distributed worldwide and is found mostly in children. The whipworm (***Trichuris***), the ***Ascaris*** (another roundworm), the hookworm (***Necator***), and the threadworm (***Strongyloides***) (Figure 8–13) also cause intestinal disorders. Nematodes may be microscopic in size, ranging from a few hundred micrometers to a macroscopic size of approximately 30 centimeters.

The flatworms or cestodes include the beef and pork tapeworms of the ***Taenia*** family and the ***Diphyllobothrium*** or fish tapeworm. These flatworms can grow to lengths of up to 20 meters and will **slough** off sections of their bodies into the stool. Other cestodes of medical importance are the dwarf tapeworm (***Hymenolepis***) and the dog tapeworm (***Echinococcus***). The presence of their eggs (Figure 8–14) in stool samples is diagnostic of infection.

The trematodes, commonly called flukes, are flat leaf-shaped helminths. They can inhabit the intestine, the liver, the lung, and the blood vessels. They vary in size from a few millimeters to a few centimeters in length. The prominent blood flukes are members of the ***Schistosoma*** group (Figure 8–15). Some of the other clinically significant flukes include the ***Fasciolopsis, Fasciola,*** and the ***Paragonimus.***

The arthropods (Figure 8–16), most often thought of as including such insects as flies, mosquitoes, true bugs, lice, and fleas, also include the **arachnids**—spiders, ticks, and mites. Some are primary or secondary hosts for other parasites, such as the mosquito, which carries the malaria protozoan, and the tick, which carries the Lyme disease bacterium. Other arthropods are directly responsible for human infections. Lice infections of

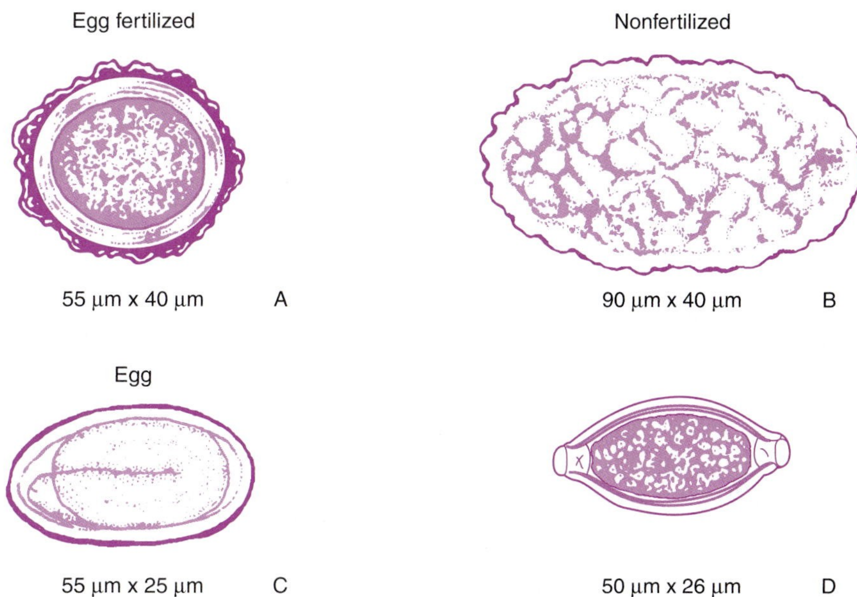

Figure 8–12 Roundworm eggs (A and B) *Ascaris lumbricoides,* (C) *Enterobius vermiculasis,* (D) *Trichuris trichuria*

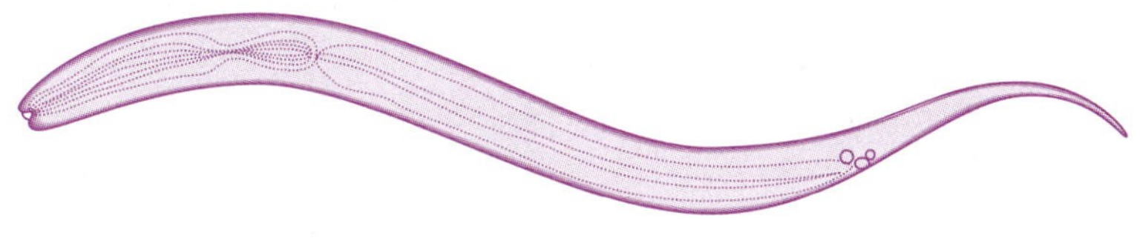

Figure 8–13 Roundworm, *Strongyloides*

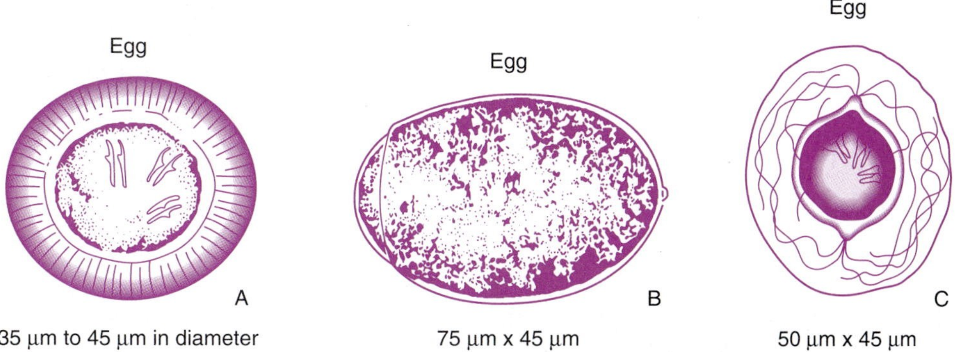

Figure 8–14 Cestode eggs (A) *Taenia* egg, (B) *Diphyllobothrium* egg, (C) *Hymenolepis* egg

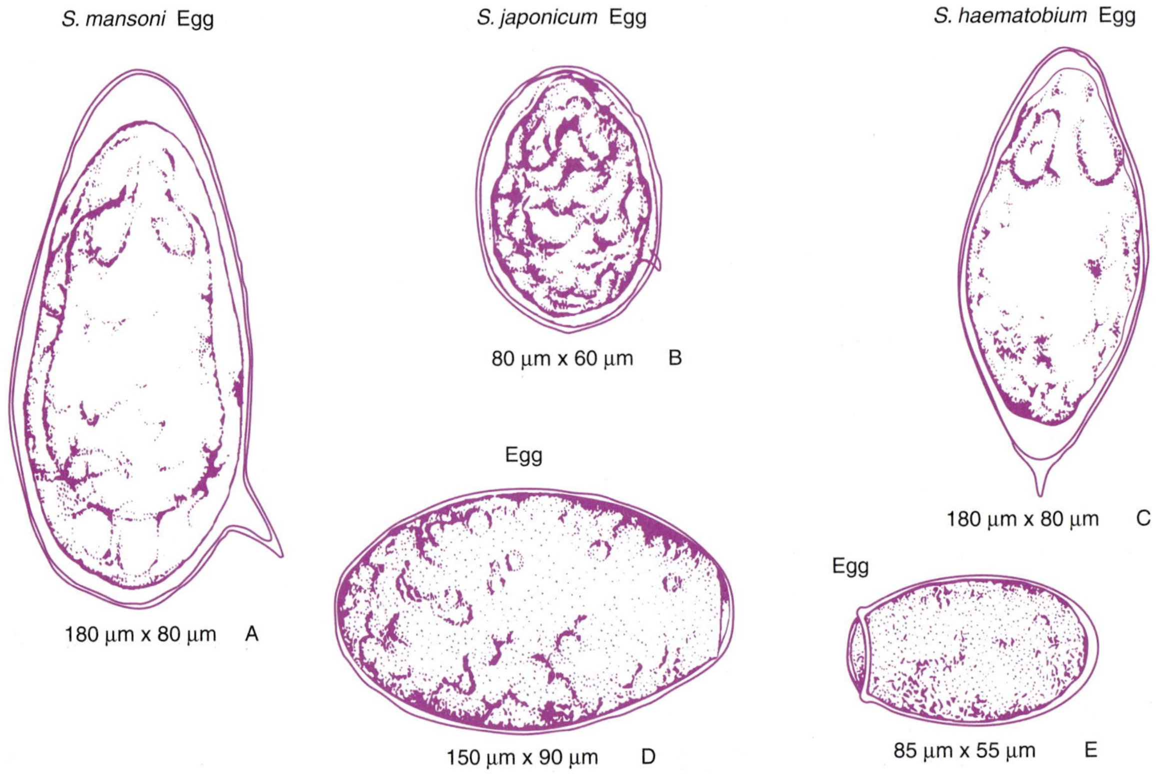

S. mansoni Egg
S. japonicum Egg
S. haematobium Egg
80 μm x 60 μm B
Egg
180 μm x 80 μm C
Egg
180 μm x 80 μm A
150 μm x 90 μm D
85 μm x 55 μm E

Figure 8–15 Trematode (fluke) eggs (A, B, C) *Schistosoma* eggs, (D) *Fasciolopsis,* (E) *Paragonimus*

A
B
C
D
Dermacentor
(Hard tick)
Sarcoptes
(Mite)
Pediculus
(Body louse)
Phthiris pubis
(Crab louse)
5.5 to 7.5 mm
Feamle 330 to 600 μm
2 to 4 mm
1 mm

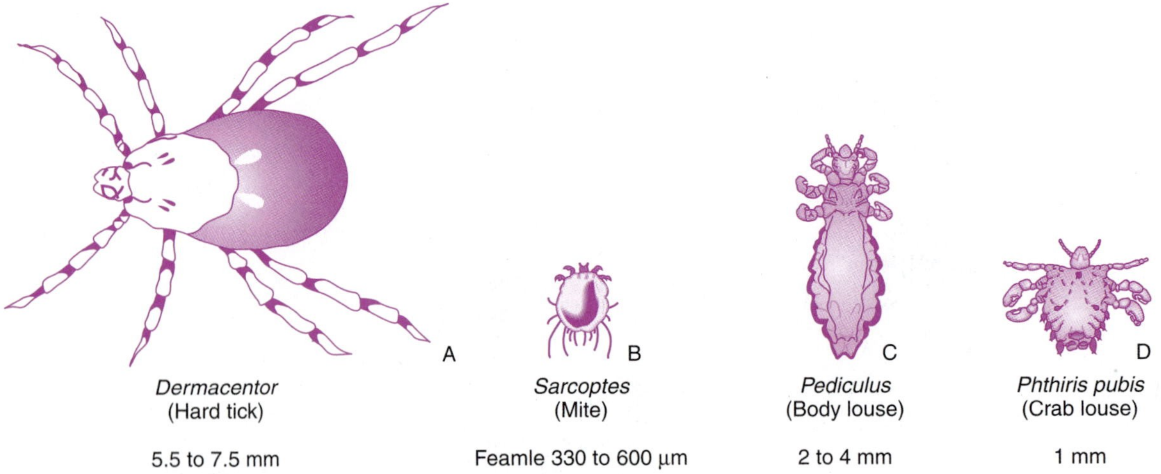

Figure 8–16 Significant arthropods (A) tick, (B) mite (*Sarcoptes*), (C) body louse (*Pediculus*), (D) pubic louse (*Phthirus pubis*)

the head and body (***Pediculus***) are easily transmitted and often cause epidemics among school children. ***Phthirus*** is the causative agent of sexually transmitted crab louse infections. Scabies is caused by the itch mite (***Sarcoptes***). Fleas are common to household pets (cats and dogs) and can infest an entire household, including carpets and furniture. Clinically significant insects include several varieties of mosquitoes that are responsible for malaria (***Anopheles*** mosquito), yellow fever (***Aedes*** mosquito), and African sleeping sickness (tsetse fly).

Bacteria

Bacteria are very small (Figure 8–17). Even under a high-power objective, they are just visible as tiny dots, rods, or spirals. The smallest of the bacterial group, the rickettsia, cannot be seen under an ordinary light microscope. Some common bacterial cells are only 1/1000 of a micrometer (μm) in diameter, meaning that about 1000 of them would reach across a pinhead. Under oil immersion, the compound microscope gives a good view of most bacteria cells. However, few details can be seen unless special stains are used in preparing the slide.

The most common stains used to begin the identification process of bacteria include the Gram stain, which categorizes bacteria by color and shape, and the acid-fast stain, in which all **Mycobacteria** are grouped. Significant gram-positive cocci include the **staphylococci** and **streptococci.** Important gram-positive rods or bacilli include the ***Bacillus*** and ***Clostridium*** groups. Gram-negative cocci important to humans belong to the ***Neisseria*** group, and significant gram-negative rods are the ***Enterobacteriaceae*** and ***Haemophilus*** groups. These and other bacteria of clinical significance will be discussed in detail in Chapter 11.

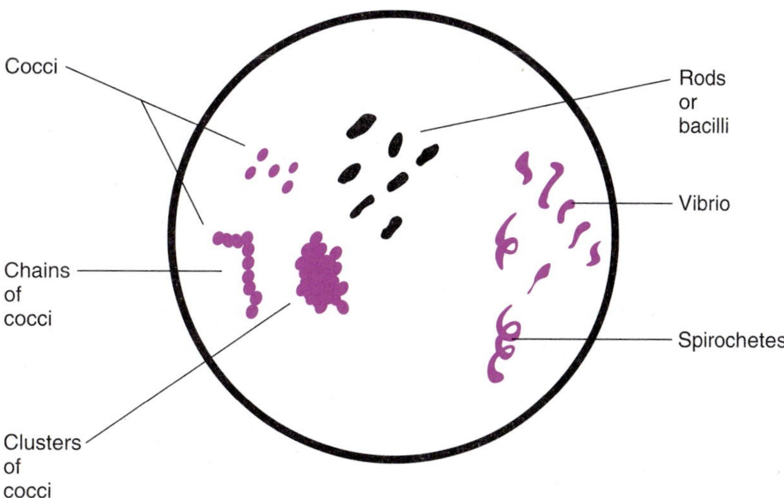

Figure 8–17 Different shapes of bacteria

Viruses

Viruses (Figure 8–18) are beyond the visibility of the compound microscope. They can be seen only with the aid of an electron microscope. Viruses are so small that a single one can pass through a porcelain filter. It would take 2500 viruses of the larger species or 40,000 viruses of the smaller species to reach across a pinhead.

The virus is a tiny, noncellular form that injects its genetic material into the cell to obtain nutrients. From there it increases in number and breaks through the cell membrane, discharging more virus particles into the bloodstream to spread to other cells. Smallpox and chicken pox are among the diseases caused by viruses.

With the exception of the viruses, all microorganisms are made up of definitely organized masses of protoplasm (cells). These cells carry on the same life activities as the cells of all other living things: obtaining food, respiration, excreting wastes, and reproducing.

The roadmap at right describes a simple scheme for the categorization and initial grouping of some members of the kingdoms Plantae, Animalia, and Protista. Once categorized, an organism can be further identified using established microbiological procedures.

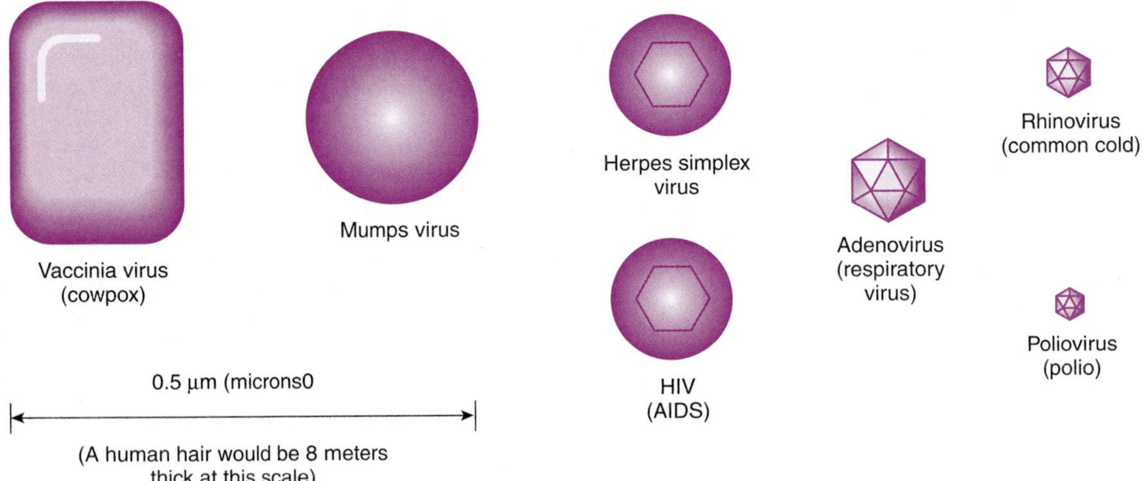

Figure 8–18 Different virus forms

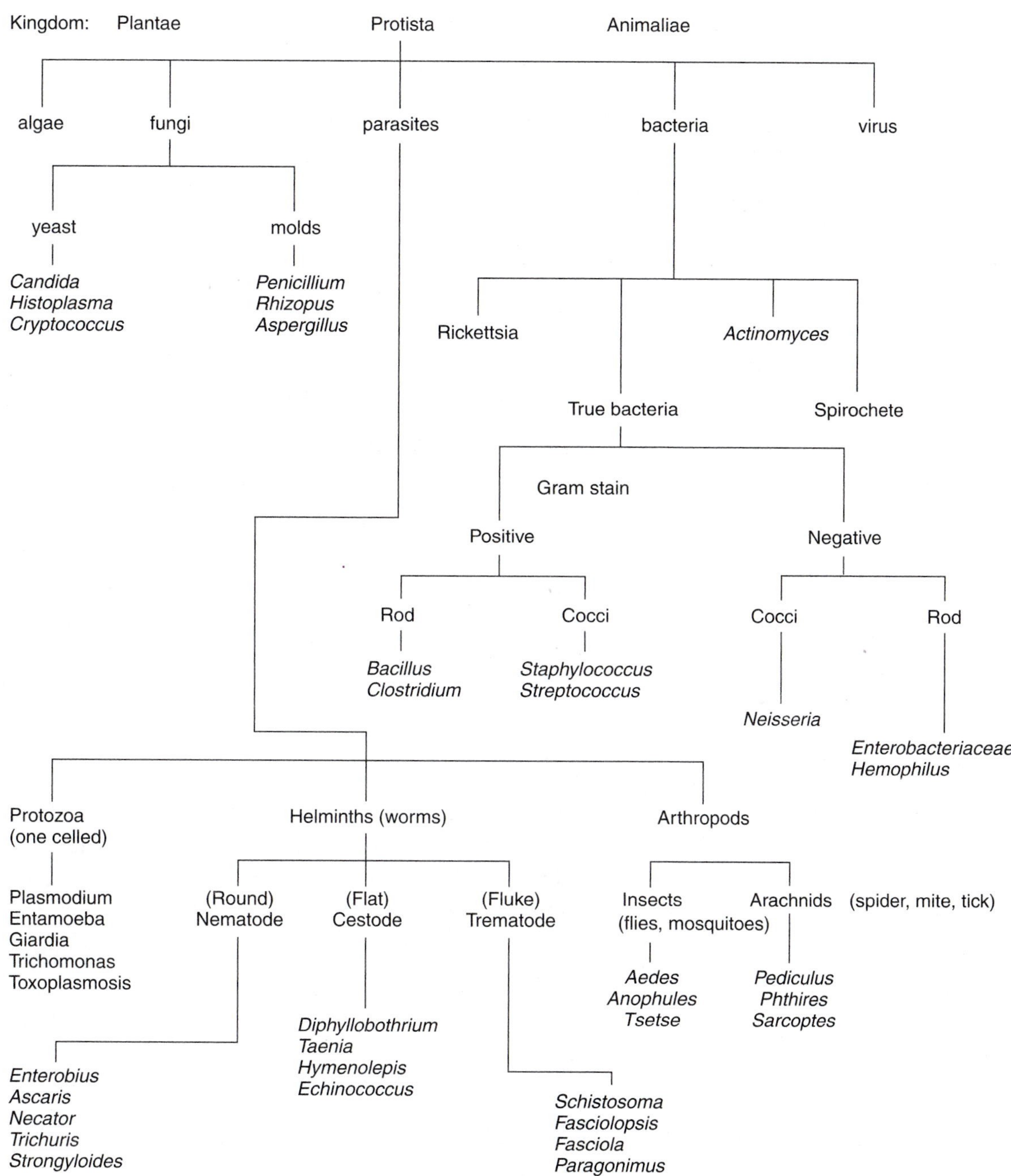

Roadmap scheme to initial categorization of microorganisms

SANITARY PRACTICES

Health care professionals must understand the nature of the diseases caused by pathogenic organisms. Only then will they fully recognize the importance of maintaining cleanliness and sterile techniques in the home, hospital, private medical and dental offices, and the community. With the advent of the bloodborne **pathogenicity** of the **acquired immunodeficiency syndrome** (**AIDS**) and **hepatitis B** viruses, the issue of laboratory safety has come into prominence. In June 1992 **OSHA** issued its Potential Bloodborne Pathogen Rule, which directs, among other requirements, that all health care workers handling any body fluids or products thereof wear protective gloves, protective clothing, and protective eyeware, if applicable, when handling specimens or blood. Additionally, frequent handwashing and the cleaning of spills with a strong disinfectant, such as a 10% solution of bleach, will increase one's protection. These are the most basic precautions in preventing the growth and spread of disease-producing microorganisms. A case in point is the virus that causes infectious hepatitis (hepatitis A). This virus is transmitted through the oral–anal route and may be excreted through the bowels. Contaminated food, milk, and water carry the virus, and infection can result in a serious liver condition. In a well-documented case that occurred some 50 years ago in a well-known hotel, many patrons came down with **typhoid fever.** In tracing the source of this epidemic, health officials found one of the cooks to be a **carrier** of the bacteria that causes typhoid fever who seldom washed her hands before returning to work.

Therefore, everyday sanitary practices, such as the washing of hands after elimination, should always be required and practiced by all. The practice of washing the hands thoroughly with soap and water is very important to proper cleanliness.

SUMMARY

Protists, the simplest of the plant and animal kingdoms, have been grouped into another kingdom—Protista. They are usually single-celled with no complex tissues or organs. Most are microscopic. Subgroups of protists include the algae, fungi, parasites, and bacteria. Viruses may also be included, even though they are not cellular.

Algae are simple plant structures that undergo photosynthesis and contain chlorophyll. They live in water, soil, rocks, plants, and trees. They aid in soil fertility, serve as food for marine life, have several commercial uses, and are a source of some vitamins. Generally nonpathogenic, some are indirectly toxic to humans, animals, and birds.

Fungi include the unicellular yeast of the *Candida* group (which reproduce by budding), the dermatophyte skin and nail fungi, and the deep-seated fungi that cause lung and meningocococcal infection, as well as the molds that are filamentous and multicellular. Molds may be seen on bread, cheese, and fruit. Many are important for their use as antibiotics.

Parasites include protozoa (the single-celled members), the wormlike helminths, and the arthropodic insects and arachnids. The protozoa are much larger than most other protists and can usually be seen with just the low-power objective. They are parasitic in that they live off a host. Paramecium, amoeba, volvox, and euglena are biological examples living in pond water. Clinically significant protozoan infections include those of the *Plasmodium, Entamoeba, Giardia, Trichomonas,* and *Toxoplasma* groups.

The important helminths include the roundworms, or nematodes; the tapeworms, or cestodes; and the trematodes, or flukes. Examples of nematodes include the roundworm (*Ascaris*), pinworm (*Enterobius*), whipworm (*Trichuris*), hookworm (*Necator*), and threadworm (*Strongyloides*). Cestodes of importance are the beef and pork tapeworms (*Taenia*) as well as the fish tapeworm (*Diphyllobothrium*). The dwarf tapeworm (*Hymenolepis*) is also included in this group. The tremetodes or flukes are flat and leaf shaped. They can be found in blood (*Schistosoma*) as well as in the intestine (*Fasciolopsis*), liver (*Fasciola*), and lung (*Paragonimus*). The arthropods include the insect class of bugs, flies, mosquitoes (carrier for malaria), lice (*Pediculus* and *Phthirus*), and fleas as well as the arachnid class of spiders, ticks (carriers for Lyme disease), and mites (*Sarcoptes*).

Bacteria are very small, single celled, and can best be seen stained under the oil-immersion objective. They range widely in size, with the rickettsia being the smallest. Bacteria are best grouped by their gram staining properties as gram-positive cocci (staphylococci and streptococci), gram-positive bacilli (*Bacillus* and *Clostridium*), gram-negative cocci (*Neisseria*), and gram-negative bacilli (*Enterobacteriacae* and *Haemophilus*). A special stain (acid-fast) identifies the mycobacteria.

Viruses, which are noncellular, can be seen only with an electron microscope. Viruses invade cells by injecting their genetic material into the cell to gain nutrients for themselves. Many diseases are caused by viruses, including chicken pox, AIDS, hepatitis B, and smallpox.

All microorganisms (except viruses) are made up of organized protoplasm or cells. These cells carry on the same life activities as cells of other living things, including obtaining food, respiration, excreting wastes, and reproducing.

STUDY AND DISCUSSION

- Prepare a chart to outline the main differences among yeasts, molds, protozoa, bacteria, and the viruses.
- Explain how algae are different from the other protists. Provide examples of their usefulness to humans.
- List some useful activities of each type of protist.
- List some harmful activities of each type of protist.

REVIEW QUESTIONS

A. General Questions: Provide complete answers to each of the following.

1. Where are microorganisms found?

2. What are single-celled animals called?

3. What are organisms with more than one cell called?

4. What are simple plants called?

5. What is the average size of bacteria? To what may this measurement be compared?

6. Explain the chief difference between bacteria and protozoa.

7. Explain why a virus is called a "filterable virus."

8. Name two diseases caused by viruses.

9. Name three diseases caused by bacteria.

10. Name two diseases caused by a protozoan.

11. Fill in the blanks for the following schematic diagram.

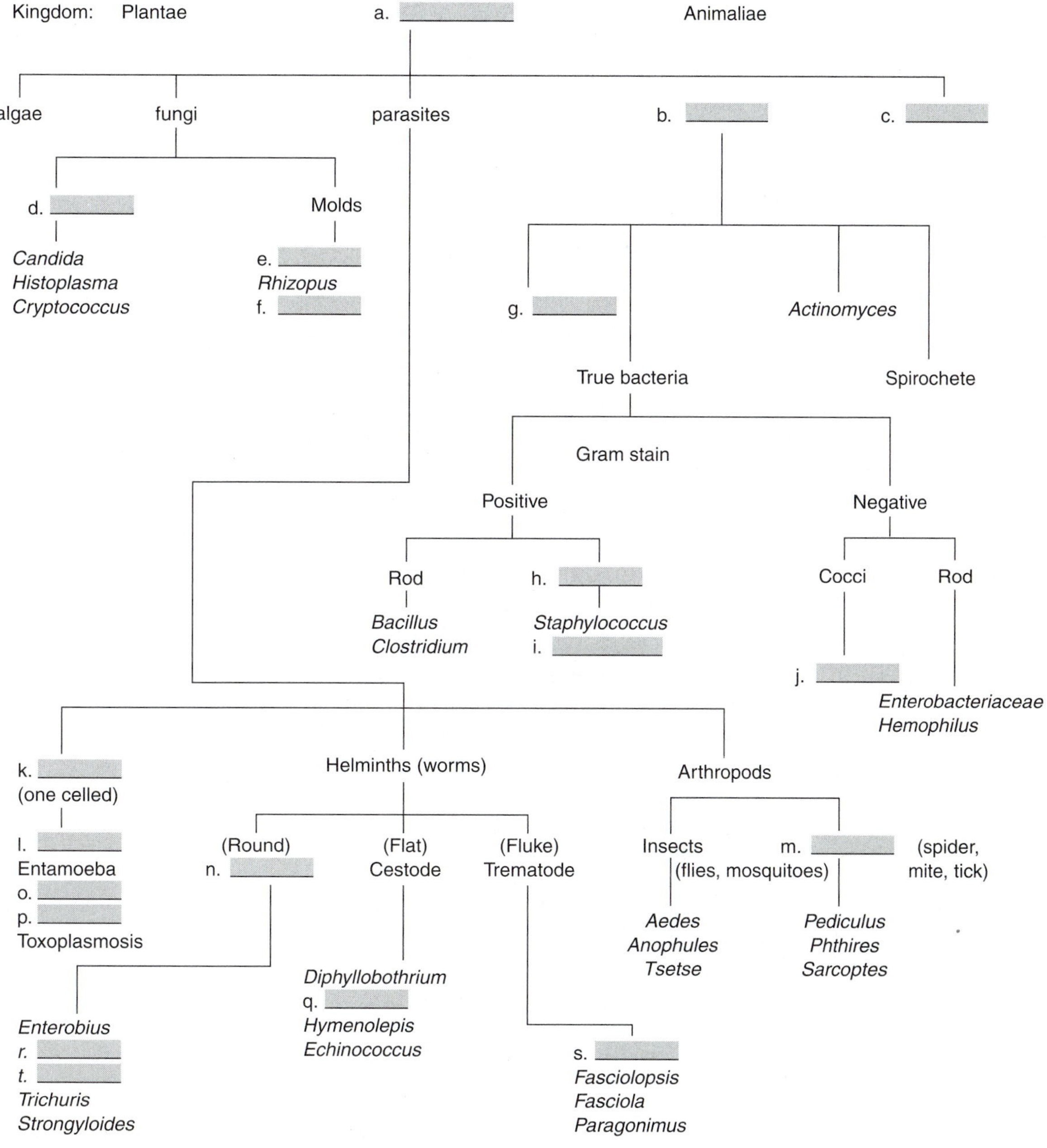

B. Multiple-Choice Questions: Select the letter of the choice that best answers the question or completes the sentence.

1. Linnaeus developed the classification system that used
   a. dissimilar characteristics.
   b. one English name.
   c. conservation of energy.
   d. binomial nomenclature.
2. The branch of biology that deals with classification is
   a. microbiology.
   b. taxonomy.
   c. cytology.
   d. botany.
3. Of the following, the most closely related group of organisms is called a(n)
   a. kingdom.
   b. genus.
   c. species.
   d. order.
4. Protists include
   a. algae and protozoa.
   b. algae and mosses.
   c. protozoa and mammals.
   d. birds and reptiles.
5. The number of protista kingdom is
   a. 2.
   b. 3.
   c. 4.
   d. 5.
6. The Latin classification for humans is *Homo sapiens*, which is the
   a. kingdom and phylum.
   b. phylum and class.
   c. genus and species.
   d. genus and family.
7. The correct arrangement of the following groups from the highest to the lowest (1 = class; 2 = family; 3 = phylum; 4 = order; 5 = genus; 6 = species) is
   a. 3-2-4-1-5-6.
   b. 3-4-1-6-5-2.
   c. 3-4-1-5-6-2.
   d. 3-1-4-2-5-6.
8. The kingdom containing organisms that are neither plants nor animals is
   a. fungi.
   b. protists.
   c. slime molds.
   d. mosses.
9. Two organisms are in the same species if they
   a. can mate and produce fertile offspring.
   b. can live together in a similar environment.
   c. can eat the same foods.
   d. are dissimilar.
10. Which of the following are recognized groups of kingdoms?
    a. plants, animals, protists
    b. protists, fungi, bacteria
    c. plants, protists, monera
    d. plants, animals, fungi, protists, monera
    e. a and d are correct
11. Yeastlike fungi include _____.
    a. *Candida, Penicillium, Cryptococcus*
    b. *Histoplasma, Candida, Cryptococcus*
    c. *Aspergillus, Candida, Histoplasma*
    d. *Candida, Histoplasma, Rhizopus*
12. The *Anopheles* is a _____.
    a. mite
    b. flea
    c. mosquito
    d. spider

13. Flukes are _____.
    a. flatworms
    b. roundworms
    c. protozoans
    d. leaflike worms
14. *Taenia* is a member of the _____ class.
    a. cestode
    b. trematode
    c. nematode
    d. arachnid
15. True bacteria are _____ shaped.
    a. rod and bacillus
    b. rod and coccoid
    c. rod and spiral
    d. filamentous
16. *Ascaris* is a _____.
    a. protozoa
    b. bacteria
    c. fungus
    d. parasite
17. Which of the following groups are roundworms?
    a. *Fasciola, Diphyllobothrium, Hymenolepis, Giardia*
    b. *Schistosoma, Taenia, Paragonimus, Trichuris*
    c. *Ascaris, Necator, Enterobius, Strongyloides*
    d. *Entamoeba, Taenia, Giardia, Trichomonas*
18. *Enterobacteriaceae* are normally found in/on the _____.
    a. urinary tract
    b. bowel
    c. upper respiratory tract
    d. skin

C. Completion Questions: From the following list of terms fill in the blanks with the correct choice.

roundworms	whipworms	insect	*Cryptococcus*
tapeworms	*Ascaris*	tsetse	*Pediculus*
pinworms	*Necator*	*Staphylococcus*	*Phthirus*
Echinococcus	*Aedes*	*Streptococcus*	*Sarcoptes*
Hymenolepis	trematode	*Bacillus*	*Schistosoma*
Anopheles	nematode	*Clostridium*	*Fasciola*
hookworms	cestode	*Neisseria*	*Candida*
threadworms	arachnid		

1. Some nematodes can be microscopic in size, but most _____________ are visible to the naked eye and grow to 30 centimeters.

2. Cestodes are _____________ that often grow to be 20 meters long.

3. Common in children, _____________ are found worldwide.

4. The dog tapeworm is called _____________, and the dwarf tapeworm is the _____________.

5. Flukes are flat leaflike _____________.

6. The cause of head lice is _____________.

7. The sexually transmitted crab louse is ______________.

8. Yellow fever is carried by the ______________ mosquito.

9. Gram-positive rods include ______________ and ______________.

10. The common thrush infection is caused by ______________.

D. Matching Questions: Match the terms in Column I with their corresponding terms in Column II.

Column I		Column II
_______	1. *Enterobacteriaceae*	a. blood fluke
_______	2. *Taenia*	b. fish tapeworm
_______	3. *Candida*	c. beef tapeworm
_______	4. *Schistosoma*	d. scabies
_______	5. Mycobacteria	e. malaria
_______	6. *Penicillium*	f. black mold
_______	7. *Diphyllobothrium*	g. viruslike bacteria
_______	8. *Neisseria*	h. gram-negative rod
_______	9. *Sarcoptes*	i. genital protozoa
_______	10. *Rhizopus*	j. yeast
_______	11. rickettsia	k. antibiotic
_______	12. *Plasmodium*	l. acid-fast
_______	13. *Strongyloides*	m. dysentary
_______	14. *Trichomonas*	n. threadworm
_______	15. *Giardia*	o. gram-negative cocci

CHAPTER

9 Fungi

OBJECTIVES

After completing this chapter, you will be able to:

- explain the structure and types of yeasts.
- identify the beneficial and harmful activities of yeasts.
- define mold and describe its composition.
- explain and provide examples of how molds affect a person's health and well-being.

KEY WORDS

aerial mycelium
Blastomyces
budding
Candida albicans
chlamydospores
Coccidioides immitis
conidia
Cryptococcus
Cryptococcus neoformans
daughter cell
dermatophytes
dimorphism
Epidermophyton
Histoplasma capsulatum
hypha
immunosuppression
macroconidia
microconidia
Microsporum
molds
mycelium
normal flora
opportunistic infection
parasites
Penicillium notatum
rhizoids
Saccharomyces cerevisiae
sphagnum moss
sporangia
spores
Sporothrix schenckii
Trichophyton

YEASTS

The study of fungi, including the yeasts, is called mycology. *Mycoses* is a term used for "fungi," as in *superficial mycoses,* meaning "fungi of the skin." Yeasts are microscopic, single-celled members of the fungi division (Figure 9–1). They are found on fruit and vegetable skins, on grain, and in water and soil. The yeasts are spherical or oval-shaped plant cells that lack chlorophyll. Because they cannot manufacture their own food, they depend upon other organic matter for nutrition. When the organic material is removed from the area, the yeasts and fungi no longer thrive.

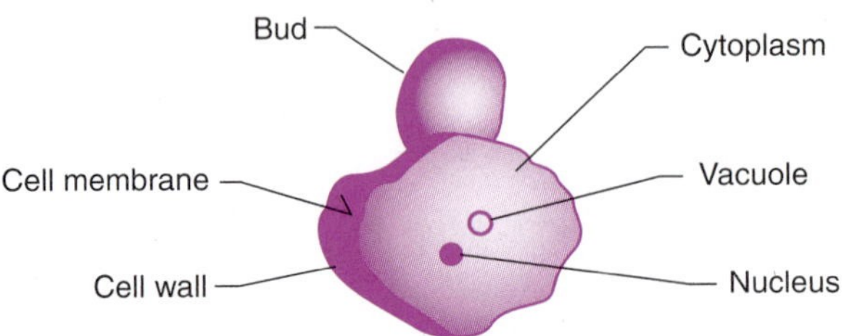

CELL WALL - Strong, ridged outside covering of the cell
CELL MEMBRANE - Thickened edge of the cytoplasm found just inside the cell wall
CYTOPLASM - Living substance within the cell outside of the nucleus
NUCLEUS - Round structure within the cell that is essential to the life activities and reproduction of the cell
VACUOLES - One or two large cavities containing fluid
SPORES - Four to eight resistant bodies within the yeast cell that enable yeasts to survive unfavorable conditions
BUDS - Projections containing cytoplasm and nuclear material

Figure 9–1 Single yeast cell with a bud

When organisms depend upon nonliving organic matter for food, they are called saprophytes. Yeasts that live on the various sugars (such as those found in fruits) are usually saprophytes. If they depend upon living organisms for their food they are called **parasites.** ***Candida albicans,*** a yeast that invades the mucous membranes of the mouth, throat, and vagina, is a parasite. It can cause an ulcerative condition known as thrush.

The yeast cell reproduces by a process known as **budding** (Figure 9–2). Each cell produces a cytoplasmic protrusion, or bud (blastopore), which is called a **daughter cell.** This later breaks off from the mother cell and reproduces in the same manner. Like other plant cells, yeasts have a cell wall, a cell membrane, cytoplasm, a nucleus, and a vacuole.

Yeasts grow quickly in a warm temperature and are killed at boiling temperature. They can reproduce very fast in a sugary solution. Yeast cells reproduce themselves about every 20 minutes when the growth conditions, including food, moisture, and temperature, are favorable. The yeast ***Saccharomyces cerevisiae*** causes the sugars to ferment into alcohol and carbon dioxide, so yeast enables us to make wine from grape sugars, cider from apple sugar, and beer from malt and hops. The carbon dioxide released by this process is also responsible for the rising of dough in breadmaking.

Saccharomyces cerevisiae has many beneficial uses and is not considered pathogenic to humans. An exception would be in an immunosuppressed patient, whose immune system is incapable of preventing such normal flora from becoming an opportunistic infection. Some activities of *Saccharomyces,* however, are harmful, including the spoilage of fruits, syrups, and jellies by fermentation.

Wild yeast found in the skin of fruits is called "grape yeast." Yeast cakes are referred to as baker's or brewer's yeast; they are used in the making of bread and beer. Yeast is a rich source of vitamin B and proteins.

The pathogenic yeast *Candida albicans* is differentiated from the nonpathogenic varieties by demonstrating its ability to produce germ tubes (Figure 9–3), when a small

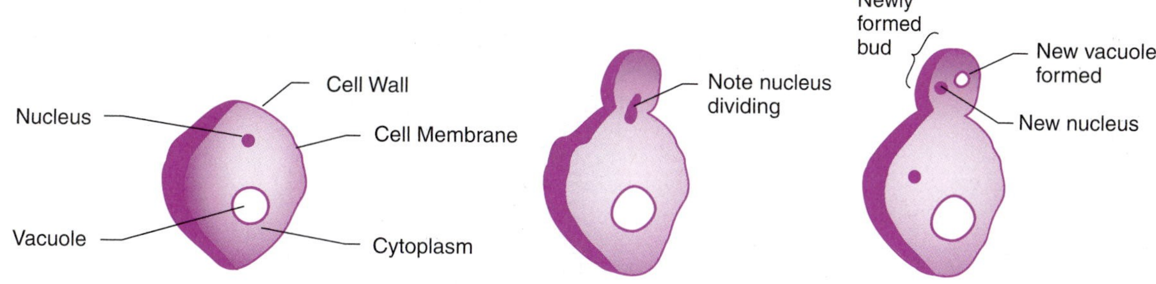

YEAST cell in the process of budding

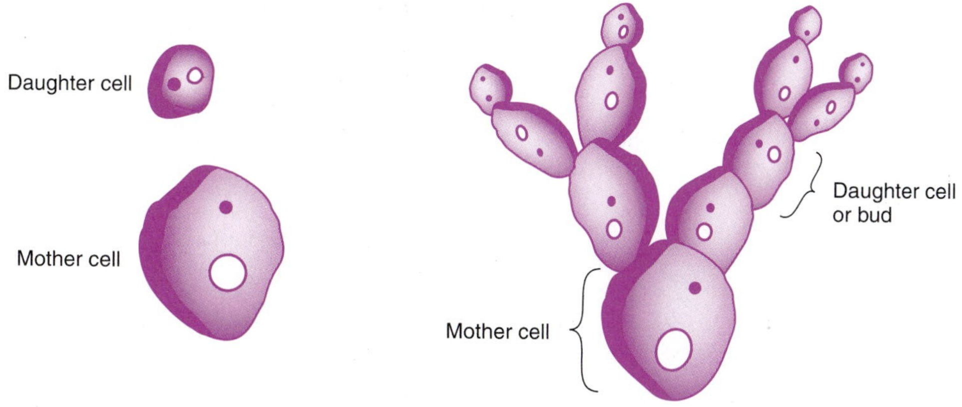

CHAIN of yeast cells as a result of budding

Figure 9–2 Budding yeasts

inoculum of the yeast colony is incubated in a test tube of fresh serum for up to 2 hours. A second identifying characteristic of *Candida albicans* is its ability to form **chlamydospores** (large spores) (Figure 9–4) when a straight wire loop of the organism is inoculated onto cornmeal agar and incubated in a bacteriological incubator at 37°C for up to 48 hours. A small chunk of the media taken along the line of inoculation is placed onto a clean glass slide and pressed under a coverslip. The material is then examined microscopically for the diagnostic chlamydospores.

Another pathogenic yeast, ***Cryptococcus neoformans,*** may be tentatively identified by adding india ink to freshly spun cerebrospinal fluid and observing microscopically for the typical encapsulated yeast cells, which have a black ring around the edge of the budding yeast cells and are surrounded by a colorless capsule against the black background of india ink. Some fungi can live as yeasts or molds depending upon the environmental growth conditions. In living tissues at body temperature (37°C) these parasitic fungi

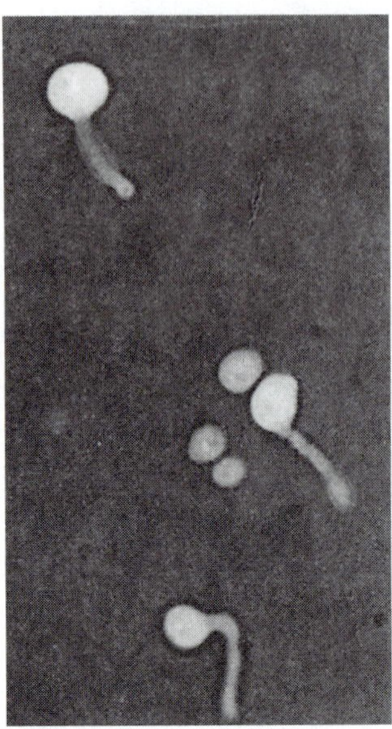

Figure 9–3 *Candida albicans* (yeast), germ tube formation in serum (*Visuals Unlimited/G. Musil © 1985*)

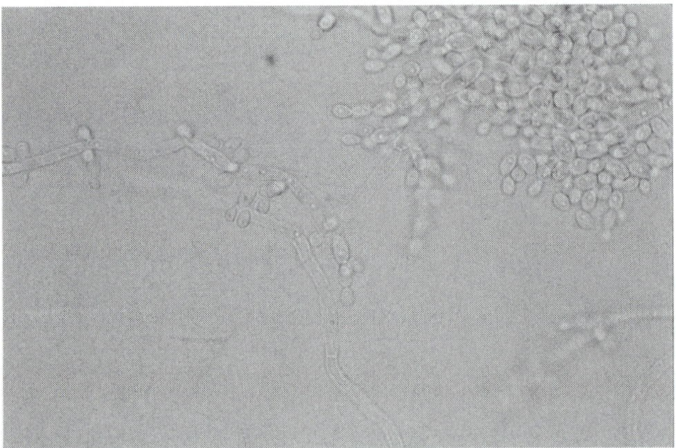

Figure 9–4 *Candida albicans*, chlamydospores (*Visuals Unlimited/E. Chan © 1985*)

appear as unicellular yeasts. If grown at room temperature (20° to 25°C) or in soil, these same organisms grow as saprophytic molds, forming hyphae and spores. This characteristic is known as **dimorphism.** Several of the pathogenic fungi known to humans are capable of this phenomenon. They include ***Histoplasma capsulatum,*** which causes the disease histoplasmosis. Histoplasmosis is obtained by breathing air containing the small spore forms, which may be found in excavation sites or areas where birds or bats have long roosted. The spores are carried for miles so one seldom recalls exposure. This disease is usually self-limiting, but with patients who are immunocompromised it may progress to death if untreated. This fungus typically causes a pneumonialike infection in the lungs and lymph glands of the lungs and responds well to antifungal drugs. ***Sporothrix schenckii,*** a soil fungus, causes a skin infection called sporotrichosis. This disease can involve the lymph system, lungs, joints, and rarely the bones. Lesions, ulcers, and abscesses form on the skin at the site where the skin is penetrated by thorns, barberry bushes, or **sphagnum moss** contaminated with the fungus. Its dimorphism is evidenced when, in cultures from skin lesions, it grows as a yeast and as mold from soil cultures. This fungus responds well to oral treatment of potassium iodide added to juices. A third dimorphic soil organism, ***Coccidioides immitis,*** causes coccidioidomycosis or San Joaquin Valley fever. This disease tends to be limited to the southwestern United States, Mexico, and Central and South America, and comes from breathing the spores found in the desert soil. Most infections are symptomless, but for those who are immunocompromised, this disease can be disseminated throughout the body and be fatal. Antifungal drugs such as amphotericin B, itraconazole, and fluconazole are usually successful treatments, although with a variety of unwanted side effects.

Fungal diseases are usually categorized by the depth of their infection. Superficial or cutaneous fungi are caused by **dermatophytes** that live on skin or mucous membranes. These fungal infections cause athlete's foot, ringworm, and infections of the hair, skin, and scalp. *Candida albicans* is an opportunistic fungus that, given the opportunity of lowered resistance or an immunocompromised immune system as in patients with the acquired immunodeficiency syndrome (AIDS), will cause infections of the mouth (oral thrush), skin, rectal area, genitalia, and vagina (vaginal candidiasis). These inlets can then be the route of entry for the spread of a generalized systemic yeast infection. Deep-seated or systemic fungi include the dimorphs, *Histoplasma* (histoplasmosis), and *Coccidiodes* (coccidioidomycosis) as well as ***Blastomyces*** (blastomycosis) and ***Cryptococcus*** (cryptococcosis). In all cases, as the infection invades beyond the superficial levels, treatment and cure are impossible or difficult to obtain. Some skin tests are available to determine susceptibility. Most mycotic infections are treated with ketoconazole, nystatin, amphotericin B, or 5-fluorocytosine, which are toxic to humans; therefore, careful monitoring and caution must be used in prescribing these chemotherapeutic drugs.

MOLDS

Molds are multicellular, filamentous fungi. They are the most familiar of all the microorganisms and are so common in our environment that anything exposed to the air is likely to collect molds. Who has not seen moldy bread, fruits, and vegetables? Many students have observed molds as contaminants in culture media. Everyone is familiar with their characteristic "moldy" odor.

To the naked eye, molds can look like a fuzzy mass, a sooty black area, or a tuft of cotton variously colored. Examined under the microscope, however, molds are seen to be made up of long filaments of protoplasm. Each of the individual threads is called a **hypha.** When considered together, these hyphae are called a **mycelium,** or plant body. When the hyphae are ripe, they form tiny knobs at their tips called **sporangia.**

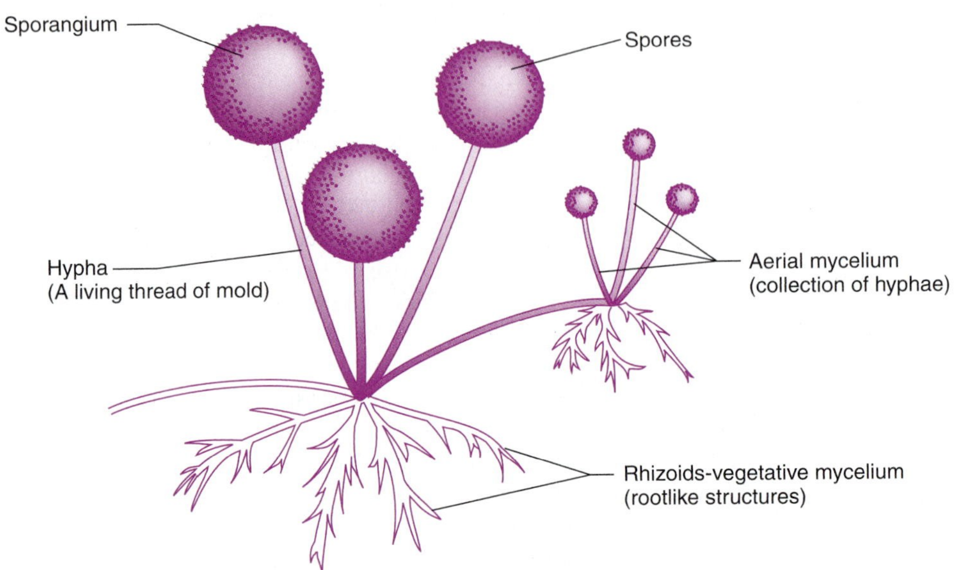

Figure 9–5 Black mold or bread mold of the *Rhizopus* genus

Each sporangium, when broken, releases thousands of microscopic **spores** into the air. In certain types of bacteria spores are entities found within the bacterial cell itself; they differ from spores shed by molds. Bacterial spores allow the bacterial cell to "hibernate" when growth conditions are not favorable. These spores may be centrally or terminally located on the bacterial cell. When the optimal growth conditions (food, warmth, moisture) are not available, the bacterium reverts to its spore stage and can then exist until the return of favorable conditions, such as when the bacterium enters a body. These more ideal growth conditions of food, warmth, and moisture allow the bacterium to exit its spore stage to begin its multiplication stage. These may later start mold growths when they come in contact with pieces of bread and other substances that can nourish them. Like seeds, this is how a mold reproduces. In addition, the spores also determine the characteristic colors (white, blue-green, red, brown, or black) of the different types of molds (Figure 9–5).

The mycelium grows like a mass of cobwebs (Figure 9–6). It sends short, rootlike branches into food. These rootlike structures are called **rhizoids.** These branches secrete enzymes that digest the food. Eventually, the digested food is absorbed by the mold, resulting in growth. The part of the mycelium that grows on the food's surface is the **aerial mycelium,** which gives mold its fuzzy appearance.

Molds require air, food, warmth, moisture, and darkness to thrive. To prevent the growth of a mold, the substance in question must be deprived of one or more of these conditions. For example, allowing direct sunlight to fall on an object will prevent mold growth. When molds attack materials that are not very nourishing, their growth is stunted; this is referred to as mildew.

There are both harmful and useful molds. Harmful molds include those that cause athlete's foot, ringworm, and food spoilage. Molds that grow on crop plants not only kill

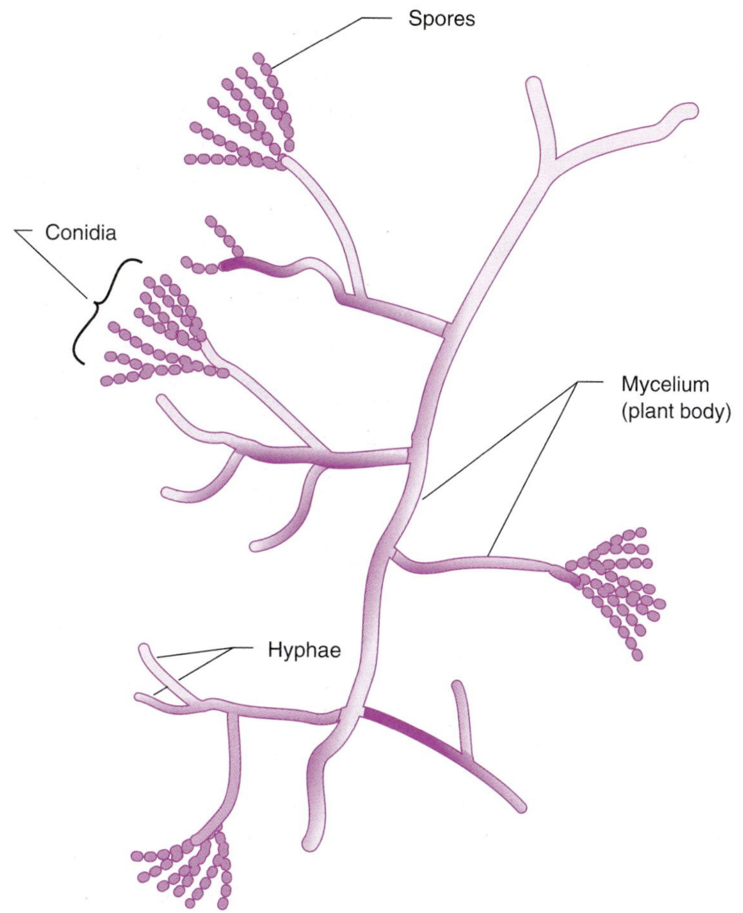

Figure 9–6 Mycelium showing the typical conidia of the *Penicillium* genus

their hosts but may be toxic to the crop's users as well. The ergot mold, which grows on wheat and rye, and the aflatoxin from the *Aspergillus* mold found on cottonseed and peanuts, are very harmful to animals and humans. Besides being toxic, aflatoxin is also a carcinogen.

The penicillin family includes useful molds (Figure 9–7). The antibiotic penicillin, developed by Sir Alexander Fleming, results from the mold ***Penicillium notatum.*** Some species of *Penicillium,* including *Penicillium notatum,* can be **opportunistic infections,** especially to patients suffering from **immunosuppression** diseases such as AIDS, lymphoma, leukemia, and diabetes. Such infections may cause respiratory, genitourinary, and skin infections. Other molds grow on cheeses, resulting in the distinctive flavors of Roquefort, Gorgonzola, Stilton, and Camembert cheeses.

Molds are also important to the nation's agricultural and food industry. They are responsible for most crop and food spoilage, which results in the loss of millions of dollars each year to the food industry.

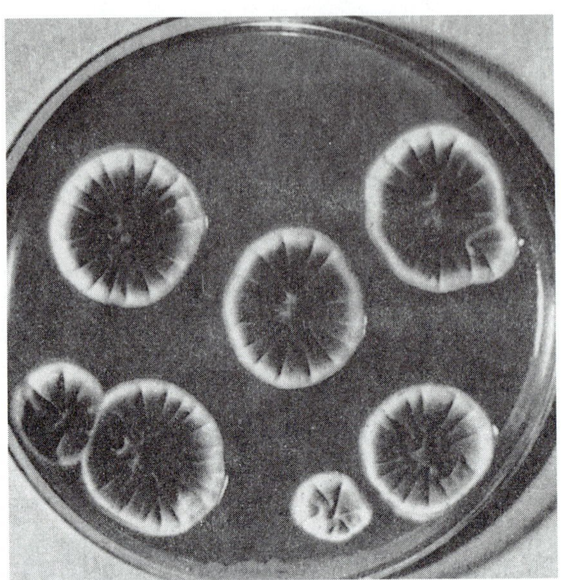

Figure 9–7 This green mold is *Penicillium chrysogenum,* a form of which now produces almost all of the world's commercial penicillin (*Courtesy of Pfizer, Inc.*)

There are many genera of molds that can cause crop and food damage. The following is a brief listing and discussion of some of these molds.

- *Mucor* are found in manure and soil and on fruits, vegetables, and starchy foods. Most of the genus are responsible for food spoilage.
- *Rhizopus* is the genus that causes the common bread mold. These grow on bread, fruits, vegetables, and other foods. The most common species is *Rhizopus stolonifer.*
- *Aspergillus* are widespread. They are found on fruits, vegetables, and many other food products. *Aspergillus* can cause molds on bread, cured meat, maple sap, and syrup.
- *Cladosporium* causes vegetables to decay. It is found in and on the soil.
- *Fusarium* is widespread in nature, found on decaying vegetation, foods, and in soil.
- *Neurospora* have some members that cause food spoilage. The type of mold they cause is red or pink in color. They are commonly called "pink bread molds."
- Certain members of the genus *Penicillium* cause spoilage or rot on fruits, grains, grasses, preserves, and vegetables.
- *Sporothrix* has one species (*Sporothrix carnis*) that causes the "white spots" on refrigerated meats.

Of the above molds found on foods and crops, members of the *Aspergillus* group are most frequently found to cause infections in humans. The *Aspergillus* molds may be recognized by their blue-green or black colors as they grow on breads, fruits, and other crops. Confirmation is made by microscopic examination of a wet mount of the mycelium. Typical conidia resemble the flower of a dandelion as it is ready to disperse it seeds to the wind.

Other clinically significant molds include the dermatophytes, which live on or within the skin. These cause ringworm of the skin, athlete's foot, and infections of the nails, scalp, and hair follicles. Among the most common dermatophytes encountered

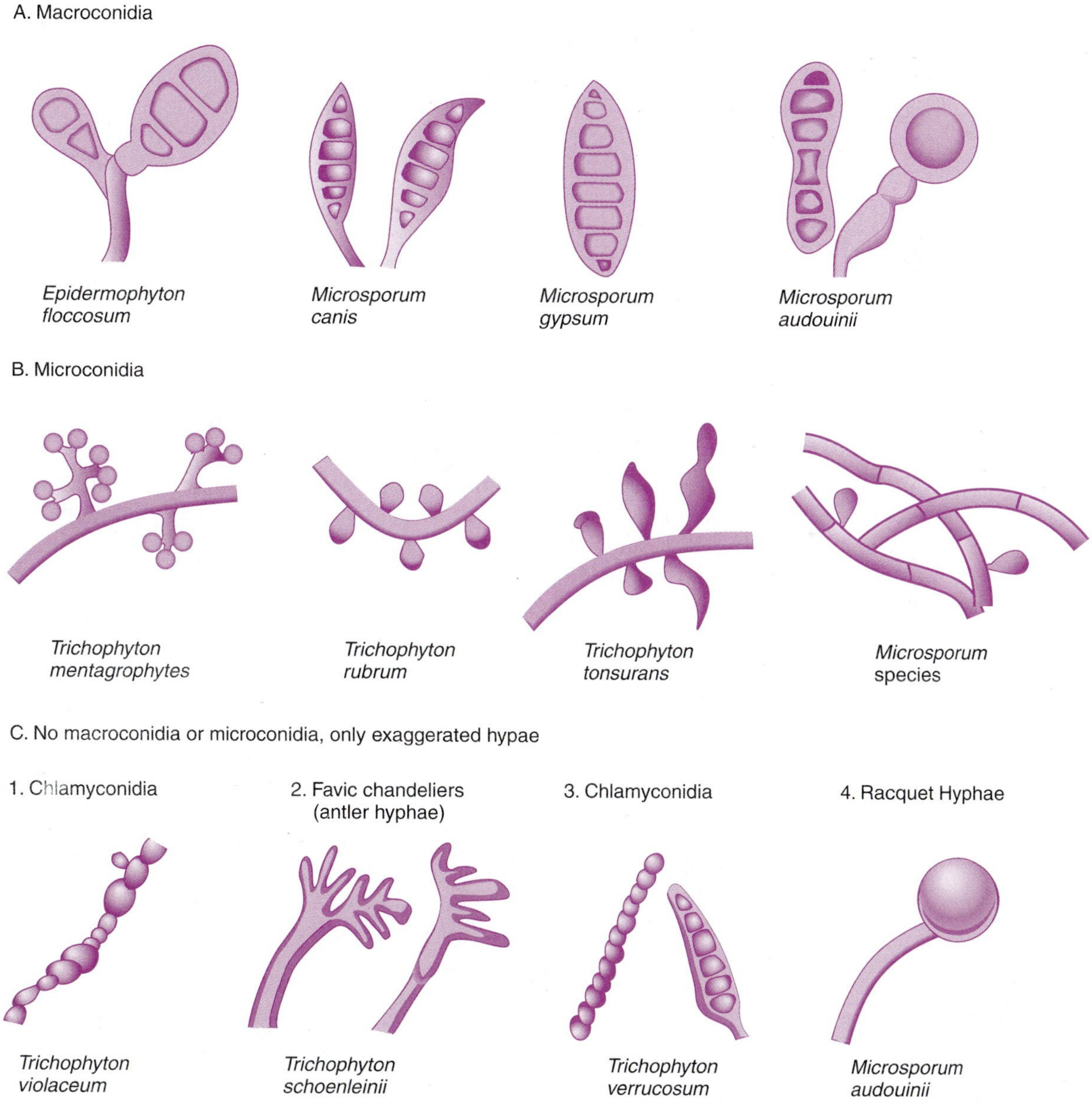

A. Macroconidia

Epidermophyton floccosum
Microsporum canis
Microsporum gypsum
Microsporum audouinii

B. Microconidia

Trichophyton mentagrophytes
Trichophyton rubrum
Trichophyton tonsurans
Microsporum species

C. No macroconidia or microconidia, only exaggerated hypae

1. Chlamyconidia
2. Favic chandeliers (antler hyphae)
3. Chlamyconidia
4. Racquet Hyphae

Trichophyton violaceum
Trichophyton schoenleinii
Trichophyton verrucosum
Microsporum audouinii

Figure 9–8 Microscopic identification features of a selection of various (A) macroconidia, (B) microconidia, and (C) hyphae for some of the dermatophytes

are the ***Trichophyton*** (hair, skin, nails), ***Microsporum*** (hair, skin), and ***Epidermophyton*** (skin, nails) genera. These are identified by their different-shaped **conidia,** as seen microscopically, and their colony appearance when grown on culture media. Conidia are described as being **macroconidia** (very large spores), **microconidia** (tiny spores), and conidia. Figure 9–8 shows examples of the diagnostic features of some of the conidia of the dermatophytes.

Besides the molds that cause superficial or cutaneous infections, another group of fungi is involved in deep-seated and systemic infections. Spores of these fungi may be inhaled with dust, may be picked up in the air from bird droppings (*Cryptococcus*), or may enter via open cuts or sores. They can be found in the lungs, lymph nodes, bones, and internal organs. As previously mentioned, these dimorphs (those that can live as molds or yeasts), can produce deep-seated systemic infections. *Histoplasma capsulatum, Candida albicans, Blastomyces dermatitidis,* and *Coccidioidomyces immitis* all cause serious pulmonary infections. Blastomycosis has been associated more often with those who work outdoors, whereas coccidioidomycosis occurs most frequently in persons of dark-skinned races. Histoplasmosis, the most widespread and common of these systemic infections, may be found in barns, chicken coops, and undisturbed places. Diagnostic microscopic fungal elements are shown in Figure 9–9. *Cryptococcus neoformans,* usually associated with cryptococcal meningitis, is frequently seen as a systemic infection in persons who are immunocompromised.

Some of the yeasts and molds that are commonly found in the environment such as *Candida, Aspergillus,* and *Cryptococcus* may be opportunistic mycoses. This means that when a person has a serious disease in which the immune system has been impaired, these normally harmless fungi can cause life-threatening infections because the immune system is not able to make antibodies. Standard antifungal treatments seem to have no effect on these types of infections and often unconventional chemotherapy that may have toxic side effects must be tried.

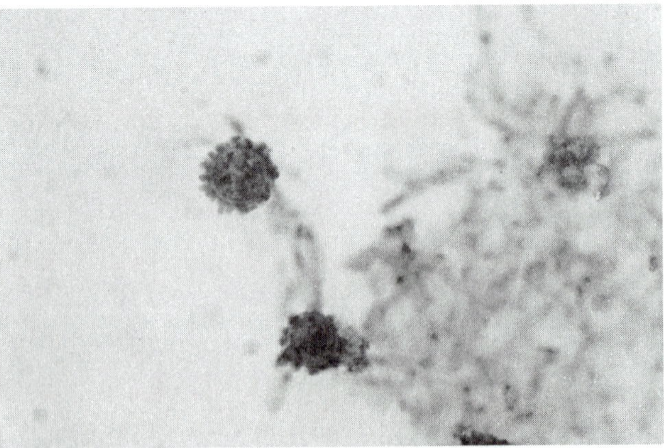

Figure 9–9 *Histoplasma capsulatum* showing characteristic macroconidia (*Visuals Unlimited © Arthur M. Siegelman*)

STUDY AND DISCUSSION

- Discuss the difference between saprophytes and parasites.
- List the precautions that must be taken in the care of patients who suffer from diseases caused by molds.
- Provide examples of symptoms of mold-caused diseases such as ringworm and athlete's foot.
- Examine the structure of molds under the microscope by performing the experiment on microscopic examination of molds.
- Study yeast cells using the following procedure.

Procedure 9–1 Microscopic Examination of Yeast

Equipment and Materials Needed

Microscope	Cover glasses
Yeast cake	Inoculating needle
Molasses	Petri dishes
Slides	Dilute 6.2% iodine solution

Method

1. Dissolve a small amount of yeast cake in tepid water in a petri dish.

2. Add a small amount of molasses, honey, or corn syrup to the solution.

3. Allow the mixture to stand overnight in a warm place.

4. With an inoculating needle, place a drop of the yeast mixture on a clean slide and cover it with a coverslip.

5. Examine and study the yeast cells under the microscope. Notice the budding of yeast cells.

6. Repeat the same procedure as before, adding a few drops of iodine solution. Examine it.

Observations and Conclusions

1. What shape are the yeast cells? Are the yeast cells arranged singularly or in clumps?

2. Identify the parts of the yeast cell shown.

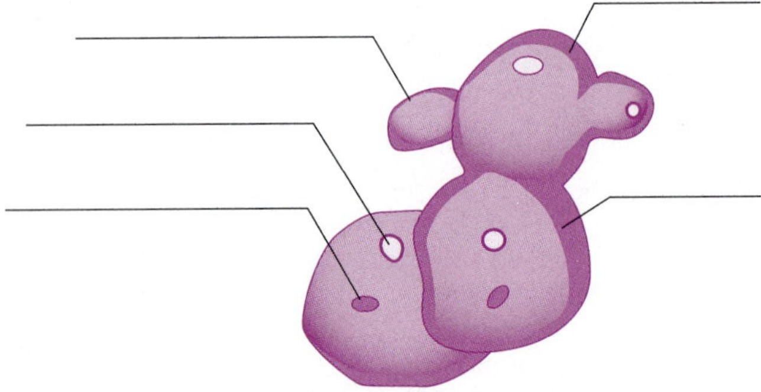

3. By what process do yeast cells reproduce? Describe this process and draw a series of simple diagrams to illustrate it.

- Examine the process of fermentation by performing the experiment on fermentation.

Procedure 9–2 Fermentation

Equipment and Materials Needed

Molasses
Yeast cake
Fermentation tube
Limewater
Rubber stopper
Distillation flask
Cotton
Water
Glass delivery tube
Flask
Test tubes

Method

1. Mix some molasses, water, and yeast and pour into a flask.
2. Put a rubber stopper on the flask, after having first inserted a glass delivery tube. Permit the free end of the delivery tube to dip into a test tube of clear limewater. (Limewater is a solution of calcium hydroxide. It will form a white precipitate of calcium carbonate when it reacts with carbon dioxide.)
3. Let the experiment stand overnight at room temperature.

Observations and Conclusions

1. What happened to the clear limewater after it stood overnight?

2. What caused the change in appearance of the limewater?

3. What two products are produced as a result of yeast fermentation?

Procedure 9–3 Microscopic Examination of Molds

Equipment and Materials Needed

Microscope	Bread
Hand lens	Orange
Petri dishes	Jam
Filter paper	Cheese

Method

1. Line several petri dishes with moist filter paper.
2. Place a piece of bread in one dish; put pieces of orange, cheese, and jam in the other dishes.
3. Place a piece of dry bread in a petri dish without moist filter paper. In other unlined petri dishes, place bits of orange, cheese, and jam.
4. Place all petri dishes, lined and unlined, in a dark closet at room temperature.
5. After 48 or 72 hours, remove all dishes from the closet. Examine the contents of each, first with a hand lens and then under a microscope.

Observations and Conclusions

1. Complete the following table:

Mold Found On:	Orange	Cheese	Bread	Jam
Type of mold:				
Color of mold:				

2. What do you notice about the pieces of food that were moist?

3. What do you notice about the foods that were not moist?

4. Do you note any molds in which fuzzy threads are seen? What are these threads called? What observations can you make about these threads?

5. Sketch and label a simple diagram of a mold.

6. What two conditions does this laboratory experiment show to be necessary for the growth of molds?

7. Are molds unicellular or multicellular plants?

SUMMARY

Fungi are divided into two groups, yeasts and molds. Yeasts reproduce by budding, are single celled, and grow as distinct colonies on culture media similar to bacterial colonies. Molds, on the other hand, are multicellular, filamentous, and reproduce by releasing millions of tiny spores from the sporangia, which are located at the tips of the long filamentous hyphea, referred to as mycelium when a mass of hyphae are considered in a unit. Some yeasts can be dimorphic, meaning they can show characteristics of a yeast and later reproduce as a mold. *Candida albicans, Cryptococcus,* and *Histoplasma* all have this characteristic. Some yeasts are associated with AIDS as opportunistic infections, including *Candida, Cryptococcus, Histoplasma,* and *Blastomycoces.* These yeasts can cause serious life-threatening pulmonary infections. Other common environmental fungi, including *Aspergillus* and *Penicillium,* can invade the human body to cause pulmonary infections.

Molds are identified by the microscopic appearance of the different types of spores, conidia, and mycelium. Physical characteristics, such as the color, texture, and growth rate, as well as some biochemical tests assist in the identification process.

Clinically important fungi can cause ringworm, athletes foot, and infections of the nail, hair, and scalp. These infections, if not treated early, will be difficult and lengthy in curing—months to years in some cases. Conversely, they also may take years to grow to be observable or discomforting. Most important are *Trichophyton, Microsporum,* and *Epidermophyton* genera for skin, hair, and nail diseases.

Fungi are ever present in the atmosphere and they prefer a sugary warm and moist environment for growth, which probably explains why, when fruits spoil, they do not exhibit bacterial growth, but rather a fuzzy fungal growth.

REVIEW QUESTIONS

A. General Questions: Provide complete answers to each of the following.

1. What is the difference between a saprophyte and a parasite?

2. List three beneficial uses of yeast.

3. Describe two harmful activities of yeast.

4. What are the conditions necessary for growth of the yeast plant?

5. What conditions would be effective to prevent the growth of yeast?

6. What are molds?

7. What conditions are needed for the growth of molds?

8. Where are molds found?

9. Do molds ever form on materials other than foods? Give some examples.

10. What gives the characteristic color to molds?

11. What gives the fuzzy appearance to molds?

12. What are some diseases caused by molds?

13. Why are molds belonging to the *Penicillium* genus beneficial?

14. Circle the letter before each of the following procedures that prevents or inhibits the growth of molds.
    a. Store in refrigerator
    b. Store in warm, dark place
    c. Store in direct sunlight
    d. Keep airtight
    e. Sterilize by boiling
    f. Store at room temperature

B. Multiple Choice Questions: Select the letter of the choice that best completes the sentence.

1. All of the following fungi are implicated in infections of hair except _____ .
   a. *Microsporum*
   b. *Epidermophyton*
   c. *Trichophyton*
2. All of the following fungi are implicated in infections of nails except _____ .
   a. *Microsporum*
   b. *Epidermophyton*
   c. *Trichophyton*
3. The ability to produce germ tubes is a characteristic of _____ .
   a. *Histoplasma*
   b. *Saccharomyces*
   c. *Candida*
   d. *Sporothrix*
4. Dimorphism means to have two _____ .
   a. shapes
   b. life cycles
   c. sizes
   d. different colors
5. A mass of hyphae is called _____ .
   a. spores
   b. conidia
   c. sporangia
   d. mycelium
6. The fungus _____ is sometimes diagnosed from an india ink stain performed directly on the spinal fluid.
   a. *Candida albicans*
   b. *Cryptococcus neoformans*
   c. *Histoplasma capsulatum*
   d. *Aspergillus niger*

C. Completion Questions: From the following list of terms fill in the blanks with the correct choice.

Saccharomyces cerevisiae	*Sporothrix*	yeast
Candida albicans	*Coccidioides*	germ tube
Histoplasma	mold	chlamydospores
dermatophytes	*Cryptococcus*	macroconidia

1. Fungi that cause superficial infections of the skin are called _______________ .

2. _______________ is used to make dough rise in bread.

3. At room temperature dimorphs grow as ______________ while at body temperature they grow as ______________ .

4. Fungi that cause deep-seated pulmonary or lung infections include ______________, ______________, and ______________ .

5. Thrush is caused by ______________.

6. A fungus that may be isolated from cerebrospinal fluid and the cause of meningitis is______________ .

7. When grown in cornmeal agar the presence of large spores called ______________ are also used to confirm *Candida albicans.*

D. Matching Questions: Match the terms in Column I with their corresponding terms in Column II.

Column I		Column II
_______	1. *Candida albicans*	a. hair, skin, nails
_______	2. nystatin	b. green mold
_______	3. dermatophyte	c. white spots on meat
_______	4. *Mucor*	d. pink bread mold
_______	5. *Penicillium*	e. antifungal
_______	6. histoplasmosis	f. food spoilage
_______	7. *Aspergillus*	g. bird droppings
_______	8. *Sporotrichum*	h. germ tubes
_______	9. *Neurospora*	i. dandelionlike conidia
_______	10. *Cryptococcus*	j. barns, chicken coops

CHAPTER

10

Parasites

OBJECTIVES

After completing this chapter, you will be able to:

- define the characteristics of parasites and the nature of their activities.
- name and describe some diseases caused by parasites.
- describe the way a parasite gets its nourishment for growth and development.

KEY WORDS

amoeboid movement
Anopheles
antibiosis
arachnids
Balantidium coli
cestodes
cilia
ciliates
contractile vacuoles
cyst
Diphyllobothrium latum
Dipylidium caninum
Endolimax nana
Entamoeba coli
Entamoeba hartmanni
Entamoeba histolytica
fission
flagella
flagellates
food vacuoles
gametocytes
Giardia intestinalis
Giardia lamblia
helminths
hookworm
hosts
infection
infestation
macronucleus
Mastigophora
microfilaria
micronucleus
nematodes
neutralism
organelles
parasites
parasitism
Pediculus
pellicle
Phthirus
Plasmodium falciparum
Plasmodium malariae
Plasmodium ovale
Plasmodium vivax
Pneumocystis carinii
proglottids
protozoa
pseudopodia
schizonts
symbiosis
Taenia
tapeworm
Toxoplasma gondii
trematodes
trichina
trichocysts
Trichomonas vaginalis
trophozoite
Trypanosoma cruzi
Trypanosoma gambiense
Trypanosoma rhodesiense
Wuchereria bancrofti

Organisms that nourish themselves at the expense of other living things and cause them damage are called **parasites. Parasitism,** as a mode of life, is characteristic of many microorganisms and also of some relatively large organisms, including worms and insects.

When the invasion and growth of unicellular, microscopic parasites in an organism cause a disease, it is commonly known as an **infection. Infestation,** on the other hand, refers to the presence in or on the host of animal parasites such as ticks, lice, and flatworms.

Symbiosis is a condition in nature in which two organisms live together with benefits to both. For example, a lichen is a combination of an alga and a fungus living together in a symbiotic relationship. The green alga provides food for the fungus, and the fungus absorbs and stores water for the alga.

When organisms coexist in the same habitat with neither a harmful nor a beneficial effect upon one another, a condition called **neutralism** exists. Bacteria living in the human intestine and mouth are examples of neutralism.

Antibiosis is a condition in which two organisms cannot coexist. In this case, one of the two microorganisms will produce an antibiotic to kill off the other. For example, a penicillium mold growing on the same agar plate as certain strains of staphylococci will kill off the bacteria by producing penicillin.

Living plants or animals from which the parasite receives nourishment are called **hosts.** Most living forms serve as hosts for other living forms. Health care professionals are mainly interested in parasites that affect people by causing disease.

Many parts of the human body encourage the growth of parasitic microorganisms by supplying food, moisture, and warmth. Parasites are constantly present in the intestine and on the skin and mucous membranes of the nose and throat. The colon always contains great numbers of bacterial flora and sometimes protozoa and **helminths** or worms. Most parasites, like normal bacterial flora, cause no harm, however.

PROTOZOA

Protozoa are microscopic, one-celled animals. They are the lowest classified forms of life in the animal kingdom. Generally larger than the fungus, the protozoan has a more complex and detailed internal structure.

Many protozoa have **organelles,** which are the specialized cellular parts that perform metabolic functions. For example, one organelle serves to ingest solid food; another gets rid of undigested particles. Other organelles perform additional metabolic functions.

Different parts of these unicellular animals, such as **contractile vacuoles** and **food vacuoles** (organelles), often show some degree of specialization. There are 45,000 types of protozoa which differ in structure, shape, and size. These creatures are classified as ciliophora, mastigophora, and sarcodina, based on their method of locomotion.

Ciliophora (Ciliates)

Ciliates are protozoa that move by means of many short, hairlike projections (**cilia**) on their surfaces (Figure 10–1). These cilia beat rhythmically to move the ciliates backward or forward.

The paramecium has an outer covering, the **pellicle,** which is strong enough to maintain its elongated, slipperlike shape. Paramecia are animals that have cilia and contain:

- semifluid, granular cytoplasm, which is differentiated into two nuclei: the macronucleus and the micronucleus; and
- organelles: the food and contractile vacuoles, the trichocysts, and the mouth and gullet.

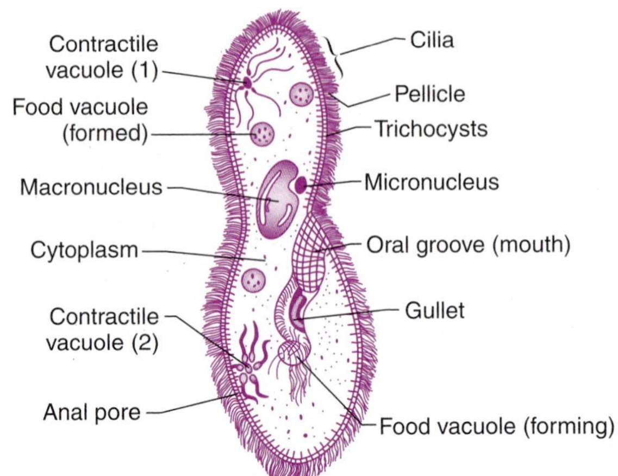

Figure 10–1 Paramecium—a ciliate

The **macronucleus** is the large nucleus, which controls the paramecium's metabolism. Its smaller nucleus, the **micronucleus,** is involved with reproduction. The food and contractile vacuoles of the paramecium function like those of the amoeba.

Beneath the pellicle are the **trichocysts**—small vesicles arranged in a layer with a hairlike thread. This thread may be discharged to sting or capture prey. The beating cilia direct prey and food into the mouth and down into the gullet. ***Balantidium coli*** is the only parasitic ciliated protozoan in humans. This parasite may cause dysentery, or may cause no symptoms. Abdominal discomfort with mild to moderate chronic diarrhea is seen more often than acute dysentary. Usually, illness is less likely to develop in a healthy person. This disease is transmitted by ingesting the **cysts** which may be found in feces, and on fingers, food, fomites, and flies. Diagnosis is made by finding cysts or the adult **trophozoite** in fecal eliminations. **B.coli** is the largest protozoa and the only ciliated protozoa that infects humans. Figure 10–2 shows a cyst and adult trophozoite *Balantidium coli.*

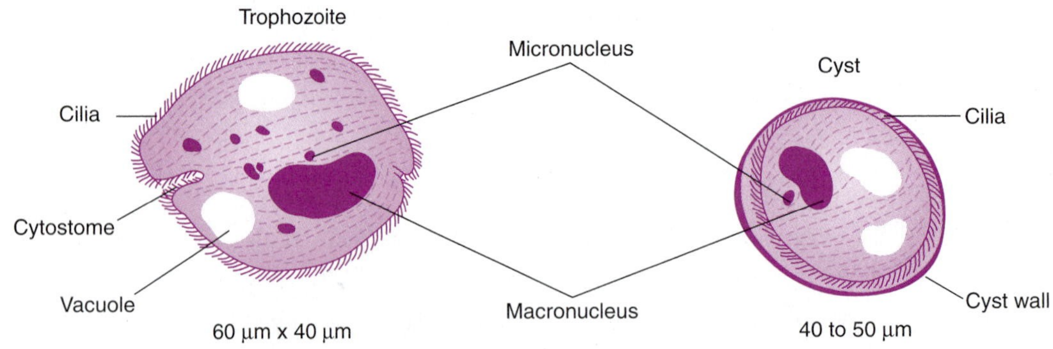

Figure 10–2 *Balantidium coli* and trophozoite

Mastigophora

Mastigophora (flagellates) move by one or more long, whiplike projections, or **flagella,** usually found at one end of the cell. Several flagellated protozoans cause disease in humans. ***Giardia lamblia*** and ***Giardia intestinalis*** are parasites found in the human intestine that cause dysentery. Another is ***Trypanosoma rhodesiense,*** the cause of African sleeping sickness. A third parasite is ***Trypanosoma cruzi,*** which causes South American trypanosomiasis or Chagas' disease.

Giardia lamblia is the most common intestinal parasite in the United States. Often referred to as traveller's diarrhea, it is easily picked up from cross-contaminated spring waters and sewage systems. *Giardia* is usually transmitted to humans when they drink contaminated, untreated water. However, it can also be transmitted through improperly treated swimming pools, water slides, or residential water supplies. *Giardia* can also be transmitted by food handlers who practice improper handwashing or by washing foods in contaminated water. A number of outbreaks of *Giardia* have been reported in nursing homes and in day-care settings. Wild animals such as the beaver are suspected to be reservoir hosts for the transmission of this parasite to humans. Additionally, a wide range of mammals, including cats, dogs, and muskrats, are also infected with *Giardia* species. *Giardia* is easily diagnosed by demonstrating the cysts or trophozoites in feces or duodenal contents (Figure 10–3).

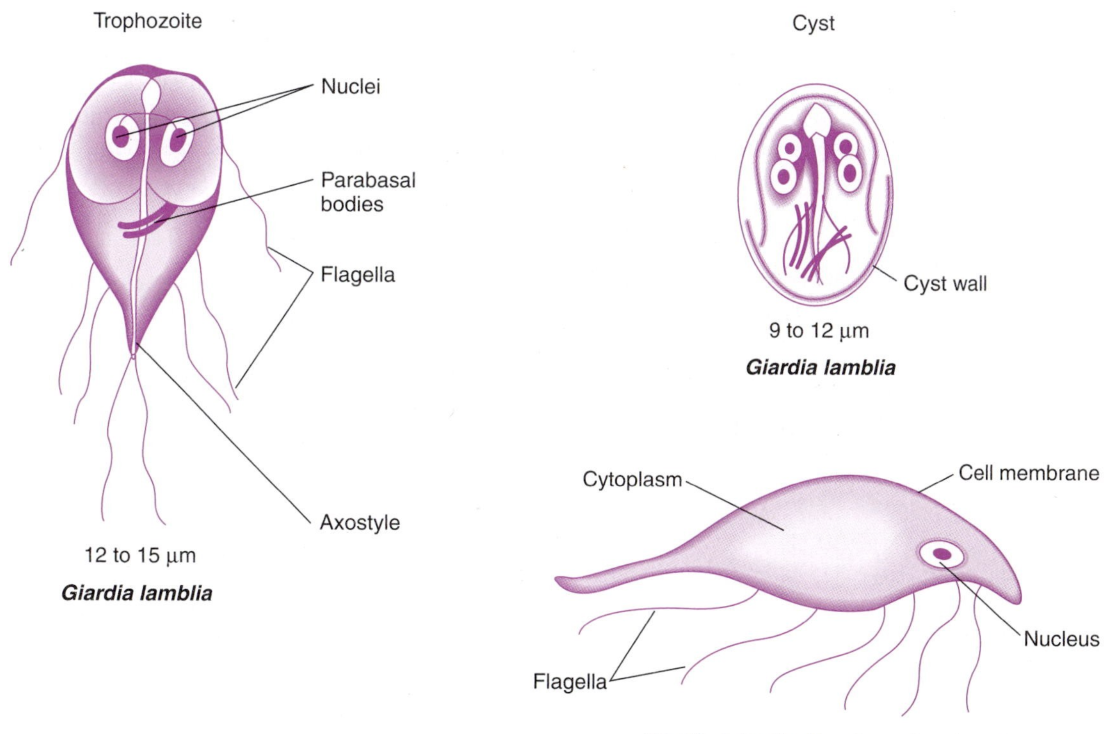

Figure 10–3 Cyst and trophozoite of *Giardia lamblia*

The trypanosomes infect humans via a secondary host, the tsetse fly. The infected fly deposits the trypanosomes into a bite site. The flagellates then multiply in the blood, where they move to the lymph nodes and the central nervous system. ***Trypanosoma gambiense*** causes African sleeping sickness, a fatal disease. *Trypanosoma cruzi* attacks the heart muscle and central nervous system and causes Chagas' disease, which also involves liver, spleen, and lymph nodes. Both diseases usually result in death (Figures 10–4 and 10–5).

Another flagellate, ***Trichomonas vaginalis,*** is a sexually transmitted disease. It may be recovered from vaginal secretions, the urethra, the epididymis, and the prostate. It is often seen on microscopic examination of urine when evaluating a patient for a urinary tract infection. A routine Papanicolaou (Pap) smear of vaginal secretions will also clearly demonstrate the trophozoite. This parasite does not produce a cyst stage. Women are more likely to demonstrate the typical symptoms of vaginal inflammation, yellowish foul discharge, and burning urination with itching and irritation. Figure 10–6 shows the *Trichomonas vaginalis* trophozoite.

Sarcodina

Sarcodina or amoeba have neither cilia nor flagella. Instead, they move by extending cytoplasmic projections, **pseudopodia.** This method of movement is called **amoeboid movement.** ***Entamoeba histolytica*** is a pathogenic amoeba that causes dysentery in humans.

The amoeba is a primitive protozoan cell found wherever decaying materials and moisture abound. It changes its shape continuously through the process of amoeboid movement. Basically, it is a shapeless mass of cytoplasm differentiated (divided) into a nucleus, cytoplasm, a cell membrane, and two organelles: the food vacuole and the contractile vacuole. It feeds upon solid food particles by first surrounding them with

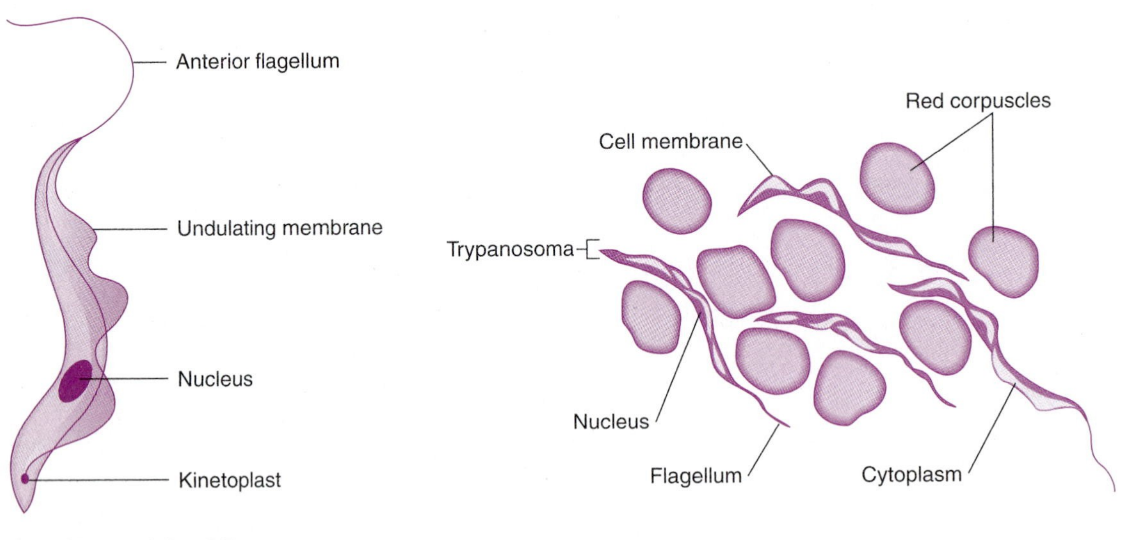

Figure 10–4 *Trypanosoma rhodesiense:* (A) Filaria (B) Filaria in the blood

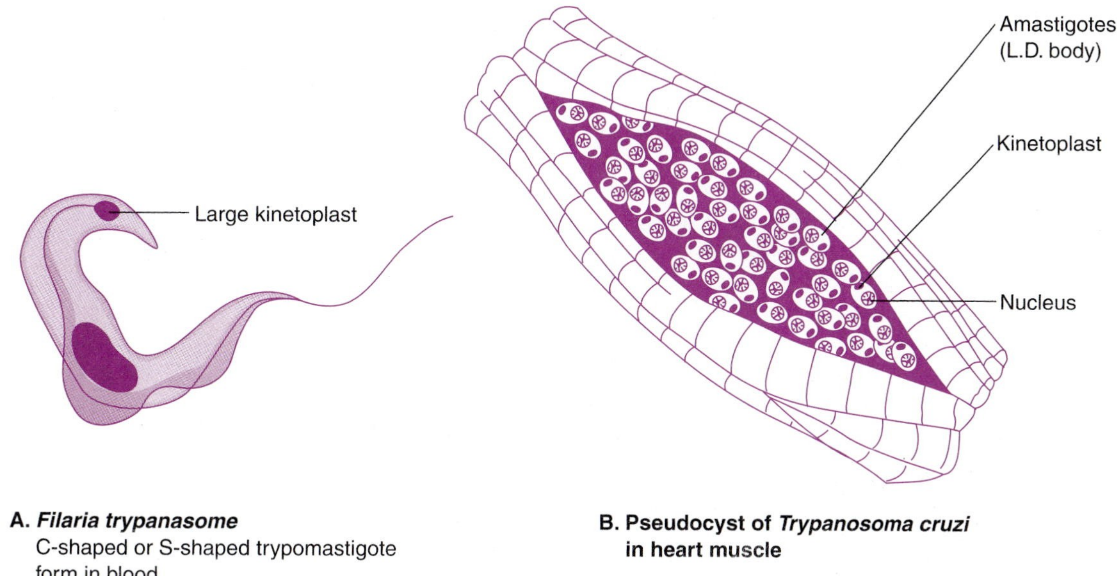

A. *Filaria trypanasome*
C-shaped or S-shaped trypomastigote form in blood

B. Pseudocyst of *Trypanosoma cruzi* in heart muscle

Figure 10–5 Cyst and trypanosome of *Trypanosoma cruzi*

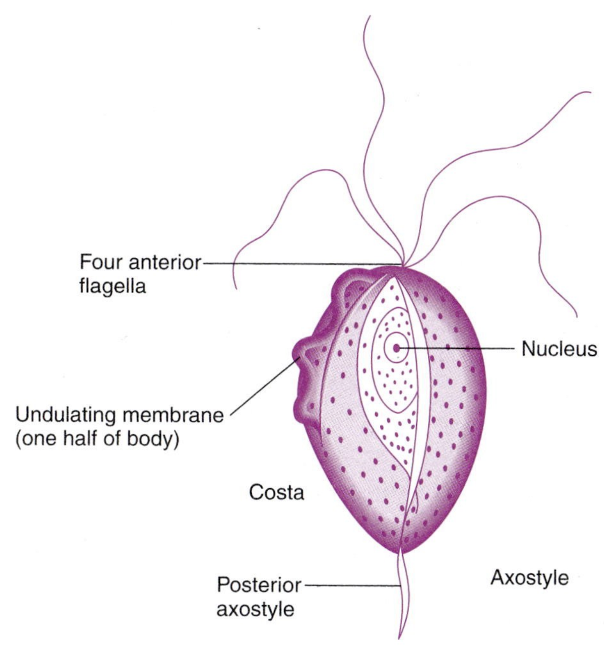

Trophozoite (no cyst stage form)
15 µm

Figure 10–6 Trophozoite of *Trichomonas vaginalis*

pseudopods; it then encloses them within a food vacuole for digestion. The amoeba excretes liquid waste products through a contractile vacuole.

The amoeba's method of reproduction is simple. The mother cell enlarges and then divides, forming two identical daughter cells. This asexual reproduction process is called **fission.** An amoeba as found in pond water is shown in Figures 10–7 and 10–8.

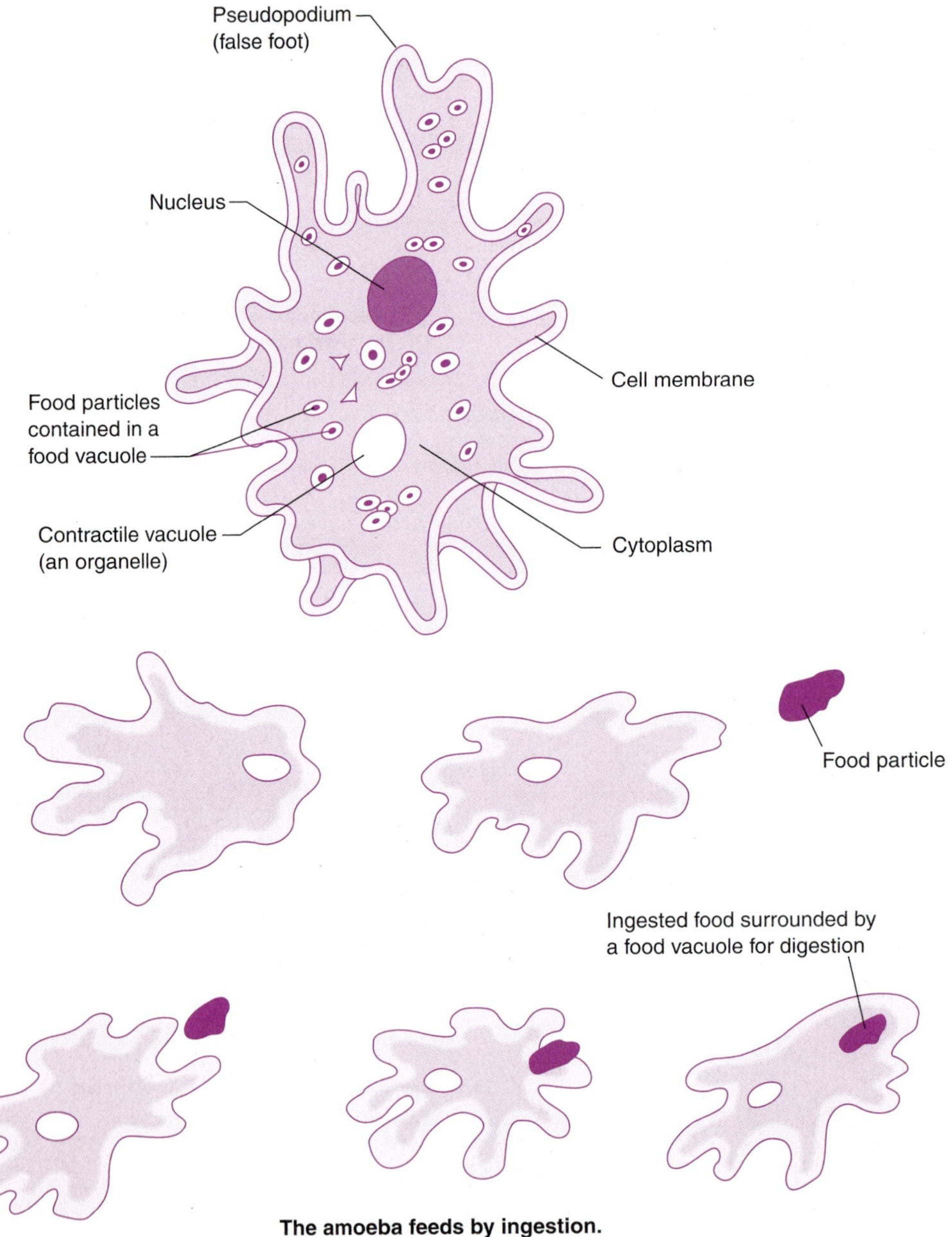

Figure 10–7 The amoeba, its parts and method of feeding

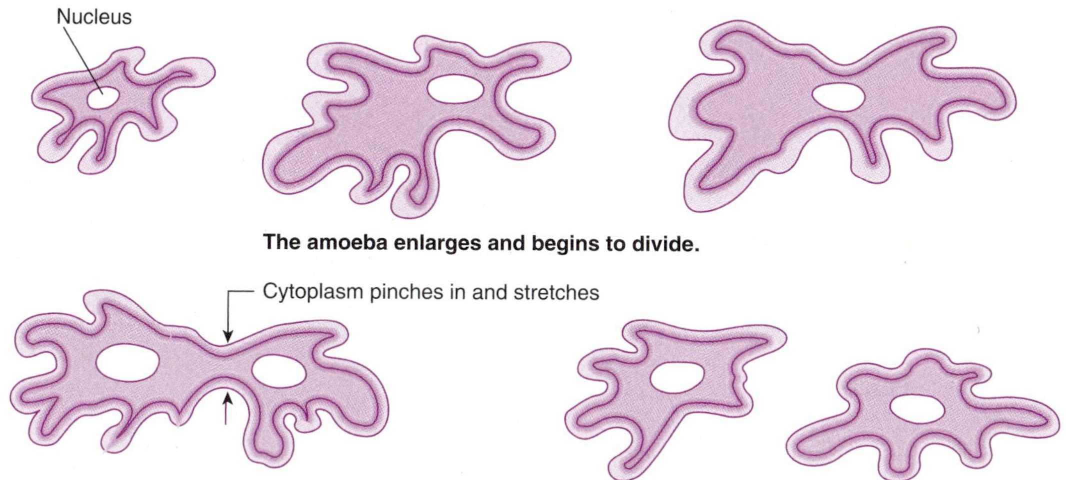

Figure 10–8 Fission: asexual reproduction of an amoeba

One specific example of a clinically significant amoeba is the *Entamoeba histolytica.* It causes amoebic dysentery in humans and is diagnosed by demonstrating the typical four nucleated cyst in feces. Occasionally, the trophozoite may also be recognized in diarrheal feces or intestinal mucosa. This parasite can invade the liver, causing amoebic hepatitis, and the infection can persist untreated for years. Other amoebic dysentaries include ***Entamoeba hartmanni,*** which produces a much smaller cyst; ***Entamoeba coli,*** which is usually differentiated from *Entamoeba histolytica* by the large number of nuclei found in the cyst (up to eight); and ***Endolimax nana,*** which produces an ovoid cyst (Figure 10–9).

OTHER SIGNIFICANT PROTOZOA

The protozoans that cause malaria and toxoplasmosis are of major importance to humans. These parasites have no apparent organelles of locomotion and are transmitted to humans by some intermediate host. The four members of the *Plasmodium* genus that cause malaria are ***Plasmodium falciparum, Plasmodium vivax, Plasmodium malariae,*** and ***Plasmodium ovale*** (Figure 10–10). All are transmitted by the bite of an infected ***Anopheles*** mosquito. In addition, *Plasmodium vivax* causes intermittent chills and fever at 48-hour intervals.

Some of the pathogenic protozoa are transmitted by blood-sucking insects such as the *Anopheles* mosquito. The protozoa that cause dysentery and diarrhea form a dormant stage, or **cyst,** when passed out of the intestinal tract. In areas of contamination, these cysts may be taken into the body through the ingestion of raw vegetables or in drinking water.

The diagnostic trophozoites, **schizonts** (asexual stage of development) and **gametocytes** (sexual stage of development) can be found in circulating blood. Special thick blood smears are taken morning and afternoon and stained to demonstrate the diagnostic

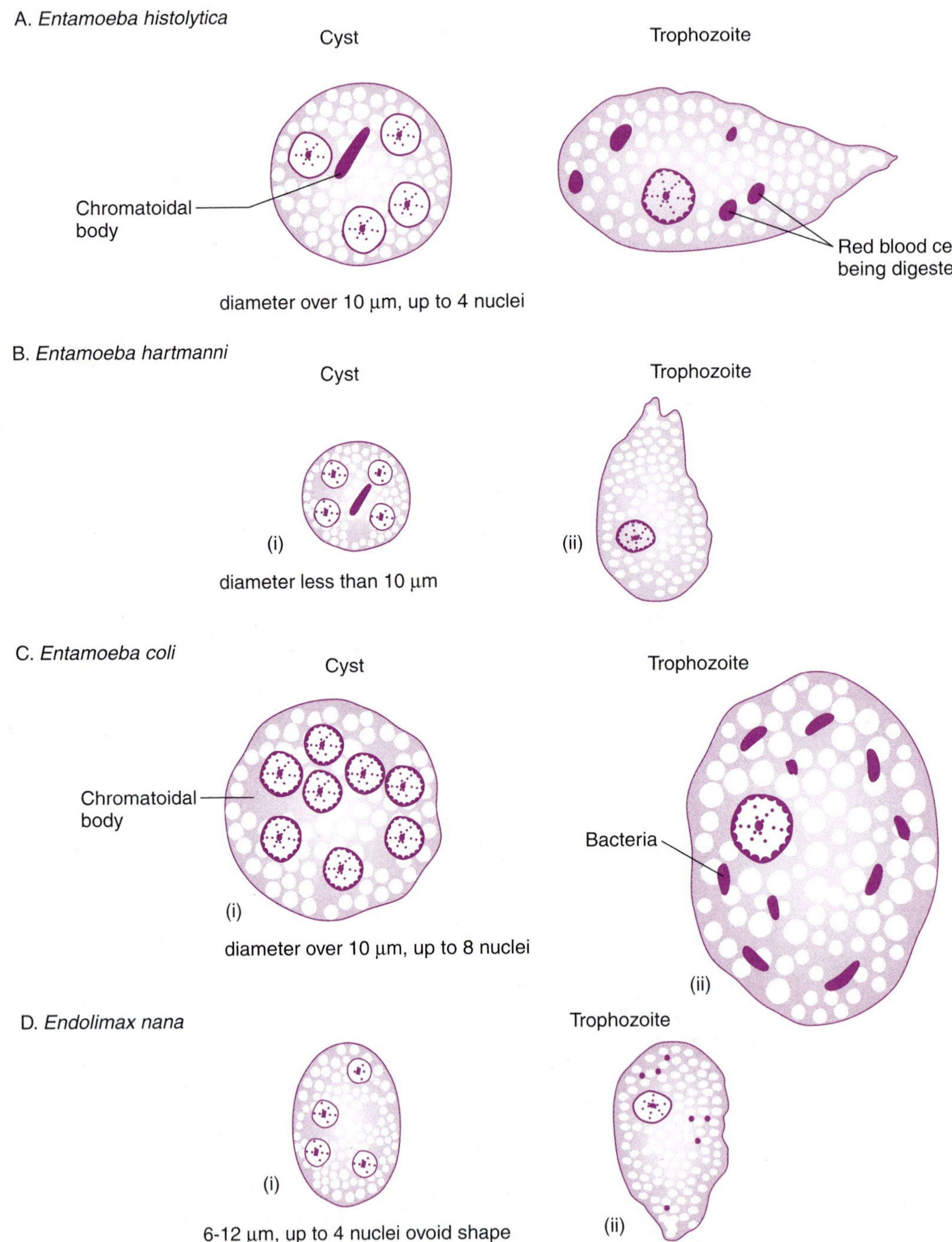

Figure 10–9 Cysts and trophozoites of amoebas significant to humans. (A) *Entamoeba histolytica*, (B) *Entamoeba hartmanni*, (C) *Entamoeba coli*, (D) *Endolimax nana*

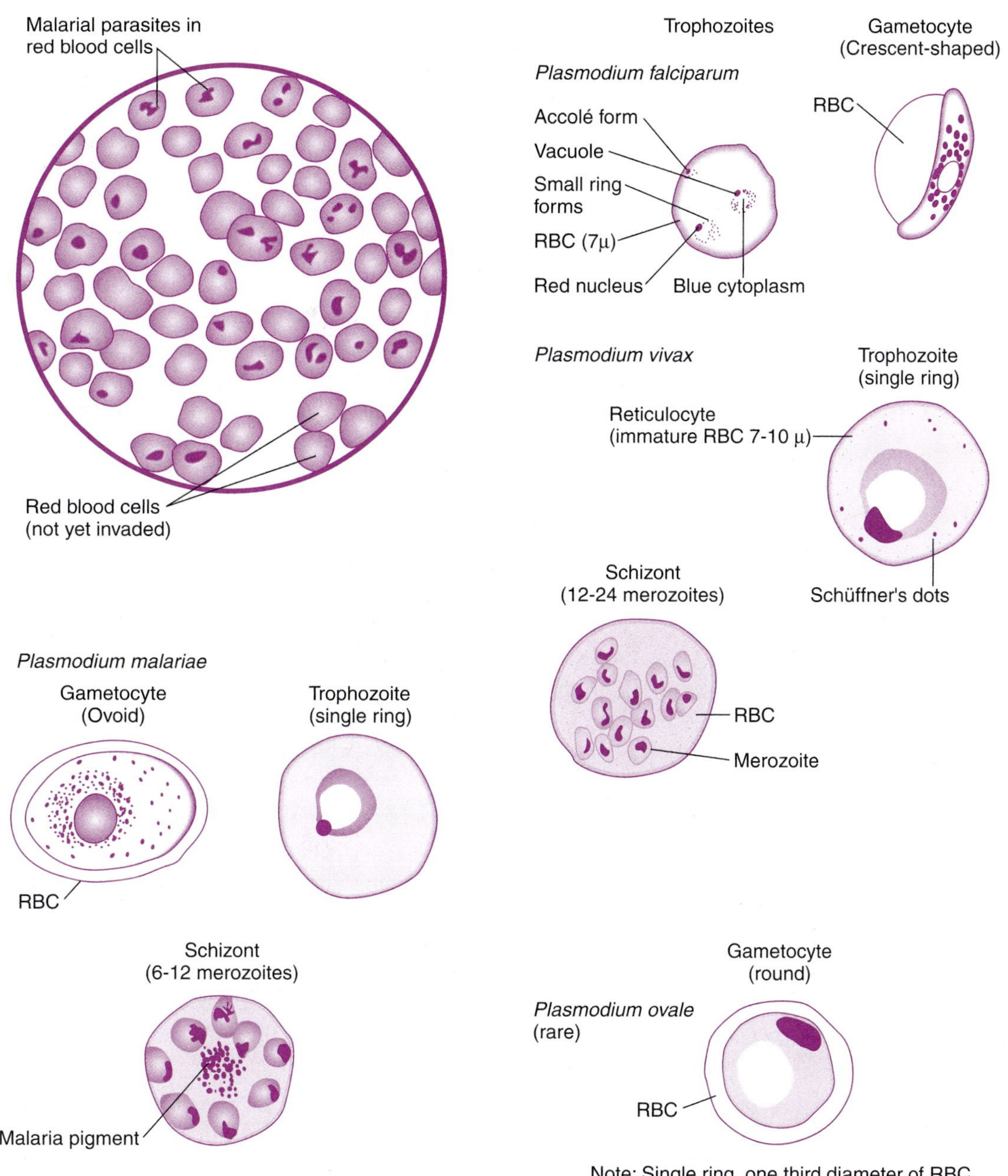

Figure 10–10 Forms of *Plasmodium* species as seen in blood

features in blood. This disease can recur years later. Quinine is still the treatment of choice. Sulfadiazine and tetracycline are also helpful.

Another protozoan, ***Toxoplasma gondii,*** which causes toxoplasmosis, is especially significant to pregnant women. This parasite can cross the placenta to the fetus, causing death, blindness, or mental retardation. The organism is found naturally in most birds and animals and their feces, but the domestic cat has been identified as the primary definitive host for *Toxoplasma.* This disease is usually identified, not by microscopic examination of material to view cysts and trophozoites but by specific serological techniques, such as a rising titer of *Toxoplasma* antibodies in the serum.

One last protozoan that has recently come into prominence is ***Pneumocystis carinii.*** It is the cause of an atypical plasma-cell pneumonia that under normal conditions never results in disease. This protozoan has come into much prominence with the emergence of AIDS, for it is an opportunistic infection and often leads to the ultimate death of the patient. *Pneumocystis* is probably transmitted via the aerosol route, and therefore can be considered to be contagious. Researchers are divided on whether this organism is a parasite or a fungus. Antibiotics including trimethoprim and sulfamethoxazole are drugs of choice. Corticosteriods may also be given.

HELMINTHS

The helminths include the roundworms (**nematodes**), the flatworms (**tapeworms** or **cestodes**), and the flukes (**trematodes**).

As a rule, worms are ingested as microscopic eggs, which later develop into mature worms in the intestine. There are many species, which vary in size from tiny flat organisms to roundworms 6 or 8 inches long to tapeworms, which attain a length of several feet. Some of the parasitic worms that cause disease include the following:

- **Hookworm** is a small, intestinal parasite that infests both people and animals (Figure 10–11). It attaches to the intestinal wall, draining blood from the host. *Necator americanus* is a common hookworm that if present in sufficient quantities can cause severe anemia.
- **Trichina** is a roundworm that causes trichinosis (Figure 10–12). Parasites are ingested by the host through insufficiently cooked pork.
- ***Wuchereria bancrofti*** is a tiny worm that causes elephantiasis, a disease characterized by enlargement of the legs. The parasite is carried by mosquitoes in tropical climates (see Figure 10–13).

Some insects act as parasites, which in turn carry other parasites, such as bacteria, protozoa, rickettsias, or viruses. For example, blood-sucking insects such as mosquitoes, flies, fleas, and lice transfer microorganisms to the larger host. Recall malaria, as one disease transmitted in this fashion.

Nematodes

The common intestinal nematode infections include the pinworm (*Enterobius vermicularis*), which is distributed worldwide, is found mostly in children, and is easily recognized on a cellophane-tape preparation by its typical ovoid egg (Figure 10–14). The whipworm

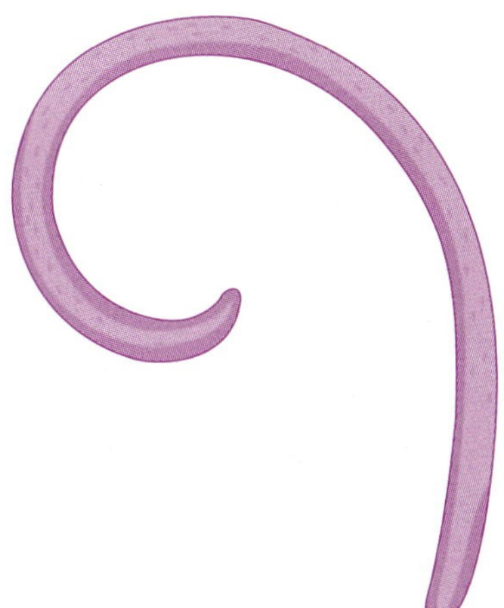

Figure 10–11 Hookworm (*Necator americanus*)

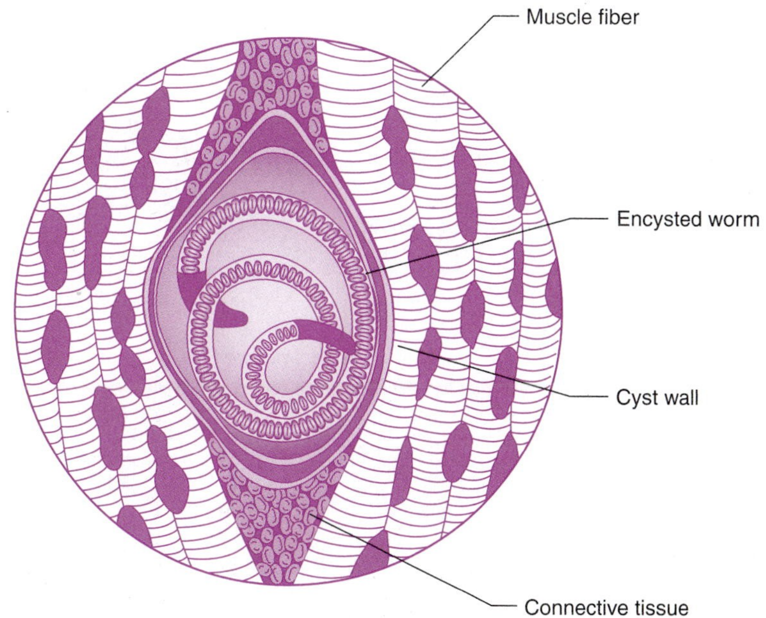

Figure 10–12 Trichina worm is enclosed in a protective casing, or cyst. The cyst is embedded in the muscles of a host organism.

egg (*Trichuris trichiura*) can be identified by its tea-tray-like handles on the eggs (Figure 10–14). *Ascaris lumbricoides,* another common roundworm that causes infection, can result in severe bowel obstructions by the adult worm if left untreated (Figures 10–14 and 10–15). *Wuchereria bancrofti* is another **microfilaria** worm that, like the *Plasmodium,* lodges in the bloodstream (Figure 10–13). Several species of mosquitoes are intermediate hosts for this tropical parasite. These mosquitoes include the *Anopheles* as well as the *Culex* and the *Aedes.*

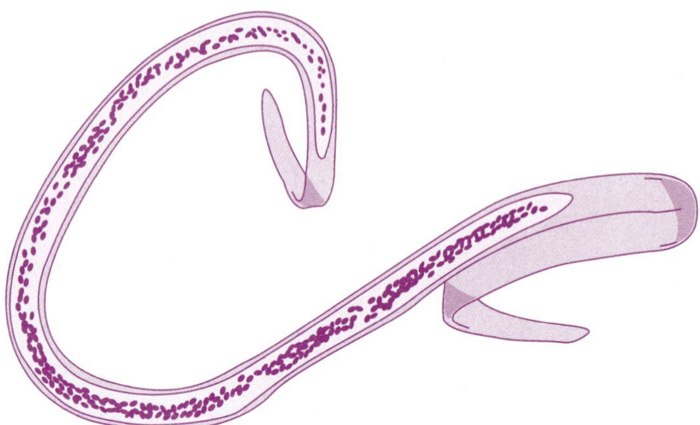

Figure 10–13 Microfilaria of *Wuchereria bancrofti* as seen in the blood

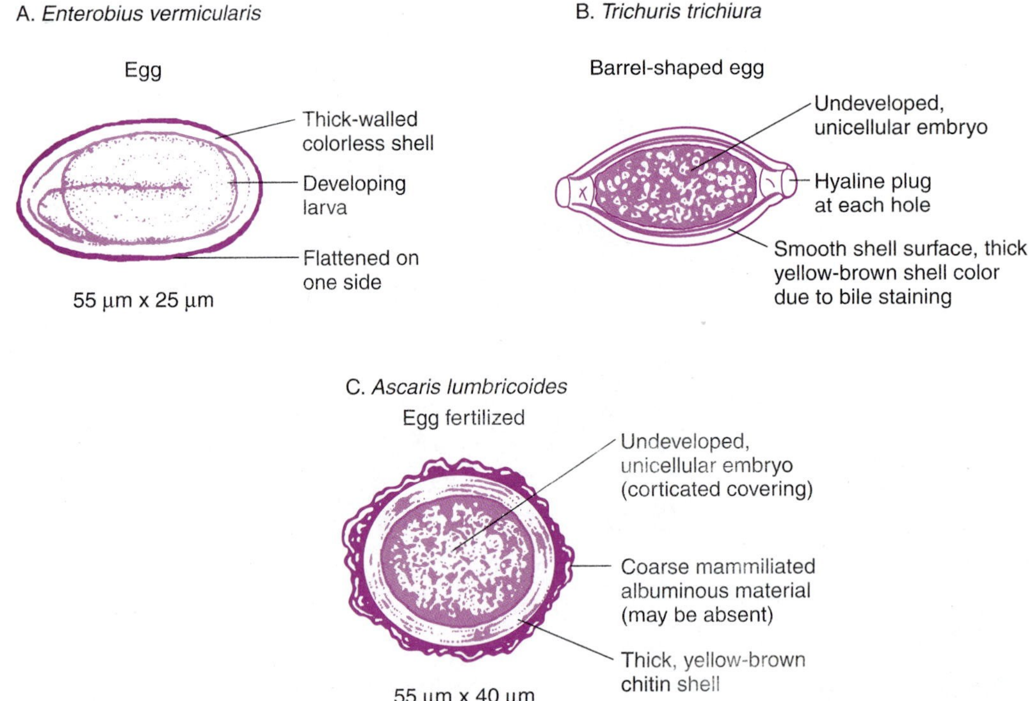

Figure 10–14 Eggs of nematodes that cause intestinal infections (A) *E. vermicularis,* (B) *T. trichiura,* (C) *A. lumbricoides*

Cestodes

The flatworms or cestodes include *Taenia saginata* (beef) and *Taenia solium* (pork) tapeworms of the ***Taenia*** family, and the ***Diphyllobothrium latum*** or fish tapeworm. These flatworms can grow to lengths of up to 20 meters and will slough off sections, called

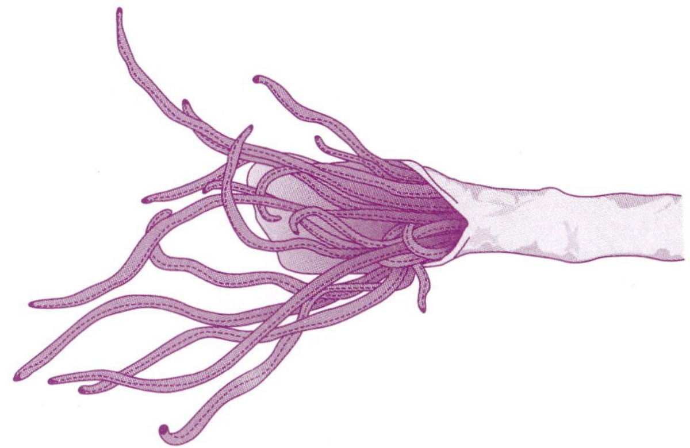

Figure 10–15 Numerous adult ascaris roundworms causing a bowel obstruction

proglottids, of their bodies into the stool. Examination of the proglottids is used as a tool to differentiate *Taenia* species. Each of these tapeworms cause intestinal disorders and one may experience severe weight loss if undiagnosed or untreated. All meat and fish should be well cooked to avoid the chance of ingesting eggs which may be found encysted in the muscle of their hosts, Figure 10–16.

Trematodes

The Trematodes, commonly called flukes, are flat leaf-shaped helminths (see Figures 10–17 through 10–20). They can inhabit the intestine, the liver, the lung, and the blood vessels. They vary in size from a few millimeters to a few centimeters in length. The prominent blood flukes are members of the *Schistosoma* group. Some of the other clinically significant flukes include the *Fasciolopsis, Fasciola,* and the *Paragonimus.*

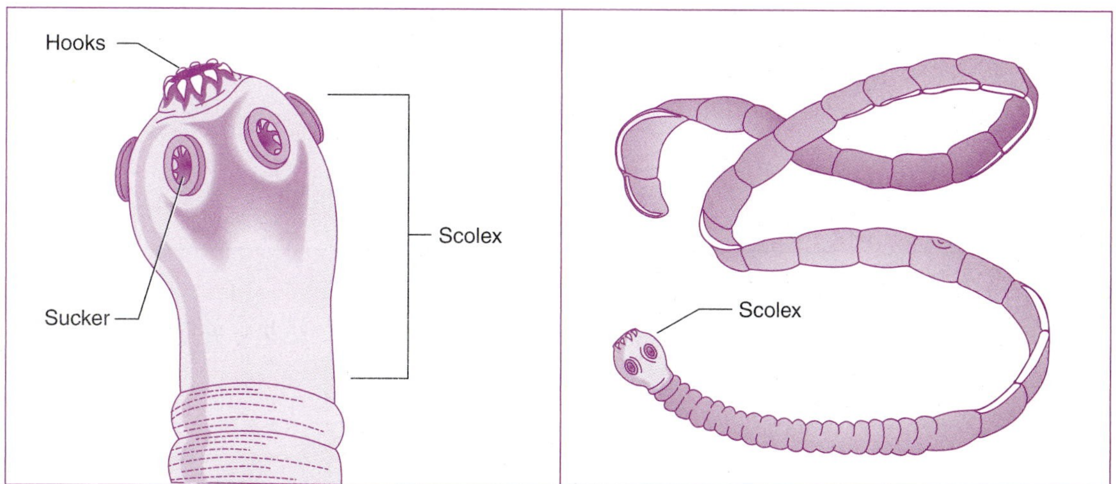

Figure 10–16 Tapeworm and an enlargement of its head or scolex containing hooks and suckers, which attach the tapeworm to the intestinal wall of its host

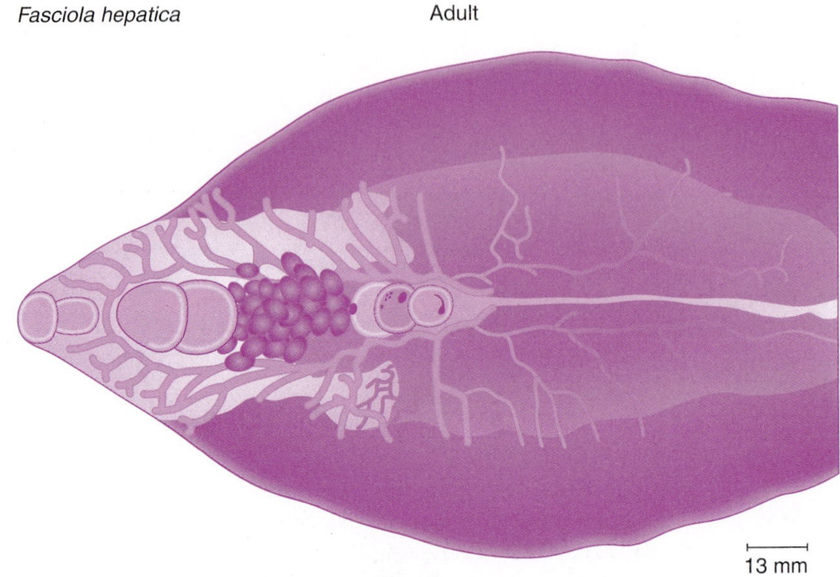

Figure 10–17 Liver fluke, *Fasciola hepatica*

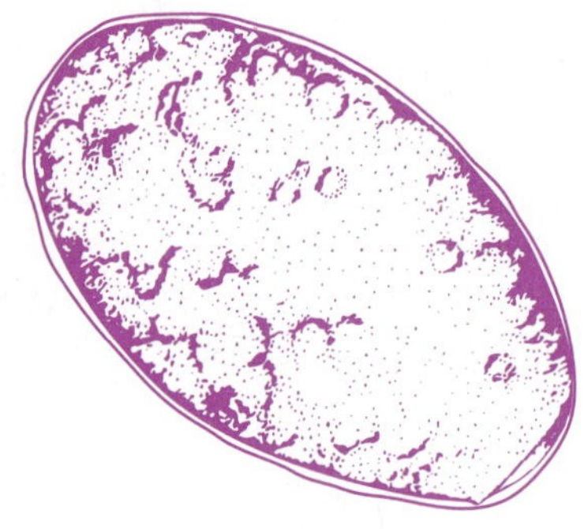

Figure 10–18 Egg of the Liver fluke, *Fasciola hepatica*

ARTHROPODS

Arthropods include the insects (flies, mosquitoes, true bugs, lice, and fleas) and the arachnids (spiders, ticks, and mites).

Insects

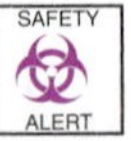

Lice infestations of the head and body (***Pediculus***) are easily transmitted and often cause epidemics among school children (Figure 10–21). The ***Phthirus,*** the causative agent of sexually transmitted crab louse infections, is found worldwide (Figure 10–22). Fleas are

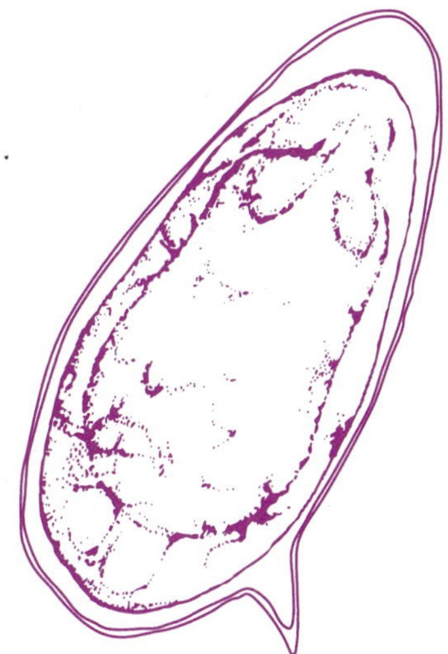

Figure 10–19 Egg of the *Schistosoma mansonii*

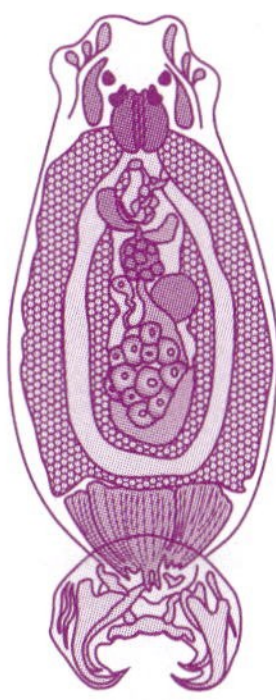

Figure 10–20 Trematode fluke (note the broad leaflike body)

common to our household pets and can infest an entire household, including carpets and furniture. Infestation of fleas by humans can lead to infection with ***Dipylidium caninum,*** the tapeworm of dogs and cats. Usually, small children become infected when they kiss or bite their pets, thus ingesting the fleas.

Arachnids

Scabies is caused by the itch mite (*Sarcoptes*) (Figure 10–23). One of the most significant arachnid infections is the one that causes Lyme disease. Ticks are the reservoir for a bac-

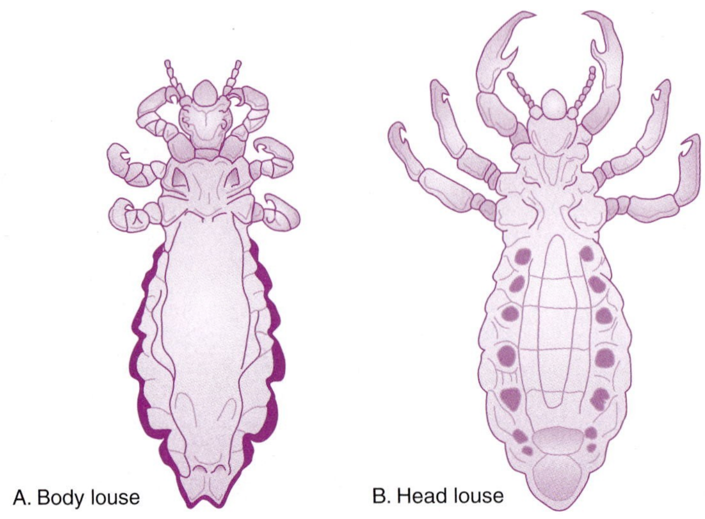

Figure 10–21 *Pediculus:* (A) Body louse, (B) head louse

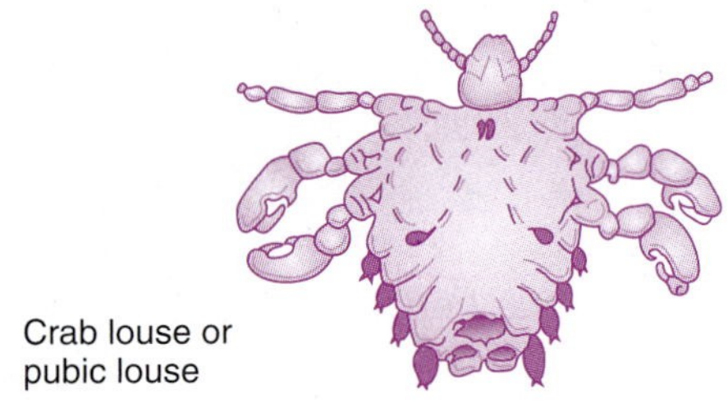

Figure 10–22 *Phthirus*

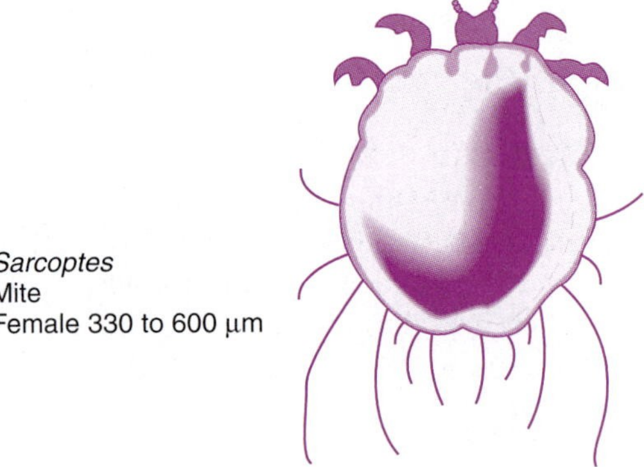

Figure 10–23 Scabies mite

terium that causes the disease. Spiders are the largest group of **arachnids.** Few transmit disease or seek human hosts. The black widow spider, brown recluse spider, and some tarantulas will bite and the toxic poison can cause serious illness.

SUMMARY

Table 10–1 categorizes the clinical parasites of interest in this chapter.

Table 10–1 Summary and Comparison of Some Parasites' Characteristics

	PROTOZOA	HELMINTHS	ARTHROPODS
Main Characteristic	Single celled	Worms, Round, Flat, Flukes	Insects, Arachnids head, thorax, abdomen, appendages
Groups	**Ciliophora** ciliated	**Nematodes** round	**Insects** flies, lice, fleas
	Mastigophora flagella	**Cestodes** flat tapeworm	**Arachnids** ticks, mites, spiders
	Sarcodina pseudopods	**Trematodes** fluke, leaflike	
	Apicomplexa Sporozoans >2 hosts		
Examples	**Cilophora** Paramecium *Balantidium coli*	**Nematodes** (roundworm) *Necator americanus* *Trichina* *Wuchereria bancrofti* *Enterobius vermicularis* *Ascaris lumbricoides* *Trichuris trichiura*	**Insects** *Anopheles:* mosquitoes *Pediculus:* head & body lice *Phthirus:* crab louse (STD)
	Mastigophora *Giardia lamblia* *Trypanosoma* sp. *Trichomonas vaginalis*	**Cestodes** (tapeworms) *Taenia saginata* (beef) *Taenia solium* (pork) *Diphyllobothrium latum* (fish)	**Arachnids** *Sarcoptes:* scabies mite
	Sarcodina Amoeba *Entamoeba histolytica* *Endolimax nana*	**Trematodes** (flukes, flatworms) *Schistosoma* sp. *Paragonimus westermani* *Fasciola hepatica*	
	Apicomplexa *Plasmodium* sp. *Toxoplasma* sp.		
Protozoan and Fungal Features	*Pneumocystis carinii*		

STUDY AND DISCUSSION

- Explain how the one-celled protozoa perform all the functions found in larger animals.
- Discuss the transmission of diseases caused by protozoa. Using library sources, prepare reports on malaria, amoebic dysentery, and African sleeping sickness.
- Using library references, explain in detail the relationships of the following:
  a. ticks and Rocky Mountain spotted fever
  b. tsetse fly and African sleeping sickness
  c. *Aedes aegypti* mosquito and yellow fever
  d. common house fly and typhoid fever or dysentery
- On a separate sheet of paper, complete a chart of parasites and the diseases caused by each. Use the following chart as a model for your work.
- Examine protozoa under the microscope following the suggested outline.

PARASITE	DISEASE	HOW TRANSMITTED
Protozoa *Giardia*		
Entamoeba		
Trichomonas		
Plasmodium		
Toxoplasma		
Helminths *Enterobius*		
Ascaris		
Taenia		
Arthropods *Phthirus*		
Pediculus		

Procedure 9–1 Microscopic Examination of Protozoa

Equipment and Materials Needed

Living cultures of paramecia and amoebae
Prepared slides of trypanosoma, *Entamoeba histolytica*, euglena, and any protozoa slides available
Slides
Coverslips
Lens paper
Pipettes

Method

1. With a pipette, place two or three drops of the living paramecium culture on one slide. Gently lower a coverslip onto the culture.
2. Repeat with the amoeba culture on another slide.
3. Examine any prepared slides of pathogenic protozoa available.

Observations and Conclusions

1. Note the size, shape, and motility of paramecia and amoebae.

2. Contrast the type of motility between paramecia and amoebae.

3. What does the amoeba use for movement? What is the type of movement called?

4. What structures are used by the paramecium for its movement?

5. Explain how the amoeba and paramecium capture food.

REVIEW QUESTIONS

A. General Questions: Provide complete answers to each of the following.

1. Describe how the paramecium and amoeba reproduce.

2. Why is it important for a health professional to understand how a paramecium carries on its life activities?

3. Using library sources, complete the following chart.

DISEASE	WHAT PROTOZOAN CAUSES IT	HOW PROTOZOAN ENTERS THE BODY	PREVENTION AND CONTROL
Malaria			
	Entamoeba histolytica		
	Giardia lamblia		
African sleeping sickness			

4. How do protozoa differ from fungi?

5. Where are protozoa found?

6. How are protozoa categorized according to their method of movement?

7. What is an amoeba?

8. Explain how an amoeba feeds.

9. How many nuclei does a paramecium have? State the name and function of each.

10. What are parasites?

11. What is a host?

12. What harm can parasites cause?

13. Give an example of a part of the body that encourages the growth of parasites, and explain why.

14. What is antibiosis?

15. Name some insects that are parasites.

16. How do most worms enter the body? Give some examples of parasitic worms.

17. Which of the parasites are the most harmful to humans, and why?

B. Multiple Choice Questions: Select the letter of the choice that best answers the question or completes the sentence.

1. Which of the following is a protozoan causing genital infections?
   a. *Trichomonas*
   b. *Taenia*
   c. *Toxoplasma*
   d. *Trypanosoma*
2. The fish tapeworm is ______.
   a. *Taenia solium*
   b. *Diphyllobothrium latum*
   c. *Necator americanus*
   d. *Trichuris trichuria*
3. Scabies is caused by ______.
   a. ticks
   b. mites
   c. lice
   d. flies
4. Malaria is identified by microscopic examination of ______.
   a. lung tissue
   b. feces
   c. blood
   d. urine
5. Arachnids include ______.
   a. mosquitoes
   b. flies
   c. spiders
   d. roaches
6. One of the most common causes of intestinal diarrhea is ______.
   a. *Ascaris*
   b. *Trichomonas*
   c. *Trypanosoma*
   d. *Pneumocystis*
7. Cats transmit ______ to children.
   a. toxoplasmosis
   b. trichomoniasis
   c. entamoebiasis
   d. trichinosis
8. The paramecium is found ______.
   a. in the gut of humans
   b. in pond water
   c. in the white-tailed deer
   d. in household pets
9. Pseudopodia are ______.
   a. organelles of movement
   b. false feet
   c. amoeboid projections
   d. all of the above
10. The largest protozoa to infect humans is ______.
    a. *Entamoeba coli*
    b. *Entamoeba histolytica*
    c. *Endolimax nana*
    d. *Balantidium coli*

C. Matching Questions: Match the terms in Column I with their corresponding terms in Column II.

Column I		Column II
_______	1. *Trichomonas vaginalis*	a. amoebic dysentary
_______	2. *Plasmodium falciparum*	b. Chagas' disease
_______	3. *Toxoplasma gondii*	c. plasma-cell pneumonia
_______	4. *Necator americanus*	d. Elephantiasis
_______	5. *Entamoeba histolytica*	e. sexually transmitted disease
_______	6. *Giardia lamblia*	f. roundworm, bowel obstructions
_______	7. *Trypanosoma cruzi*	g. infects fetuses
_______	8. *Pneumocystis carinii*	h. hookworm disease
_______	9. *Enterobius vermicularis*	i. pinworm disease
_______	10. *Ascaris lumbricoides*	j. sleeping sickness
_______	11. *Wuchereria bancrofti*	k. spring waters
_______	12. *Trichuris trichiura*	l. tea-tray-handled eggs
_______	13. *Trypanosoma gambiense*	m. tapeworm disease
_______	14. *Taenia saginata*	n. malaria

D. Completion Questions: From the following list of terms fill in the blanks with the correct choice.

trypanosomes	*Giardia lamblia*	malaria
Trypanosoma	*Entamoeba*	*Trichomonas rhodesiense*
Plasmodium	*Giardia*	*Trichomonas vaginalis*
Ascaris	*Enterobius*	sleeping sickness
Trichuris	*Taenia*	*Fasciola*

1. The most common intestinal parasite is ________________.

2. The tsetse fly hosts ________________.

3. Flagellated parasites include ________________ and ________________ genera.

4. African sleeping sickness is caused by ________________ .

5. A Papanicolaou smear easily identifies ________________.

6. Amoebic dysenteries can be caused by three species of the________________ genera.

7. The presence of *Plasmodium vivax* indicates ________________, whereas the presence of *Trypanosoma gambiense* indicates ________________ .

8. Roundworm infections are caused by ________________, ________________, and ________________.

CHAPTER

11

Bacteria, Rickettsias, Chlamydias, and Mycoplasmas

OBJECTIVES

After completing this chapter, you will be able to:

- list some structures found in a bacterial cell.
- explain how bacteria may be observed.
- give examples of bacteria that are nonpathogenic to people and those that are pathogenic to people.
- sketch a simple identification scheme for gram-negative bacteria.
- list biochemical tests that are commonly used to differentiate gram-positive and gram-negative cocci.
- describe mycoplasmas.
- explain cell structure and transmission of rickettsias.
- name the chlamydias that are considered to be sexually transmitted.

KEY WORDS

aerobe
anaerobe
Bacillus
Bacillus anthracis
Bacillus cereus
Bacillus subtilis
bacteremia
beta-lactam
Borrelia burgdorferi
Campylobacter
carbuncles
cervicitis
Chlamydia psittaci
Chlamydia trachomatis
Clostridium
Clostridium botulinum
Clostridium difficile
Clostridium perfringens
Clostridium tetani
coagulase
cold agglutinins
commensal
Corynebacterium diphtheriae
denitrifying bacteria
diplococci
energy parasites
enteric
Enterobacteriaceae
Escherichia coli
fastidious
gastritis
impetigo
intracellular
Ixodes dammini
Ixodes pacificus
meningitis
Mycoplasma pleomorphic PPLO
Mycoplasma pneumoniae
necrotizing fasciitis
Neisseria
Neisseria gonorrhoeae
Neisseria meningitidis
nitrifying bacteria
nitrogen-fixing bacteria
nonpathogenic bacteria
normal flora
nosocomial
nutrient agar
nutrient broth

KEY WORDS (cont.)

obligate intracellular parasites
opportunistic pathogens
pathogenic bacteria
penicillinase
Prosthetic
Pseudomonas aeruginosa
putrefactive bacteria
retting
Rickettsia prowazekii
Rickettsia typhi
Salmonella
Saprophytes
Shigella
Staphylococcus aureus
Staphylococcus epidermidis
Streptococcus pneumoniae
Streptococcus pyogenes
Streptococcus viridans
titer
Tracheotomy
urethritis

Bacteria are grown in the laboratory in specially prepared media such as **nutrient agar** or **nutrient broth.** When bacteria multiply to form millions of cells, they may be seen as a tiny spot, or colony. From this colony a smear may be made on a slide, permitting microscopic examination of cell structure.

PATHOGENIC AND NONPATHOGENIC BACTERIA

Bacteria may be classified as to their harmful or beneficial qualities. Two general types of bacteria are **pathogenic bacteria** and **nonpathogenic bacteria.** Pathogenic bacteria are harmful because they invade plant or animal tissue, often secreting enzymes or toxins into the host tissue. (Pathogenic bacteria are discussed in chapter 4.) Nonpathogenic bacteria perform many useful functions, such as decomposing refuse and improving the fertility of soil. Nonpathogenic bacteria are of great economic importance to the world. They aid in the processes of the **retting** of flax into linen, the curing of tobacco, tea, coffee, cocoa, and leather, and the making of sauerkraut, vinegar, yogurt, cheeses, and acidophilus milk.

In the field of medicine, bacteria are recognized as being pathogenic, **normal flora** (nonpathogenic saprophytes), or **opportunistic pathogens.** Microbiologists have increasingly found microbes of normal flora (organisms, once thought to be harmless, found in humans, soil, or air) and other infectious bacteria that normally caused uncomplicated infection-causing serious, even life-threatening, infections in patients with immunosuppression diseases such as acquired immunodeficiency syndrome (AIDS). As a result, the designation of these organisms as opportunistic pathogens becomes more common.

Even more vital to our existence is the role bacteria play in the balance of nature among living things. Without the bacteria of decay our world would soon be piled high with the dead bodies of animals and plants. The all-important element nitrogen is locked inside the dead plants and animals in the form of organic compounds. **Putrefactive bacteria** will disintegrate these dead organisms, returning carbon and nitrogen compounds to the soil. The next step is performed by the **nitrifying bacteria** in the soil, which convert ammonia into the nitrites and nitrates that plants use for food. Animals, in turn, eat the plants; when they die, nitrogen is returned to the soil through the decay caused by the putrefactive bacteria, completing the cycle. The **denitrifying bacteria** are also very beneficial because they are able to extract oxygen from nitrates, releasing free nitrogen into the atmosphere.

Finally, **nitrogen-fixing bacteria** found in the soil can build nitrates by extracting inert nitrogen from the air and returning nitrates to the soil. This fact is especially true of nitrogen-fixing bacteria on the roots of leguminous plants such as peas, clover, alfalfa, and peanuts. For this reason, leguminous plants are used by farmers in crop rotation to enrich the nitrogen of the soil. Animals and plants are, therefore, dependent upon bacteria for their food supply.

Health care professionals must understand the nature of bacteria, their activities, and how to control them, because bacterial growth is the greatest cause of infectious disease. Aseptic procedures, sterilization, disinfection, and isolation techniques are all important procedures practiced to control bacterial growth.

In the bacteriology laboratory, the identification process begins with the performance of a Gram stain. Bacteria are grouped by their staining reaction with crystal violet and safranin dyes, a decolorizing agent, and fixative agent. Bacteria that stain purple are said to be gram positive; those that stain pink or red are gram negative. Additionally, stained bacteria are described by their basic shapes. The round spherelike bacterial cells are cocci and the rectangular rod-shaped ones are bacilli (sing., coccus, bacillus). A common cause of boils, **carbuncles, impetigo,** postoperative wound infections, toxic shock syndrome, and **nosocomial** hospital infections is a gram-positive coccus called ***Staphylococcus aureus.*** Its normal flora "cousin," ***Staphylococcus epidermidis,*** found on skin and rarely causing disease, is also a gram-positive coccus and is distinguished from the pathogen *Staphylococcus aureus* by comparing the color of colonies on culture media containing blood and their clumping reaction with fresh plasma in the **coagulase** test (Table 11–1).

Other common gram-positive cocci include ***Streptococcus viridans,*** which is usually found as a normal flora of the upper respiratory tract, but can cause the serious complication subacute bacterial endocarditis (SBE), and ***Streptococcus pyogenes,*** also known as group A streptococcus—the cause of strep throat, rheumatic fever, and scarlet fever (Table 11–1). Other members of the *Streptococcus* genus cause genitourinary and intestinal infections. One strain of ***Streptococcus pneumoniae*** causes a bacterial pneumonia that is the second most common cause of bacterial meningitis. This pathogen contains a capsule that is shiny and mucoid in appearance. Its noncapsulated cousin is dry and pitted, and is most often a cause of pneumonia. It is less virulent than the capsulated form.

Commonly encountered gram-positive bacilli or rods include the ***Bacillus*** species and the ***Clostridium*** species. Both groups tend to form spores, and these may be seen in the Gram stain as terminal or subterminal spores in the bacilli. The groups are easily differentiated by their growth needs.

Bacillus species, normal soil contaminants found in air and on bench tops, are strict or obligate **aerobes,** and *Clostridia* are obligate **anaerobes.** Typical ***Bacillus subtilis*** organisms will grow on minimally enriched culture media and appear as large spreading flat, beta-hemolytic colonies. ***Bacillus cereus*** causes food poisoning and has been associated with warmed-over fried rice. Most notable among this group is the organism that causes anthrax in cattle. ***Bacillus anthracis*** is deadly to humans and is the organism referred to in biological warfare concerns. Fortunately, penicillin, the drug of choice, is successful in treating the disease. Today members of the *Bacillus* species are implicated as opportunistic pathogens in immunocompromised patients. Pneumonias caused by *Bacillus cereus* and *Bacillus subtilis* can be devastating.

The anaerobic gram-positive bacilli have three clinically important members, ***Clostridium perfringens,*** which causes gas gangrene; ***Clostridium tetani,*** which causes

Table 11–1 Differentiation of the *Staphylococcus*, *Streptococcus*, *Neisseria*, and *Moraxella* Species

	Growth on BA /Chocolate	Hemolysis	Coagulase	Mannitol Fermentation	Optochin Growth	Glucose Fermentation	Maltose Fermentation	Sucrose Fermentation
S. aureus	Yes / Yes yellow, golden creamy	Beta	Positive	Yes	N/A	N/A	N/A	N/A
S. epidermidis	Yes/Yes white creamy	Gamma	Negative	No	N/A	N/A	N/A	N/A
Strep group A	Yes/Yes tiny, pinpoint beta hemolysis	Beta	N/A	N/A	No	N/A	N/A	N/A
S. pneumoniae	Yes/Yes mucoid or dry & pitted	Alpha	N/A	N/A	Yes	N/A	N/A	N/A
S. viridans	Yes/Yes tiny, alpha hemolysis	Alpha	N/A	N/A	No	N/A	N/A	N/A
N. gonorrhoeae	No/Yes mucoid, sticky, translucent	None	N/A	N/A	N/A	Yes	No	No
N. meningitidis	No/Yes mucoid, sticky, translucent	None	N/A	N/A	N/A	Yes	Yes	No
M. catarrhalis	Yes/Yes dry, sticky, translucent	None	N/A	N/A	N/A	No	No	No

tetanus or lockjaw; and ***Clostridium botulinum*** which causes botulism or food poisoning. A fourth family member, ***Clostridium difficile,*** causes a severe colitis. All members produce spores and therefore can live in unfavorable environments such as soil, dirt, and manure for long periods. The toxins produced by *Clostridium tetani* and *Clostridium botulinum* are a million times more potent than the venom of a rattlesnake.

Other gram-positive bacilli include the organism that causes diphtheria, ***Corynebacterium diphtheriae,*** and its normal flora relative the diphtheroid, which is found on skin, nasal mucosa, and the upper respiratory tract. *Corynebacterium diphtheriae* colonies demonstrate a garliclike odor and appear blackish or gray on special media.

Gram-negative cocci generally appear as **diplococci** when examined microscopically. Notable members of the ***Neisseria*** family include ***Neisseria gonorrhoeae,*** the causative agent of the sexually transmitted disease gonorrhea, and ***Neisseria meningitidis,*** a cause of bacterial **meningitis.** In both diseases, to find the bacteria inside white blood cells (**intracellular**) of genital or spinal fluid specimens is a presumptive diagnosis. Cultural characteristics with enhanced carbon dioxide on chocolate agar and biochemical reactions confirm the diagnosis of these diseases (Table 11–1). ***Moraxella*** (formerly, *Neisseria*) ***Branhamella catarrhalis*** is considered normal flora of the upper respiratory tract but is occasionally implicated in disease, especially in immunocompromised patients, in whom it has been known to cause a severe pneumonia or respiratory tract infection.

Gram-negative bacilli or rods include those of the ***Enterobacteriaceae*** family. They are the most commonly encountered organisms in a clinical laboratory. They are often referred to as **enteric** organisms or coliforms because of their affinity for habitation in the lower intestinal tract and bowel. Enteric organisms are **commensal** inhabitants of the bowel and may be readily grouped as such by their growth on differential media containing bile salts and their characteristic odors. They can cause urinary tract infections, intestinal diarrhea, gastroenteritis, and dysentery. Identification is based on their biochemical reactions in sugars and enzymes. Schema to identify this group are complex, but several simple kit methods are available when modern automated methods are not feasible. The Enterotube system requires a 24-hour growth of the organism in pure culture. Once inoculated, the tube's chambers contain eight to ten different fermentation reactions. Color changes are noted as positive or negative, and the assigned score for each and the number are then compared with the keybook provided by the manufacturer. The API system (color plate 28) requires the making of a broth suspension of a pure culture of the unknown organism and dropping one drop of the suspension into each small chamber containing a different biochemical. Color changes are then read the next day and results tabulated. The RB system requires inoculation methodology similar to the Enterotube system.

The most common organism, ***Escherichia coli,*** is implicated in urinary tract infections and intestinal disorders of infants. Members of the *Proteus* species and ***Pseudomonas aeruginosa*** join *E. coli* in being causative agents in appendicitis, peritonitis, and wound infections in the hospital. Pneumonias and middle-ear infections are often linked to the *Pseudomonas* species. *Pseudomonas aeruginosa* has a characteristic grapejuicelike, or musty, odor and has a greenish pigment on culture media. This organism is a normal inhabitant of the bowel and soil but can cause life-threatening secondary infections in burn patients and pneumonia in elderly and immunocompromised patients as well as nosocomial infections. Members of the ***Salmonella*** and ***Shigella*** groups are important enteric organisms whose pathogenic activity is usually confined to the intestinal tract as a result of dysentery or food poisoning. *Salmonella typhi,* however, causes typhoid fever, which can result in septicemia.

Microbiologists perform numerous simple biochemical tests to identify an organism. Figure 11–1 demonstrates a typical flowchart pattern used to identify enteric organisms. This chart is not a complete one, but the novice bacteriologist can use this pattern as a guide. A wide range of antibiotics are marketed for the express purpose of treating enteric infections. To assist physicians in determining the best drug to treat a disorder, antibiotic susceptibility testing is performed on all enteric pathogens to determine the least amount of an antibiotic needed to kill the organism or inhibit any further growth.

New bacteria are constantly being added to the list of organisms and names and classifications change as new features about an organism are recognized. One recent addition is the ***Campylobacter*** genera, which are transmitted via contaminated food, milk, or water. It is increasingly being diagnosed in patients with AIDS. It may also be the etiologic agent of **gastritis** and probably peptic ulcers.

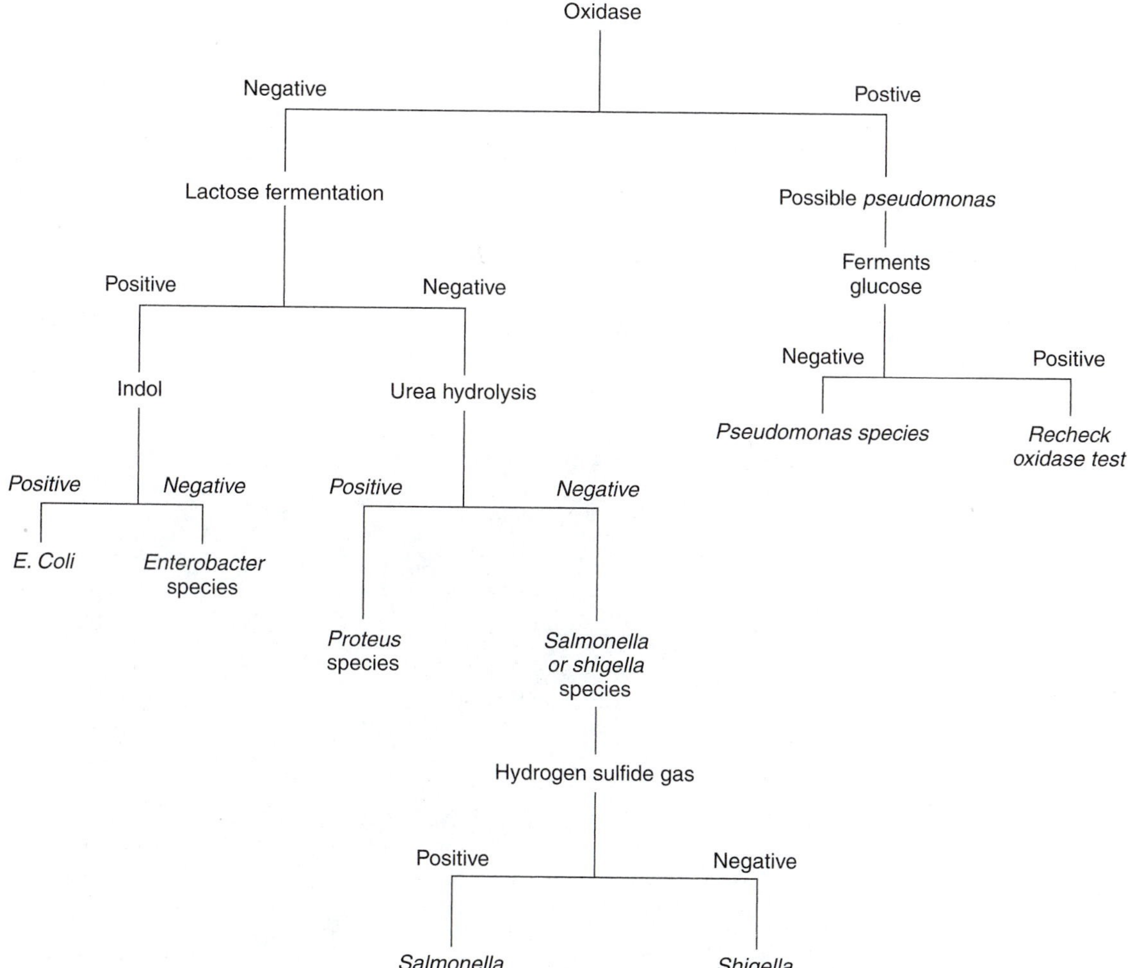

Figure 11–1 Typical pathway for the partial identification of some enteric organisms

LYME DISEASE

Lyme disease is actually a bacterial disease caused by ***Borrelia burgdorferi*** (see Figure 11–2), a spirochete bacterium, but the bacteria is transmitted to humans via the bite of a tick from the Ixodes genus (***Ixodes dammini*** in the Northeast and Midwest and ***Ixodes pacificus*** in the western United States). The natural hosts for this tick are deer and rodents. All stages of the tick life cycle can transmit the disease, including the nymph, which is very active in the spring and summer months, the time of year when people are lightly dressed and often out in the woods. This disease can also be passed on via the milk of infected mammals who are intermediate hosts. This disease causes a serious pseudorheumatoid arthritis, which was first described in young boys living in Lyme, Connecticut. First, a reddish ring-shaped rash or lesion appears at the site where the tick was attached, followed by skin blotches. Several weeks or months later symptoms of arthritis, malaise, myalgia, and neurologic and cardiac involvement appear. The rash may not always be present; therefore, detection could be missed. When recognized early, antibiotic therapy with penicillin, tetracycline, or erythromycin is usually quite successful. Today, the disease is endemic in most northern, central, and eastern parts of the United States, where white-tailed deer are found. Campers, hikers, and hunters are advised to not go into the woods without wearing light-colored clothing that covers and seals the arms and legs and to use a tick repellent such as DEET.

ATYPICAL BACTERIA

Rickettsia, *Chlamydia*, and *Mycoplasma* are prokaryotic organisms that differ from most other bacteria in that they are much smaller than most and they have an unusual cell wall structure. *Rickettsia* cannot live outside cells of living organisms and *Chlamydia* and

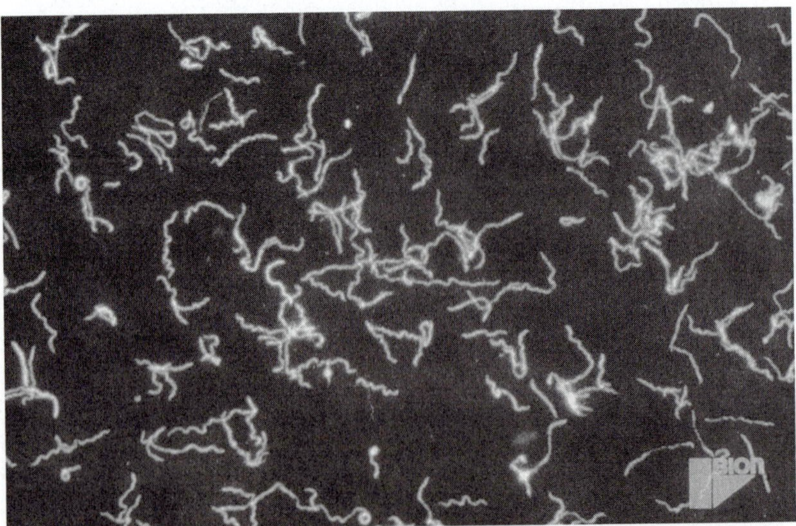

Figure 11–2 *Borrelia burgdorferi*, the spirochete that causes Lyme disease

Mycoplasma genera each include members that cause pneumonia as well as sexually transmitted diseases (STDs). These organisms are most **fastidious** in that they are difficult to grow and require special growth nutrients to demonstrate them in culture. The *Rickettsia* group is extremely difficult and hazardous to work with and thus is most often identified by serological testing methods.

Antibiotic-resistant bacteria, and those causing necrotizing fasciitis, are not themselves so atypical, as in the cases of Rickettsias, Chlamydias, and Mycoplasma. Such bacteria are easy to grow on routine culture media, are found frequently in infections, and look and chemical react just as the less virulent strains of the same bacteria. It is the adaptation to the enviornment that results in genetic changes of common *Staphylococci* and *Streptococci* to resist destruction due to overuse by antibiotics.

Rickettsias

Until recently, it was thought that rickettsias were microorganisms between bacteria and viruses. Rickettsias are much smaller than the smallest bacteria, and are only barely visible as tiny specks under oil immersion. Electron microscopic studies show that they have the cell structure of true bacteria and occur in rod and spherical forms. They are both nonmotile and gram negative. All rickettsias are **obligate intracellular parasites** (like the viruses), which means they cannot live outside the cells of another living organism, and they are widely distributed in nature, infecting many species of animals that form their natural reservoir. Transmitted by the bites of fleas, lice, ticks, and mites, they cause several types of typhus fever, Rocky Mountain spotted fever, and the relatively mild rickettsial pox. The latter is carried by a mite found on house mice.

Epidemic typhus fever is the only rickettsial infection in which humans form the reservoir. Rickettsials get their name from the physician who first identified the causative agent of Rocky Mountain spotted fever, Dr. Howard T. Ricketts, an American pathologist. He subsequently died from typhus, having been infected through his own research on the disease. One rarely sees this disease today, but it is transmitted when one shares a common habitation with rats, fleas, and lice. ***Rickettsia prowazekii*** is a human louseborne typhus. It was responsible for typhus epidemics during both world wars. ***Rickettsia typhi*** causes endemic fleaborne typhus and is found worldwide to be transmitted by the rat flea. Scrub typhus is a miteborne typhus. A serological laboratory test known as the Weil-Felix reaction, in which typhus antibodies will agglutinate certain strains of the enteric bacteria *Proteus*, is easy to perform, and a rising **titer** of antibodies is diagnostic. Q fever, not commonly seen in the United States, is transmitted by ticks to animals then to humans who drink contaminated milk or inhale dust contaminated with animal material.

Chlamydias

Chlamydias are intracellular, microscopic, gram-negative obligate bacteria with a coccoid (spherical) shape. These organisms were once grouped with the viruses because of their dependence on a host cell for energy. They are therefore known as **energy parasites** (see Figure 11–3). They were once regarded as viruses because of their need for host cells to reproduce. Chlamydias cause very severe infections in humans and animals, including ornithosis, a severe respiratory infection; lymphogranuloma venereum, a highly contagious tropical venereal disease; and both trachoma and conjunctivitis, which cause acute eye infections.

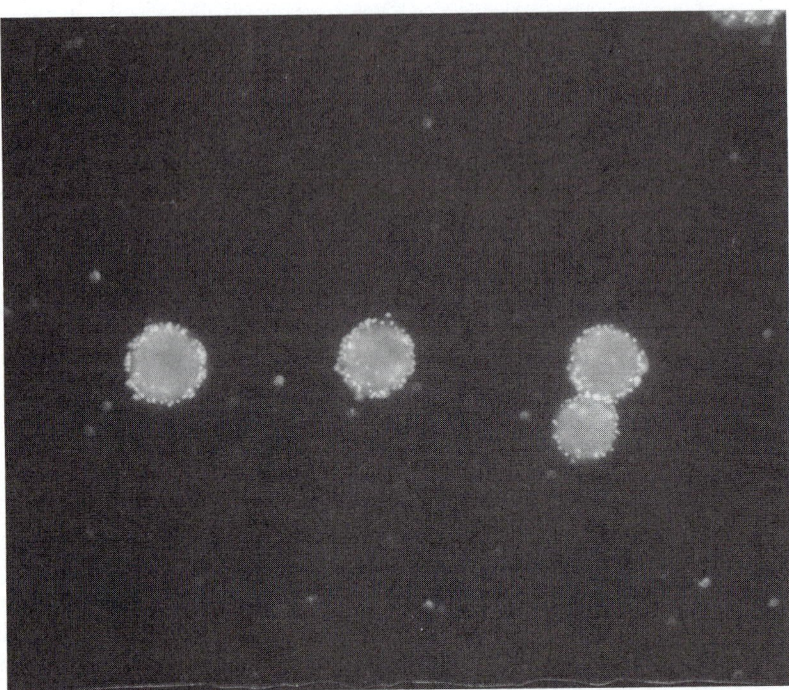

Figure 11–3 Chlamydia, free elementary bodies (Note the bodies attached to cells are close to the reticulum stage.) *(Courtesy BION Enterprises, Ltd., Park Ridge, IL).*

Psittacosis, or ornithosis, is a very severe pneumonia caused by the organism ***Chlamydia psittaci,*** which is found in close association with birds. It can also cause extended systemic infections, particularly in immunocompromised patients. Another species, ***Chlamydia trachomatis,*** causes acute eye infections that can lead to blindness, sexually transmitted chlamydial **urethritis,** and **cervicitis.** This organism, often undetected in the female genital area, is found in conjunction with the organism causing gonorrhea and is often overlooked because of the ease of identifying *Neisseria gonorrhoeae* as compared with *C. trachomatis.* Once gonorrhea has been identified, the patient is treated with penicillin and recovery is apparent. *C. trachomatis* is slow-growing and resistant to penicillin, and when postgonococcal nonspecific urethritis or cervicitis develops, chlamydial cultures are considered. This organism, often undetected in the female genital area, promotes a reservoir of infection. As many as 22% of women and 7% of men are asymptomatic carriers. It can cause pelvic inflammatory disease (PID) and can be transmitted to the eyes of babies during labor and delivery. Today, diagnostic tests are readily available. It can be identified by culture, cytology, and direct antigen detection methods in clinical genital specimens, and it can be diagnosed by serological testing of patient sera. The organism has been recovered from the urethra, cervix, nasopharynx, and rectum, as well as aspirates from fallopian tubes and the epididymis.

Another venereal disease, lymphogranuloma venerum (LGV), found only in tropical areas of Africa, Asia, and South America, is also caused by this organism. LGV can cause systemic disease, settle in the inguinal lymph nodes, and produce rectal fistulas, rectal stricture, and draining sinuses. Recovery rates from this disease are very low, and only about 30% of the patients become disease free.

Mycoplasmas

Mycoplasma organisms are very small prokaryotic microbes surrounded by a single triple-layered membrane. They do not have the typical bacterial cell wall. Their cell structure is very simple. A mycoplasma contains only a cell membrane, a prokaryotic nucleus, and some ribosomes. It is considered to be the simplest life form capable of independent growth and metabolism.

When mycoplasmas are grown on an agar medium, they display a characteristic "fried egg" appearance. They are highly **pleomorphic** (the occurrence of more than one shape in a bacterial species). They can be bulbous, coccoid, or filamentous in shape for the same species, because they lack cell walls.

Mycoplasmas are classified under class Mollicutes and order Mycoplasmatales. The order is further subdivided into two families: Family I, Mycoplasmataceae (require sterol for growth) and Family II, Acholeplasmataceae (does not require sterol for growth).

Mycoplasmas were earlier named "pleuropneumonialike organisms" **(PPLO),** because they were first isolated and described at the turn of the century from cattle with lung infections. They are pathogenic to many animals and some plants. Mycoplasma strains are found among the normal flora of the genital and respiratory membranes. They have been implicated in infections of these membranes such as cervicitis, prostatitis, and urethritis. They also have been isolated in pus from deep-tissue abscesses. In laboratory animals, mycoplasmas can cause a condition similar to chronic arthritis, with lesions like those of rheumatoid arthritis in humans.

Mycoplasma pneumoniae can cause a whole range of respiratory diseases, ranging from a mild upper respiratory tract infection to severe bilateral pneumonia. Because they do not have a cell wall, they are resistant to antibiotic treatment that works by inhibiting cell wall synthesis. The drug of choice is tetracycline, unless the patient is pregnant, in which case erythromycin is preferred because it does not impair fetal tooth development as does tetracycline. Usually complete recovery is slow, and the dry, hacking cough characteristic of infection with this organism persists for months. One curious clinical laboratory feature of this disease is that **cold autoagglutinins** often develop (that is, antibodies developed to self that are apparent only at refrigerated temperatures) and that standard tests for syphilis [rapid plasma reagin (RPR), Venereal Disease Research Laboratory (VDRL)] are positive. These features disappear on recovery. The most common diagnostic tests are serological tests rather than attempts to culture this difficult-to-grow organism. *Mycoplasma pneumoniae,* or primary atypical pneumonia, is often referred to as "walking pneumonia."

Antibiotic-Resistant Bacterial Strains

Penicillin-resistant strains of *Staphylococcus aureus* have been well known for some time. Bacterial resistance has been emerging over the years due to the indiscriminate and overuse of antibiotics to treat upper respiratory infections, sexually transmitted diseases, and numerous other infections. More than 90% of all *Staphylococcus aureus* strains are resistant to penicillin today, and several strains are found to be resistant to many other antibiotics as well. Some of the more notable resistant organisms today include not only penicillin-resistant *Staphylococcus,* but also methicillin-resistant *Staphylococcus aureus* (MRSA) and methicillin-resistant *Staphylococcus epidermidis* (MRSE). These strains are resistant to all **beta-lactam** antibiotics including the semisynthetic penicillin derivatives, nafcillin, oxacillin, and cloxacillin as well as the cephalosporins and cephalomicins.* These organisms are of great concern to the modern medical community. Most nosocomial infections are a result of infections with *Staphylococcus aureus* acquired during a hospital stay. Wounds, the lower respiratory system, and blood (**bacteremia**) are most commonly the sites affected. About 45% of these infections are due to MRSA. *Staphylococcus epidermidis,* a common skin inhabitant, is most often implicated in infections related to the use of intravenous catheters and **prosthetic** devices, especially urinary infections and subacute bacterial endocarditis (SBE). Many of these *S. epidermidis* infections are also MRSE strains, and they account for upwards of 75% of the methicillin-resistant *S. epidermidis* infections. Unfortunately physicians have had to turn to a very potent, toxic, and expensive antibiotic—vancomycin—to treat MRSA and MRSE.

This toxic drug worries clinicians and scientists, for it will be only a matter of time before vancomycin resistance is widespread. Resistance to this drug has already been demonstrated by *Enterococcus* spp., a gram-positive coccus found in bowel flora and often the cause of urinary tract infections. Soon physicians will have no effective antibiotics to treat the common staphylococcal infections.

Additionally, penicillin-resistant strains are common among strains of *Neisseria gonorrhoeae* (**penicillinase** producing *N. gonorrhoeae* or PPNG), *Haemophilus influenzae,* and *Streptococcus pneumoniae,* both being common causes of pneumonia in children and the elderly. *H. influenzae* also causes bacterial meningitis and severe ear infections.

Pseudomonas aeruginosa has always been extremely resistant to antibiotics. It is a deadly organism that often causes severe secondary infections in burn patients, and lower respiratory infections in patients with **tracheotomies** or those on breathing life support. Because of its nosocomial notoriety, patients who use respirators or who require a tracheotomy are at the greatest risk.

Much has been noted in the news about the common bowel flora *Escherichia coli* as the cause of severe food poisoning. This organism includes numerous strains, most of which are harmless in the bowel, but *E. coli* strains such as the 0156, CDC-identified strain, have been isolated in fast-food restaurants and in meats, and can cause severe diarrhea and sometimes even death. This strain of *E. coli* is also very resistant to the antibiotics commonly used to treat gram-negative organisms.

Necrotizing Fasciitis

One of the deadliest organisms to be in the news lately is the fast spreading form of *Streptococcus pyogenes,* also known as beta hemolytic streptococcus or group A streptococcus (GAS). **Necrotizing fasciitis (NF),** dubbed by the press as "flesh-eating bacteria," because it literally destroys the skin and underlying tissues and muscles, can go from minor dis-

*Ref NC. Guidelines for Control of Antibiotic resistance

comfort at the site of a small cut or abrasion to a life-threatening gangrenelike disease in hours. This particularly virulent strain of bacteria produces toxins that directly kill the tissue, interfere with blood flow to the tissue, and digest materials in the tissue, all of which allow the bacteria to multiply rapidly and cause widespread systemic effects such as a toxic shock. Although most necrotizing fasciitis infections are associated with GAS, mixed infections with *Staphylococcus*, gram-negative bacilli, and anaerobes such as *Bacteriodes* are also observed.

Sometimes the initial pain is remote from the site of the minor injury, such as pain in the upper arm following a small cut on the finger. This pain may be nothing more than a muscle ache, but soon progresses to a severe pain in the area. The infection may begin with a small, harmless, reddish, painful spot or bump on the skin which quickly becomes a very painful purplish or bronzed patch that rapidly expands. The center may become black and dead (necrotic) and the skin may break open. Visible expansion of the opening can occur in less than 1 hour and may exhibit an oozing fluid that ranges from a yellowish clear or yellowish bloody to puslike substance. Very soon flulike symptoms appear, including diarrhea, fever, sweating, chills, nausea, dizziness, and general malaise followed by profound weakness until finally shock takes over. Without treatment, death occurs rapidly.

Necrotizing fasciitis is often misdiagnosed because most of the early symptoms present as other diseases, such as a carbuncle (boil), a mildly infected scratch, or a pimple. This disease is still relatively rare and often health care providers do not think of NF as a cause until the symptoms are so obvious that it may be too late for the patient. Therefore, early diagnosis is most important to begin therapy with powerful broad-spectrum antibiotics. Surgery is usually required to open and drain the infected sites and to remove (debride) the dead tissue. This operation may include amputation if a limb infection cannot be contained or controlled. Often skin grafts will be required after the infection is cleared. Approximately 15,000 cases of invasive group A streptococcus are diagnosed each year, resulting in over 2000 deaths, of which about 1500 develop necrotizing fasciitis, killing up to 300 (20%) each year. Another 3000 cases develop streptococcal toxic shock syndrome, killing almost 1800 (60%) patients each year. In contrast, several million persons get group A strep throat and impetigo each year. Invasive GAS is no doubt a killer, but is rare compared with the breadth of ordinary group A streptococcus.

Other Atypical Bacteria

Neisseria gonorrhoeae is a sexually transmitted disease and can cause serious reproductive complications if left untreated. *Neisseria meningitidis* causes meningitis, a life-threatening disease. *Moraxella catarrhalis* is normal flora of the upper respiratory tract. Of the gram-positive bacilli, the *Clostridium* are important disease-producing organisms. *Clostridium perfringens* causes gas gangrene, *Clostridium botulinum* causes food poisoning, and *Clostridium tetani* causes lockjaw. All of these organisms are strict anaerobes and are readily recognized in Gram stains as large gram-positive rods, some with spores. They cause life-threatening diseases. A fourth member, *Clostridium difficile,* causes a severe colitis. Gram-negative bacilli include the family of *Enterobacteriaceae,* or enteric organisms. These bacteria are found in the bowel and in bladder and kidney infections. Normal enteric flora can easily cause urinary tract infections, especially in females because of the proximity of the urethral opening to the anal area. *E. coli* is the most common, but there are a number of strains of this organism. One strain that causes dysentery and diarrhea is CDC-identified strain number 0156. This *E. coli,* which has been identified in numerous infections, traces back to meat sources purchased at a particular grocery store or fast-food restaurant. *Salmonella* and *Shigella* species also cause intestinal disorders, as does *Campylobacter,* which may be transferred from food, milk, or water. Other important gram-negative enteric rods include the *Proteus* species and the *Pseudomonas* organisms, which are also well known in nosocomial infections, lower respiratory infections, and in severe burn patients. This unit concludes with two introductory lab procedures to assist the student in recognizing that bacteria are everywhere and in preparing bacterial cultures for microscopic viewing.

SUMMARY

Bacterial infections will be the majority of infections encountered on a daily basis. This chapter discusses some of the most common bacteria that cause disease. Certainly *Staphylococcus aureus* is the most common and often one of the most resistant bacteria due to the overuse of antibiotics over the years. The result has been penicillin- and methicillin-resistant strains. To differentiate *Staphylococcus aureus* from other (usually) nonpathogenic staphylococcal organisms, the coagulase test and growth on mannitol salt agar are the gold standards. Staph infections often are like boils and carbuncles. They can contaminate open areas and cause the development of osteomyletis following a bone fracture.

Among the streptococcal organisms, group A streptococcus or hemolytic streptococcus is most important for causing strep throat. It can also develop complications by causing rheumatic fever, scarlet fever, septicemia, necrotizing fasciitis (destruction of fat and muscle), and rarely, streptococcal toxic shock syndrome (STSS). People with strep throat have a fever, sore throat, loss of energy, headache, and swollen lymph nodes. Streptococcus pneumoniae causes pneumonia, and it can also be implicated in bacterial meningitis, as can *Haemophilus influenzae* and *Neisseria meningitidis.* Group A strep can be identified by any of the rapid slide or kit tests on the market today, or by demonstration of its zone of inhibition of growth on blood agar around a Taxos A disk. *Streptococcus pneumoniae* is differentiated from *Streptococcus viridans* by its zone of no growth around an optochin disk. The *Neisseria* species are differentiated by their fermentative actions in glucose, maltose, and sucrose.

STUDY AND DISCUSSION

- Discuss and identify the useful activities of the following bacteria:
  a. nitrifying bacteria
  b. denitrifying bacteria
  c. putrefactive bacteria
  d. nitrogen-fixing bacteria

- Explain the relationship between bacteria and the sterilization and disinfection of dressings.
- Name several culture media used by bacteriologists in growing bacteria.

Procedure 11–1 Presence and Growth of Bacteria in Culture Media

Equipment and Materials Needed

Sterilizer (autoclave)
Petri dishes
Cotton
Culture medium for growth of bacteria (this may be nutrient broth, nutrient agar, gelatin, litmus milk, or other special media)
Test tubes
Bunsen burners
Incubator

Note: Commercially prepared plates may be purchased in lieu of making culture media.

Method

Following manufacturer's directions, weigh a measured amount of agar and heat with water to dissolve the powder, stirring constantly.

1. Sterilize the agar medium in an autoclave at 250°F (121°C) for 15 minutes; pour into sterilized petri dishes.
2. Cover the dishes immediately, and allow the culture medium to cool and harden. After cooling, keep one petri dish unopened as a control.
3. Expose other petri dishes as follows and then cover. [*Note:* Place all petri dishes lid side down in an incubator at body temperature (98.6°F; 37°C) overnight after you cover them.]
   a. Expose one to air of classroom for 3 minutes. Cover.
   b. Cough into a second one. Cover.
   c. Place a penny into a third one. Cover.
   d. Touch a handkerchief to another. Cover.
   e. Touch a comb to another. Cover.
   f. Touch your fingertip to another. Cover.
   g. Place a hair into another. Cover.
   h. While making a bed, place an open petri dish on a bedside table, being careful to not shake the bedclothes in removing and replacing them. Cover the dish.
   i. Repeat with another dish on a bedside table while making the same bed, but handle the bedclothes carelessly. Cover the dish.
   j. Open one dish in the treatment room before patient enters and before anyone else has entered. Cover.
   k. Open a second dish in the treatment room after patient has entered and been treated. Cover.

Observations and Conclusions

1. Examine all the petri dishes after their incubation for 24 hours at 98.6°F (37°C).

2. Compare the control petri dish with all the other dishes. What differences are noted? Why?

3. Compare the number of colonies found in the various dishes. Explain.

4. Compare the number of colonies in petri dish (h) with that in dish (i). Explain.

5. Compare the number of colonies in petri dishes (j) and (k). Explain.

6. Why is it necessary to sterilize the petri dishes and cover them immediately when preparing them?

7. Why did the control dish remain sterile?

Procedure 11–2 Preparation of a Smear

Equipment and Materials Needed

Microscope
Bunsen burner
Inoculating needle
Bibulous paper
Cultures of bacteria
Slides
Dyes (crystal violet, methylene blue, safranin)
Distilled water

Method

1. Wearing protective outer covering and gloves, label each slide.
2. Flame a loop and place a loopful of water on a clean slide with the inoculating needle.
3. Flame the inoculating needle in a Bunsen burner. Allow to cool.
4. Transfer a pinhead size amount of the culture to a clean slide.
5. Spread the culture over an area the size of a dime.
6. Flame the needle in the Bunsen burner.
7. Hold the slide 12 to 18 inches above the flame to dry and fix the smear.
8. Add a small amount of stain (methylene blue or safranin) to the smear and let stand for 1 minute.
9. Wash the smear with water and blot dry.
10. Examine the smear with the oil-immersion objective.

Observations and Conclusions

1. Describe what you see under the microscope.

2. Sketch and label what you see.

3. Why must the inoculating needle be flamed?

4. Why must the smear be stained?

5. What is meant by "fixing" a slide?

REVIEW QUESTIONS

A. General Questions: Provide complete answers to each of the following.

1. Where are bacteria found?

2. Explain in your own words how a bacteriologist tests for the presence of diphtheria bacilli in a child.

3. Why are culture media used?

4. How do bacteria differ from protozoa, yeasts, and molds?

5. What name is given to useful bacteria?

6. How are the useful bacteria important to us?

7. What are harmful bacteria called? What makes them harmful?

8. Why is the study of bacteria so essential for the health professional?

9. Why is it difficult to see the structure of bacteria even under the microscope?

10. What measures can be taken by the health care professional to destroy bacterial growth?

11. What are mycoplasmas?

12. Why are mycoplasmas said to be pleomorphic?

13. What conditions can *Mycoplasma pneumoniae* cause?

14. Name the clinically significant rickettsias and chlamydias.

15. Compare the growth characteristics of rickettsias and chlamydias.

B. Multiple-Choice Questions: Select the letter of the choice that best answers the question.

1. Normal flora are considered to be bacteria that _______ .
   a. cause upper respiratory infections
   b. are normal inhabitants of the body
   c. cause opportunistic infections
   d. most often cause infections
2. Opportunistic pathogens are _______ .
   a. normal flora
   b. organisms waiting to attack a healthy immune system
   c. organisms that normally do not cause disease in healthy individuals
   d. organisms that cause well-documented infections
3. *Staphylococcus aureus* has which of the following set of characteristics?
   a. golden yellow, gram-positive cocci, mannitol negative
   b. creamy white, coagulase positive, mannitol negative
   c. coagulase positive, mannitol positive, golden yellow
   d. coagulase negative, mannitol positive, golden yellow
4. *Streptococcus pyogenes* is also known as _______ .
   a. *Streptococcus viridans*
   b. *Streptococcus pneumoniae*
   c. group A streptococcus
   d. *Streptococcus fecalis*
5. *Streptococcus pneumoniae* has which of the following set of characteristics?
   a. beta hemolysis, mucoid colony, optochin positive
   b. alpha hemolysis, pitted colony, optochin negative
   c. beta hemolysis, encapsulated, optochin negative
   d. alpha hemolysis, encapsulated, mucoid colony
6. A common sexually transmitted disease (STD), the organism that can also cause blindness in newborns is _______ .
   a. *Neisseria meningitidis*
   b. *Neisseria gonorrhoeae*
   c. *Haemophilis influenzae*
   d. *Treponema pallidum*
7. Which of the following groups of organisms cause food poisoning?
   a. *Campylobacter, Clostridium, Salmonella*
   b. *Salmonella, Corynebacterium, Salmonella*
   c. *Campylobacter, Corynebacterium, Shigella*
   d. *Campylobacter, Neisseria, Salmonella*
8. Ear infections as well as secondary burn infections are caused by _______ .
   a. *Staphylococcus*
   b. *Streptococcus*
   c. *Pseudomonas*
   d. *Neisseria*

9. Nosocomial infections are those infections _______ .
   a. that manifest during the night
   b. that originate in a hospital environment
   c. in which patients always succumb to death
   d. that are noncommunicable
10. *Neisseria gonorrhoeae* ferments which of the following sugars?
    a. glucose, maltose, and sucrose
    b. glucose and sucrose
    c. glucose only
    d. maltose and glucose
    e. none of the above sugars
11. Rickettsias are actually
    a. viruses
    b. parasites
    c. fungi
    d. bacteria
12. Chlamydias were once grouped with the _______ .
    a. viruses
    b. parasites
    c. fungi
    d. bacteria
13. A clinically important sexually transmitted disease, often difficult to isolate, is the _______ .
    a. *Rickettsia prowazekii*
    b. *Chlamydia psittaci*
    c. *Chlamydia trachomatis*
    d. *Rickettsia typhi*
14. A tiny organism that has a "fried egg" appearance on culture media is the _______ organisms.
    a. rickettsia
    b. mycoplasma
    c. chlamydia
    d. herpes

C. From the following list of terms fill in the blanks with the correct choice.

urinary infections
carbuncles
typhoid fever
rheumatic fever
anthrax
abortions
Streptococcus pneumoniae
Streptococcus pyogenes
Streptococcus viridans
coliforms
Campylobacter
beta
enterics
Shigella
Pseudomonas
Salmonella
Clostridium tetani
alpha
Felix
Weil
rickettsia
louse
flea
Rickettsia Prowazekii
Mycoplasma pneumoniae
Chlamydia trachomatis

1. *Staphylococcus aureus* is a common cause of ____________________ .
2. Salmonella can cause ____________________ .
3. *Escherichia coli* is most frequently found in ____________________ .
4. ____________________ may be a complication of group A streptococcus.
5. Subacute bacterial endocarditis is often caused by ____________________ .
6. Enteric organisms that inhabit the bowel are often referred to as ______________ .

7. Grapejuice or musty odors may be attributed to the ____________________ organism.

8. Lockjaw is caused by ____________________ .

9. A *Bacillus* organism, sometimes associated with biological warfare, can cause ____________________in cattle.

10. Partial hemolysis on a blood agar plate results in a greenish zone around the bacteria. This is referred to as ____________________ hemolysis, while the clear zone or full hemolysis is referred to as ____________________ hemolysis.

11. Lymphogranuloma venerum, found only in tropical countries, is caused by ____________________ .

12. Serological identification of rickettsia infections is made using the ____________________ reactions.

13. *Rickettsia typhi* is caused by a ____________________ .

14. Q fever is caused by a ____________________ organism.

15. Patients often develop cold autoagglutinins as a curious feature of ____________________.

D. Matching Questions: Match the terms in Column I with their corresponding terms in Column II.

Column I		Column II
_______	1. *Staphylococcus aureus*	a. coagulase negative
_______	2. *Streptococcus pyogenes*	b. obligate anaerobes
_______	3. *Staphylococcus epidermidis*	c. DNAse positive
_______	4. *Streptococcus pneumoniae*	d. walking pneumonia
_______	5. *Bacillus* species	e. causes dysentery
_______	6. *Clostridia* species	f. hydrogen sulfide positive
_______	7. *Corynebacterium diphtheriae*	g. coagulase positive
_______	8. *Neisseria gonorrhoeae*	h. urease positive
_______	9. *Branhamella catarrhalis*	i. gas gangrene
_______	10. *Pseudomonas aeruginosa*	j. scrub typhus
_______	11. *Salmonella* species	k. encapsulated
_______	12. *Proteus* species	l. oxidase positive
_______	13. *Escherichia* coli	m. indol positive
_______	14. *Shigella* species	n. *Group A Streptococcus*
_______	15. *Clostridium perfringens*	o. garliclike odor
_______	16. *Mycoplasma pneumoniae*	p. obligate aerobes
_______	17. *Rickettsia*	q. gram-negative intracellular diplococci

CHAPTER

12 Viruses

OBJECTIVES

After completing this chapter, you will be able to:

- explain how viral infections occur, and explain the role of interferon.
- identify the significant characteristics of viruses.
- identify the causative agent of AIDS.
- list the symptoms of AIDS.
- describe the modes of AIDS transmission and measures used to prevent its transmission and acquisition.
- describe some of the opportunistic infections associated with HIV.
- distinguish between Hepatitis A, Hepatitis B, and Hepatitis C.
- indicate the difference between chlamydias and viruses.

KEY WORDS

acquired immunodeficiency syndrome (AIDS)
adenovirus group
afflictions
antibody
arbovirus group
asymptomatic
ataxia
bacteriophage
capsids
CD4 cells
eclipse period
enzymes
gamma globulin
geneticist
hepatomegaly
herpesvirus group
histiocytes
human immunodeficiency virus (HIV)
hypergammaglobulinemia
immunosuppressed
incubation period
interferon
Kaposi's sarcoma
latent
leukopenia
lymphadenopathy
lymphoma
lymphopenia
lyse
lysozyme
macrophage
myxovirus group
neurodegenerative
opportunistic
oral hairy leukoplakia
papovavirus group
paramyxovirus group
phage
picornavirus group
poxvirus group
Prions
prophylaxis
proteinaceous infectious particles
recipients
retrovirus
rhabdovirus group
scrapie
seroconversion
splenomegaly
spongiform encephalopathies
T-lymphocyte

VIRUSES

The smallest infectious agents are the viruses. Viruses are usually thought of as intracellular agents rather than as microorganisms. They are unlike living things in that they cannot carry on independent metabolism, and they can reproduce only by replication in a host cell (Figure 12–1).

The tobacco mosaic virus, discovered in 1892, was the first known virus. At that time the only way to identify a virus was that it (1) caused disease, (2) passed through bacteria-retaining filters, (3) was not visible with the ordinary microscope, and (4) could not be cultivated on inanimate media the way bacteria could be cultivated.

In 1931, the first means for culturing viruses using tissue culture was perfected. Using this method, although we do not see the virus itself, we are able to see the effect of viral growth on growing tissue.

Viruses are not cellular and consist only of a nucleic acid, either ribonucleic acid (RNA) or deoxyribonucleic acid (DNA), surrounded by a protein coat. RNA and DNA make up the material of the nucleus in the cells of living things. They control both the heredity and life activities of the cells. The protein coat of the virus determines what sort of cell the virus can parasitize and acts much like the cell membrane of any other kind of cell by protecting the nucleic acid inside. A virus that attacks bacterial cells is called a **phage** or **bacteriophage.** The bacteriophage has one of the most interesting shapes of all

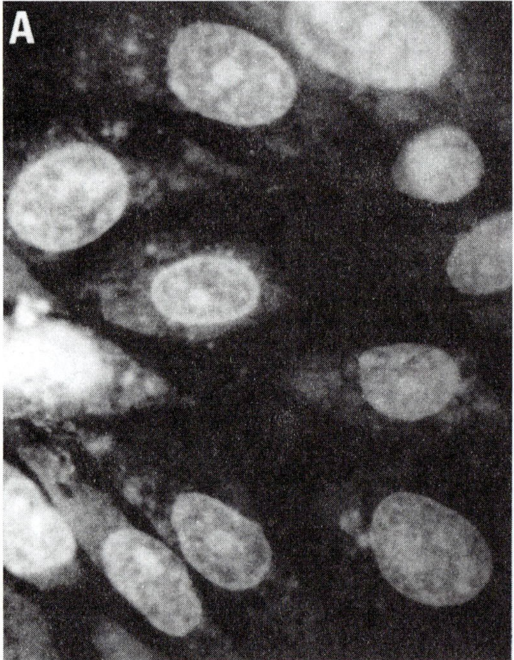

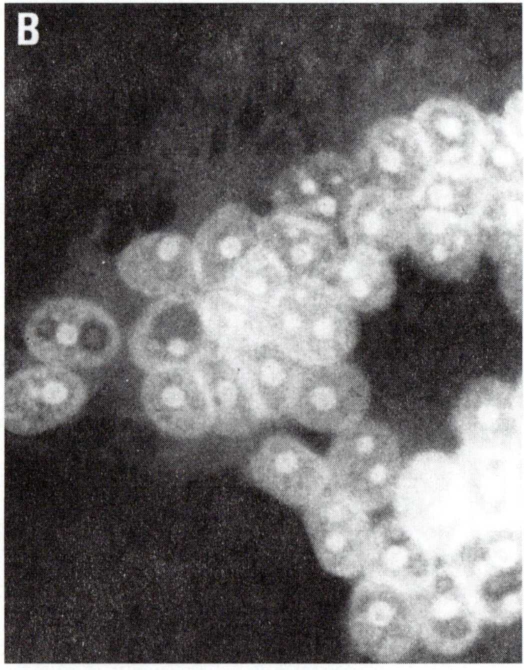

Figure 12–1 (A) Normal cells, (B) cells attacked by measles virus. The cells have clumped together into one giant cell. All the cytoplasm has fused into a single mass, and the nuclei have clustered together. (*Courtesy of Pfizer, Inc.*)

viruses (Figure 12–2). As mentioned, a phage consists of a head made from a protein membrane with twenty facets (sides) surrounding either DNA or RNA. The tail combines a collar attached to a tail sheath. The tail sheath surrounds a hollow core. At the end opposite to the collar, beneath the tail sheath, is the end plate. Extending from the end plate are six tail fibers. When a phage attacks a bacterial cell it goes through six stages. These six stages are adsorption or attachment, penetration, uncoating, protein and nucleic acid replication, maturation, and release (Figure 12–3).

Adsorption (attachment). The phage attaches itself to the bacterial cell wall by way of its tail fibers. These tail fibers attach to the bacterial cell wall. The location on the cell wall chosen by the phage seems to be the result of some affinity of the virus to attach to specific cell-receptor sites known as the CD4 receptors located on T4 lymphocytes and monocytes.

Penetration. Following adsorption, an enzyme called phage **lysozyme** is secreted from the phage tail. This enzyme digests part of the bacterial cell wall. Then the tail sheath contracts, and the tail core penetrates the cell wall, injecting the phage DNA into the bacteria.

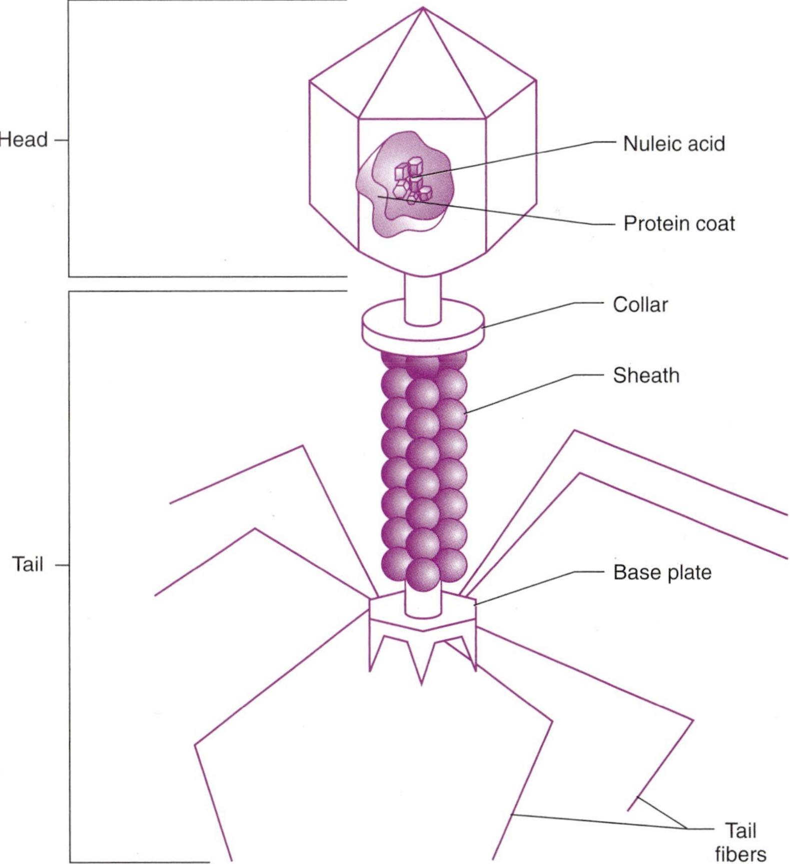

Figure 12–2 Typical bacteriophage

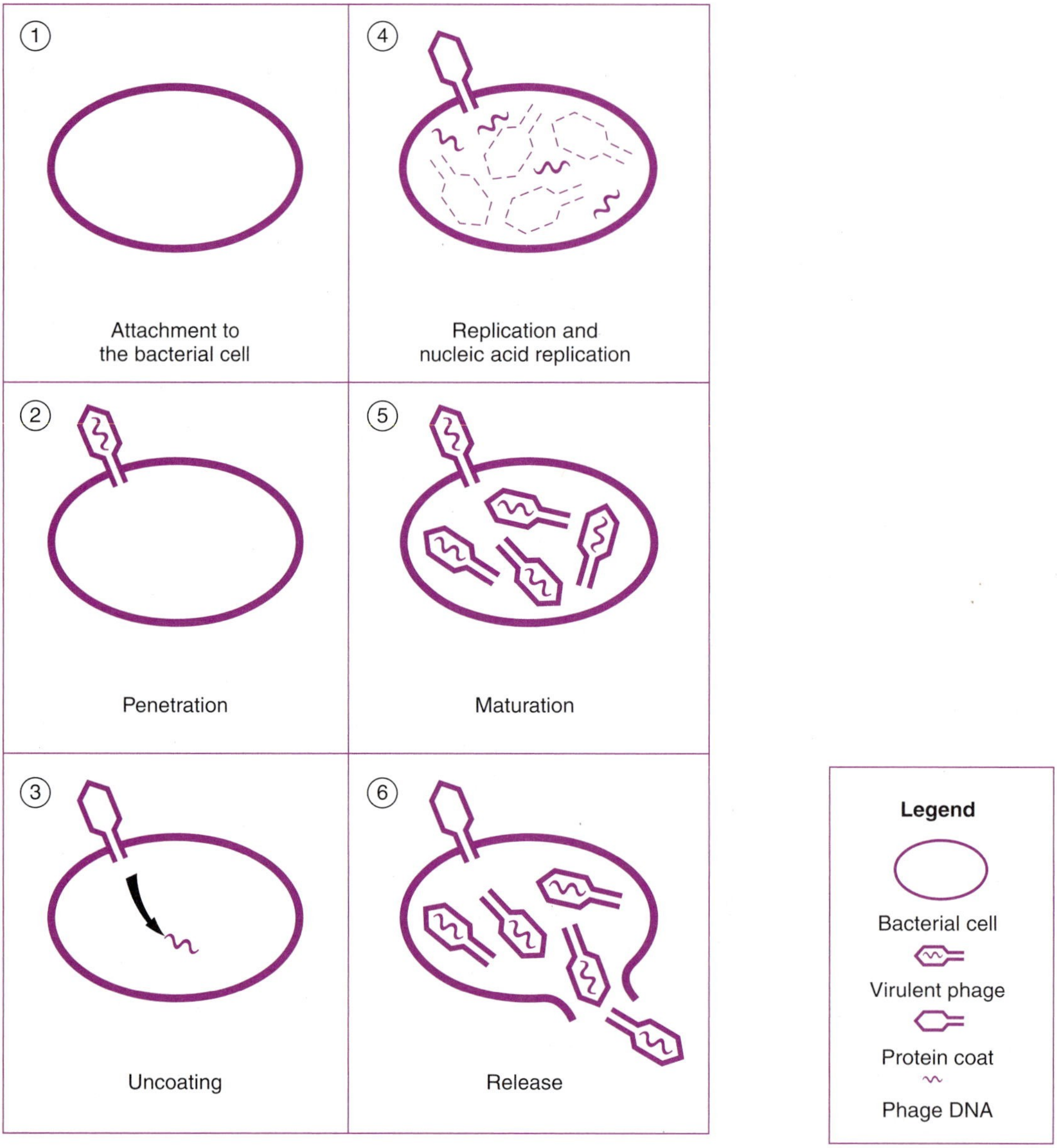

① Attachment to the bacterial cell

② Penetration

③ Uncoating

④ Replication and nucleic acid replication

⑤ Maturation

⑥ Release

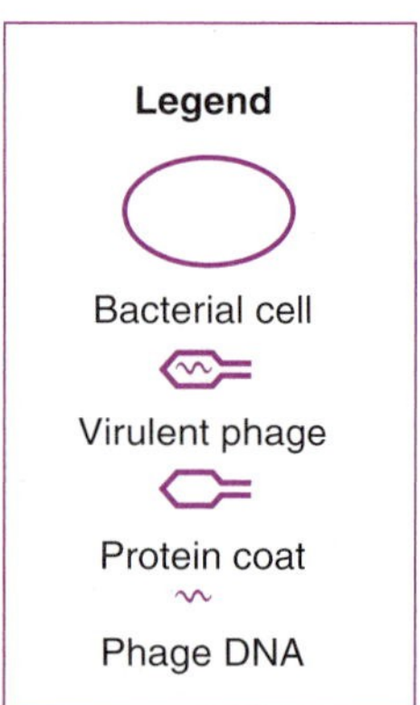

Figure 12–3 Stages in bacterial cell invasion by a virus

Uncoating. When the phage DNA is injected into the bacterial cell, the empty protein coat is left outside the bacterial cell. The protein phage head protects or "coats" the phage DNA before adsorption and penetration.

Replication and nucleic acid replication. The phage DNA takes over the biosynthetic machinery of the bacteria. It directs the bacteria to synthesize *only* phage

BACTERIAL STAINS

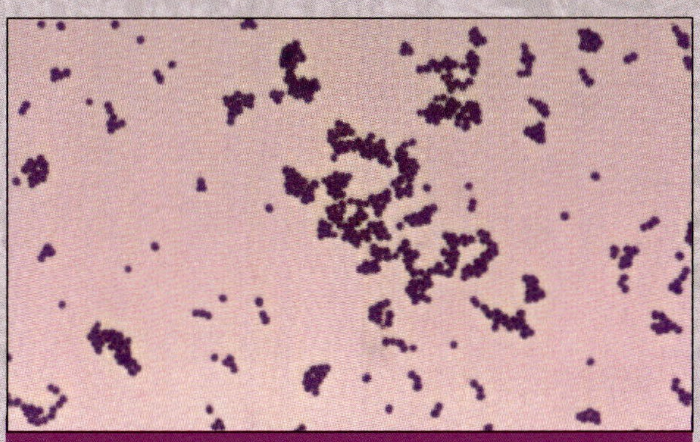

PLATE 1 *Staphylococci*, (gram positive)

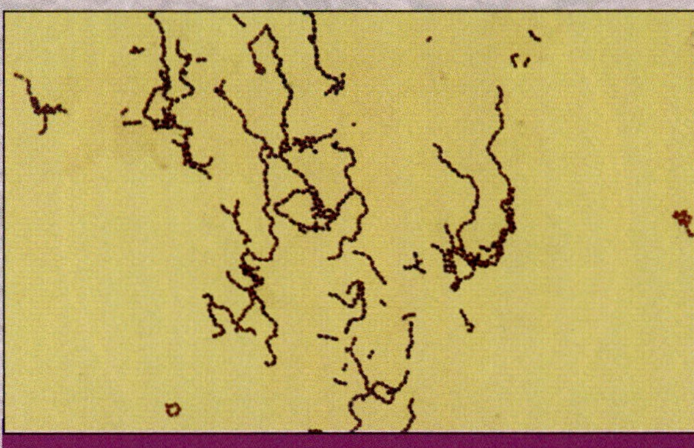

PLATE 2 *Streptococci*, (gram positive)

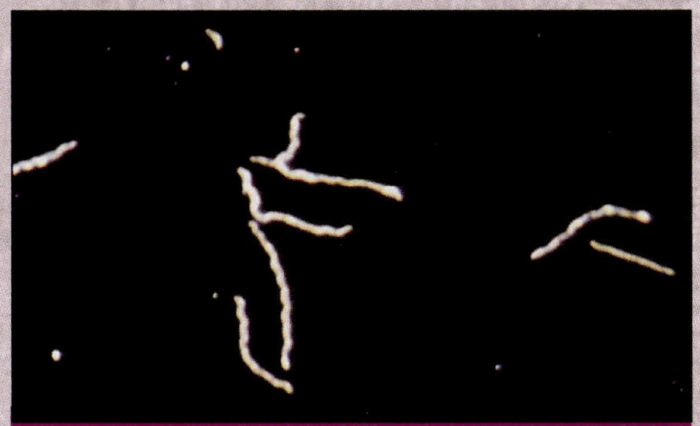

PLATE 3 Darkfield microscope preparation of *Treponema pallidum*, the causative agent of syphilis.

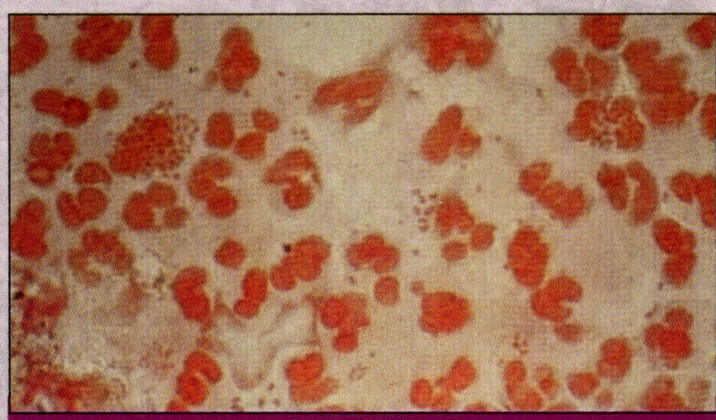

PLATE 4 Gram stain, male urethral discharge showing gram negative intracellular diplococci, resembling *N. gonorrhoeae*.

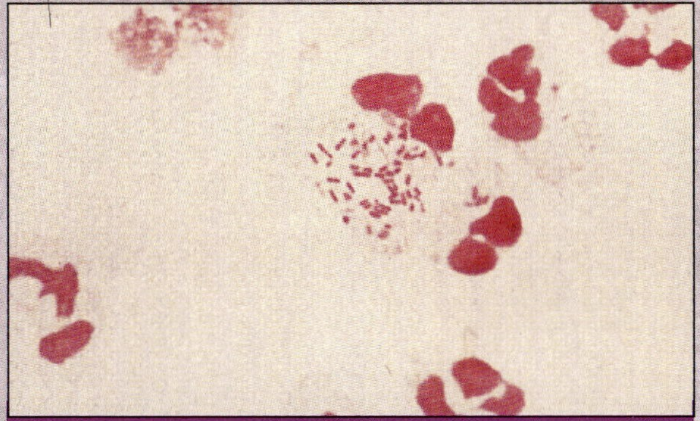

PLATE 5 Gram stain, of *Haemophilus influenzae* in cerebrospinal fluid (CSF). Bacterial Meningitis.

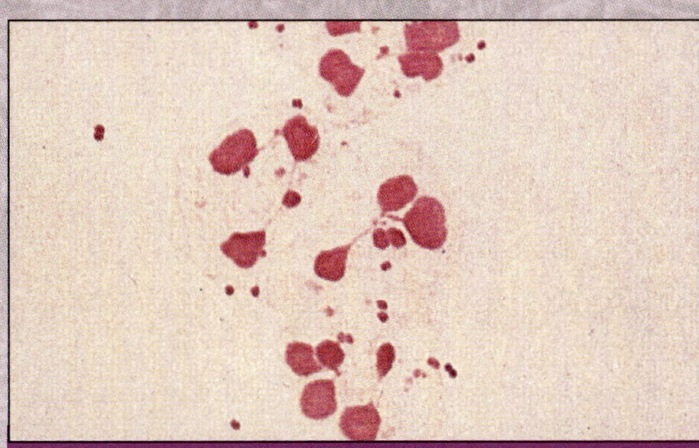

PLATE 6 Gram stain showing WBC containing *N. meningitis* in CSF. Bacterial Meningitis

BACTERIOLOGY CULTURE MEDIA

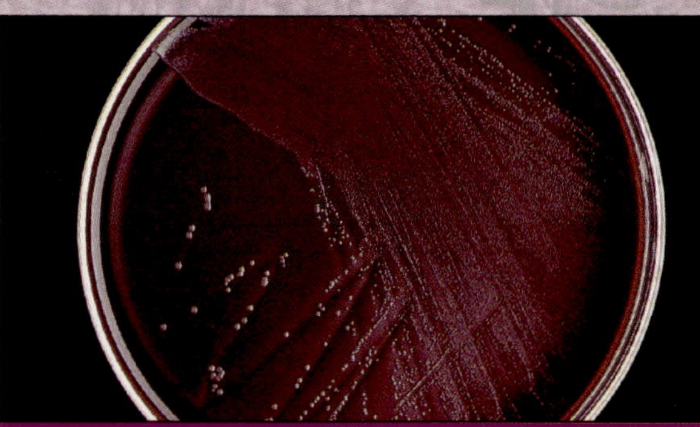

Plate 7 *Bordetella pertussis* on Regan-Lowe charcoal agar (Courtesy of Becton Dickinson Microbiology Systems, Sparks, MD)

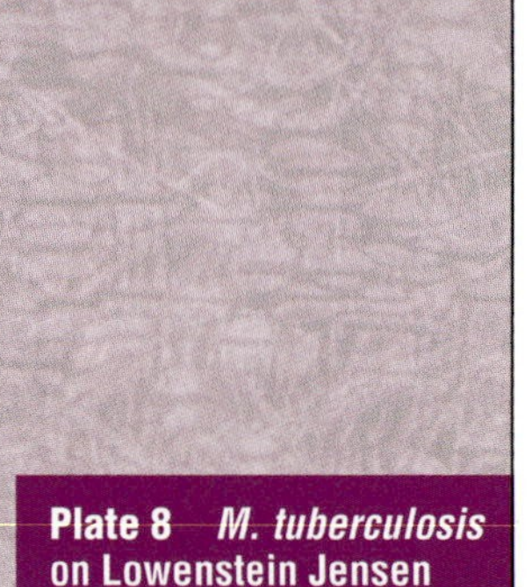

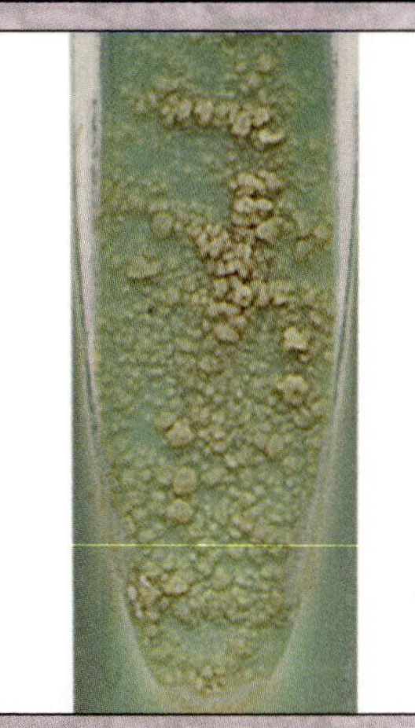

Plate 8 *M. tuberculosis* on Lowenstein Jensen media (Courtesy Remel, Inc.)

Plate 9 *Streptococcus pyogenes* (group A Strep) on blood agar

Plate 10 *Neisseria gonorrhoeae* on Thayer-Martin agar

Plate 11 *Corynebacterium diphtheriae* on blood agar

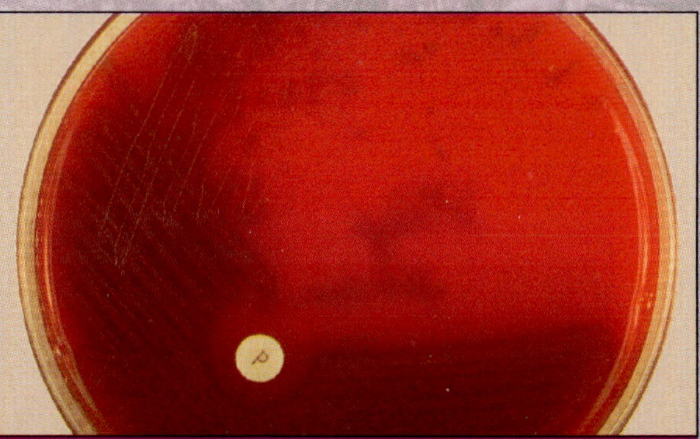

Plate 12 *Streptococcus pneumoniae* on blood agar, showing susceptibility to the optochin disk

BACTERIOLOGY CULTURE MEDIA (continued)

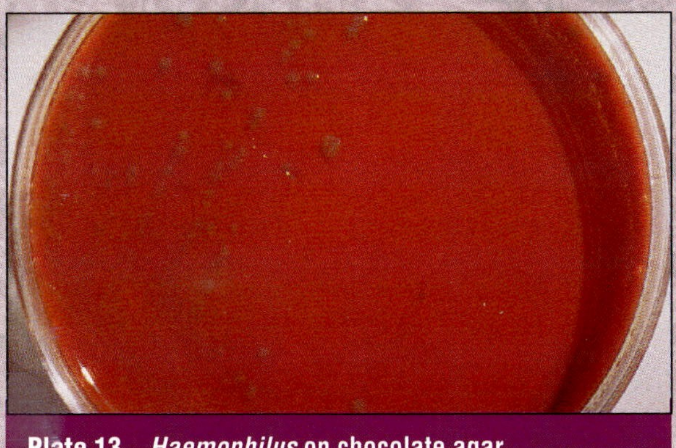

Plate 13 *Haemophilus* on chocolate agar

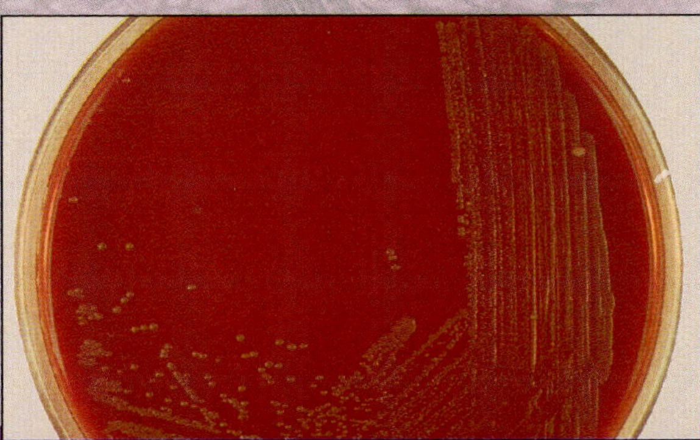

Plate 14 *Branhamella catarrhalis* on chocolate agar

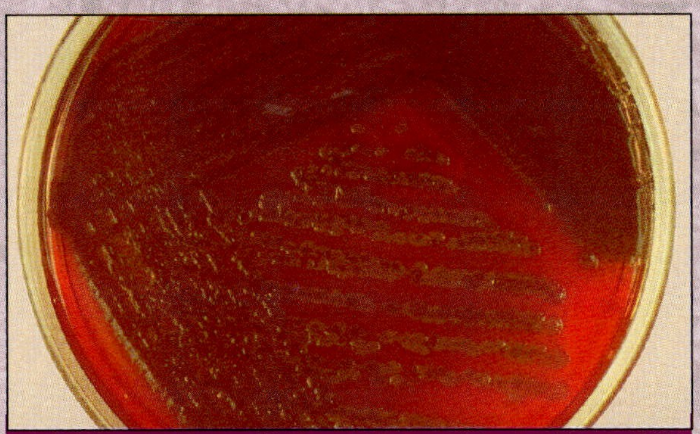

Plate 15 *Pseudomonas aeruginosa* on blood agar

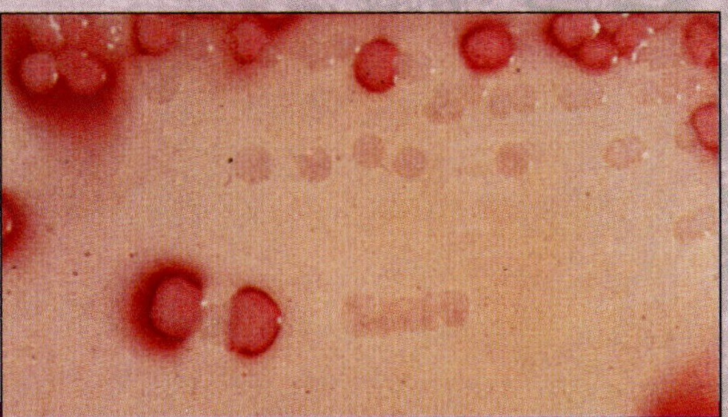

Plate 16 Bright pink lactose fermenting colonies and straw or pale non-lactose fermenting colonies on McConkey agar

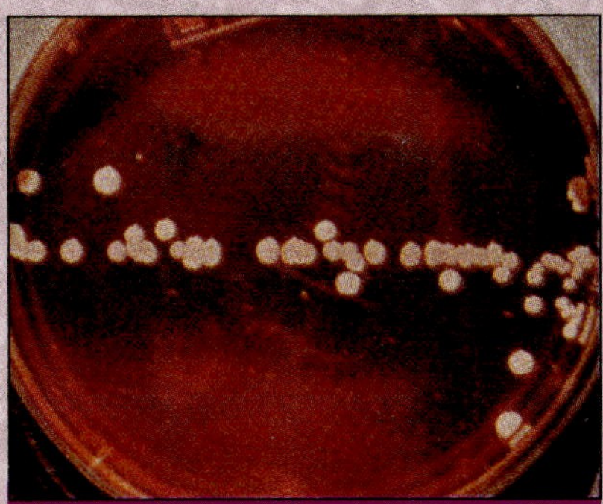

Plate 17 Blood agar plate showing isolated, golden, creamy beta hemolytic colonies

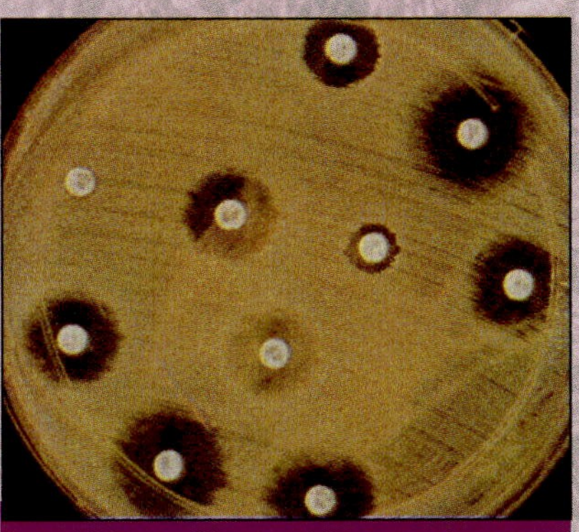

Plate 18 Kirby Bauer antibiotic sensitivity test.

BACTERIOLOGY/MYCOLOGY

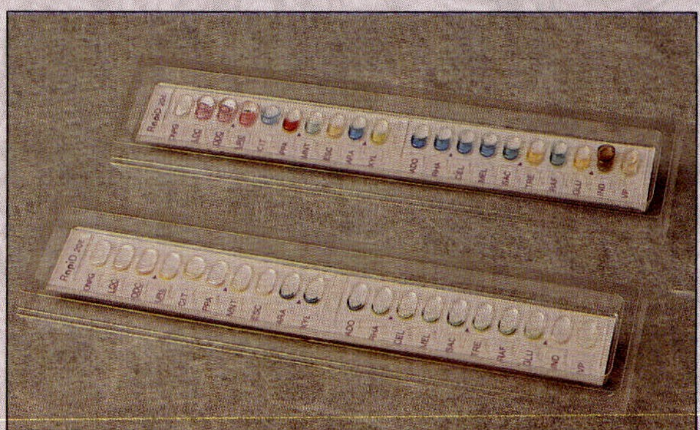

Plate 19 API Gram Negative identification system for Gram negative bacilli.

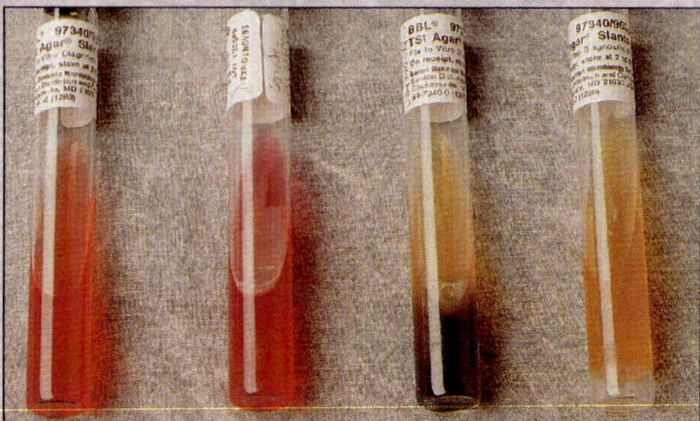

Plate 20 Triple Sugar Iron Agar reactions for the identification of gram negative enteric bacteria.

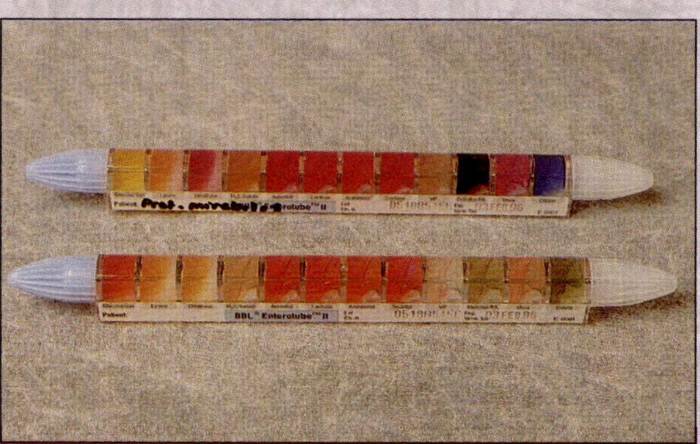

Plate 21 Enterotube system for identification of gram negative enteric bacteria.

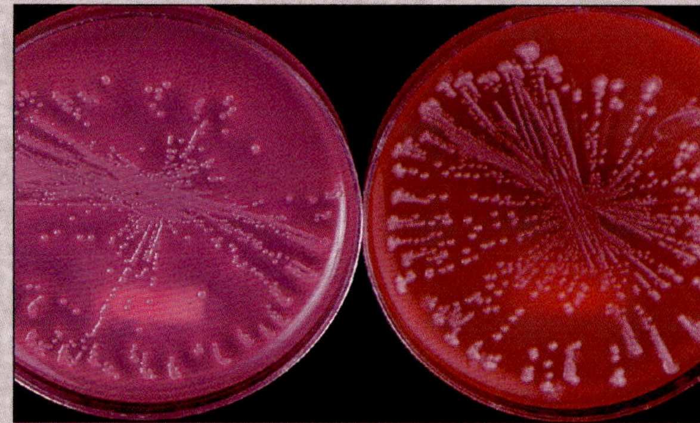

Plate 22 Blood and MacConkey Plates showing a positive streaked colony count of $>10^5$ cfu/ml of *E. coli*

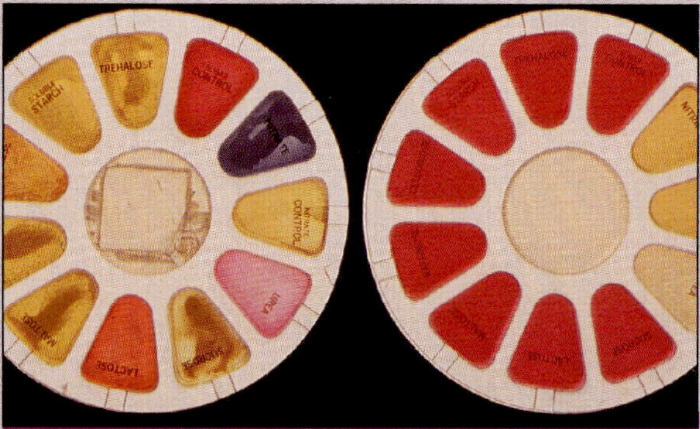

Plate 23 Uni-Yeast-Tek Plate for the identification of Yeasts and fungi. (Courtesy Remel, Inc.)

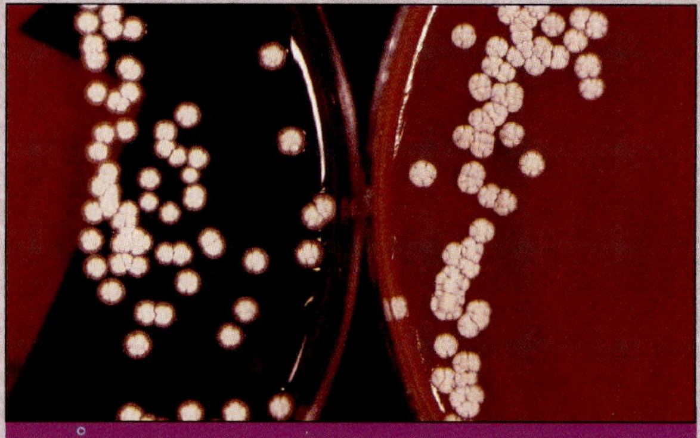

Plate 24 *Nocardia asteriodes* on blood and Chocolate agar

MYCOLOGY/HEMATOLOGY

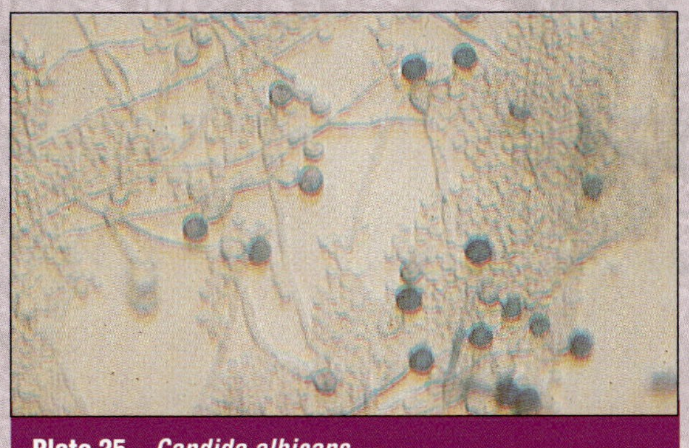

Plate 25 *Candida albicans*

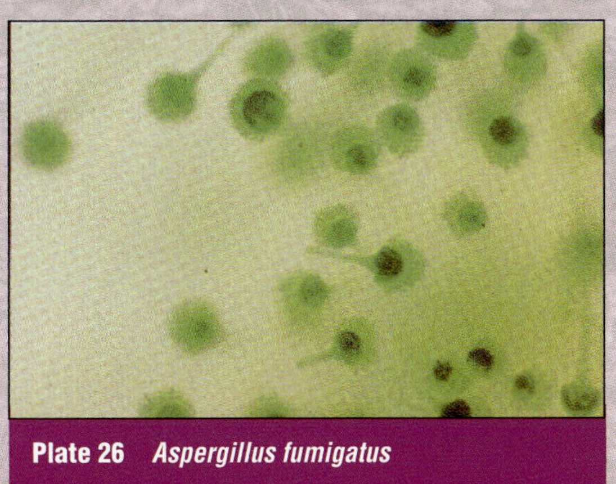

Plate 26 *Aspergillus fumigatus*

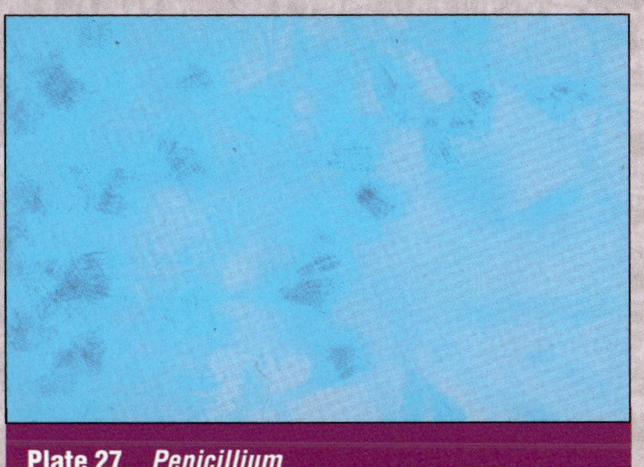

Plate 27 *Penicillium*

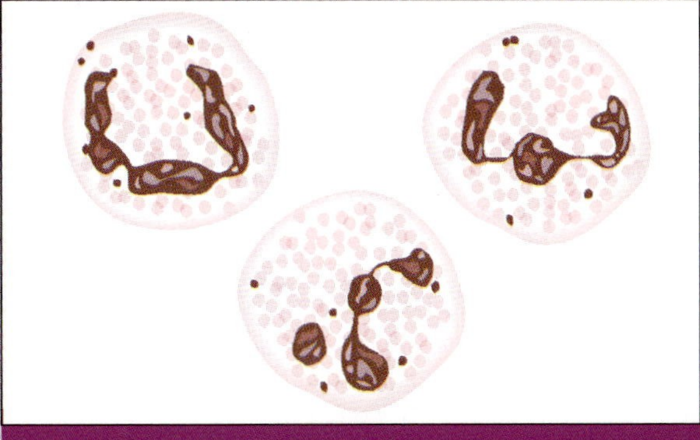

Plate 28 Segmented neutrophils (phagocytes)

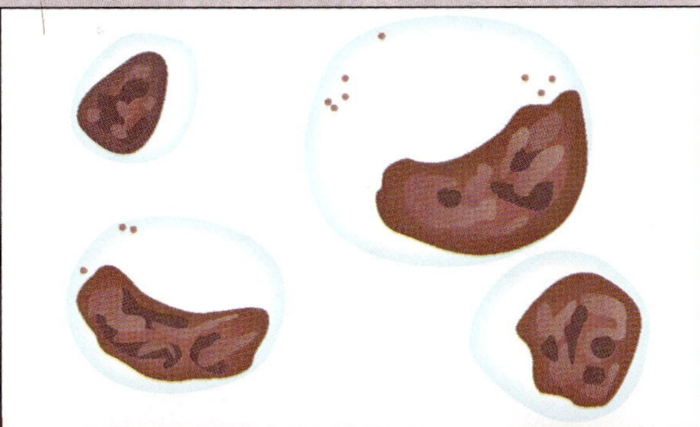

Plate 29 Lymphocytes, large and small

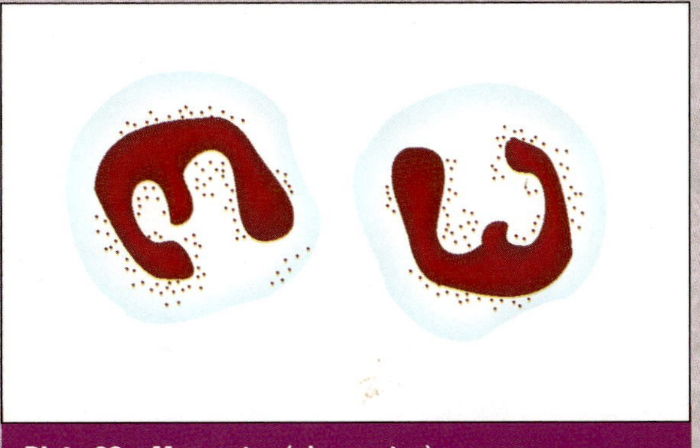

Plate 30 Monocytes (phagocytes)

BLOOD PARASITES

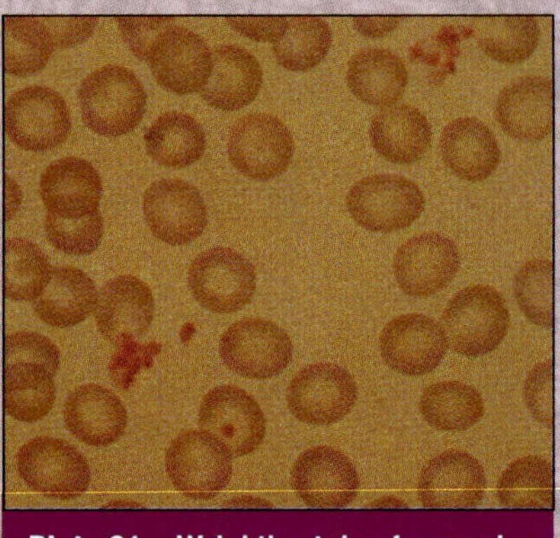

Plate 31 Wright's stain of normal red blood cells and platelets

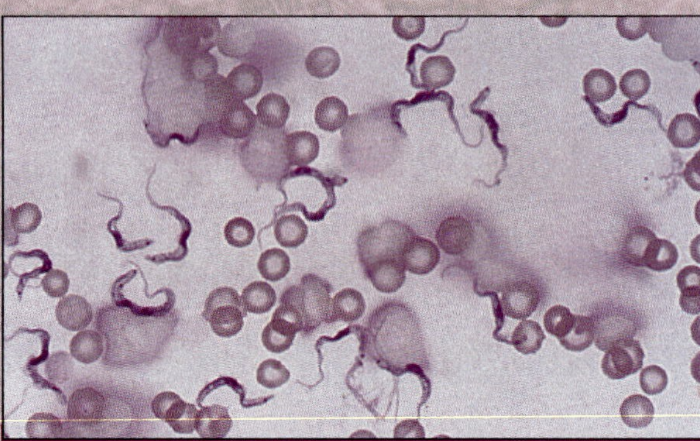

Plate 32 *Trypanosoma cruzi*, tryptomasigote in blood

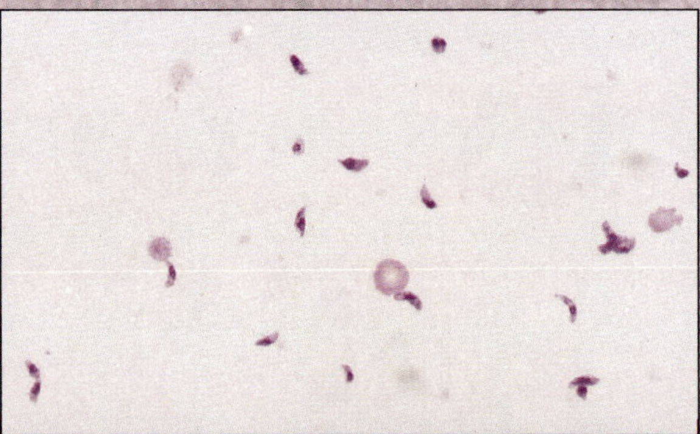

Plate 33 *Toxoplasma gondii*, trophozoite in a blood smear

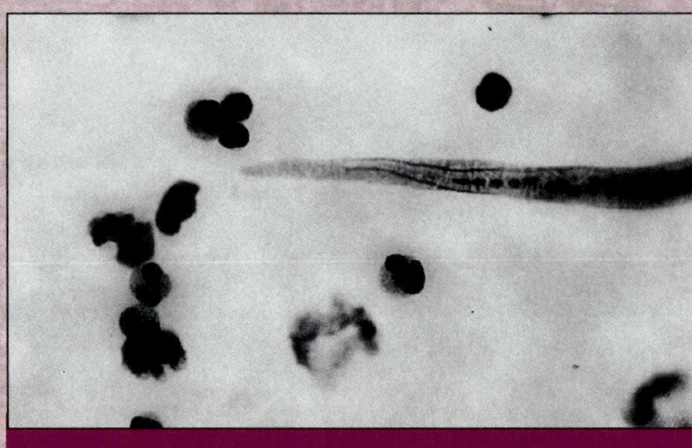

Plate 34 *Wuschereria bancrofi* microfalaries, anterior portion

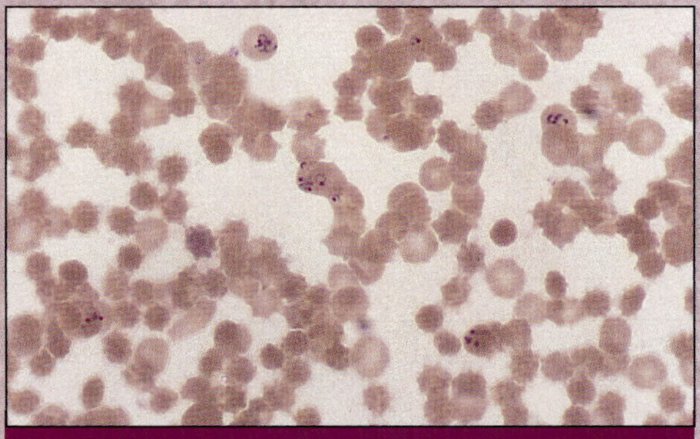

Plate 35 *P. falciparium*, ring stage

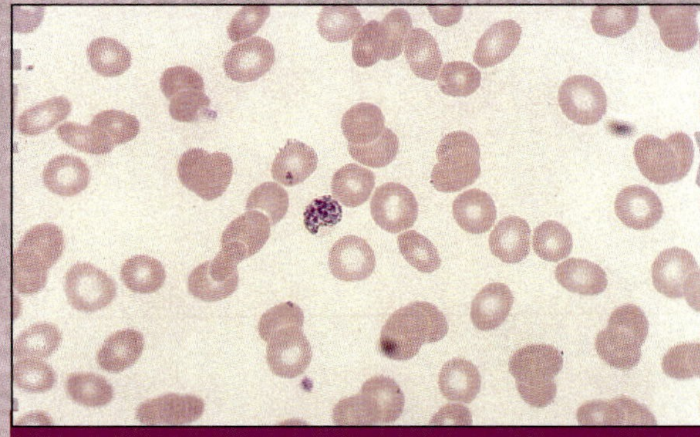

Plate 36 *P. malariae*, gametocytes.

PARASITES

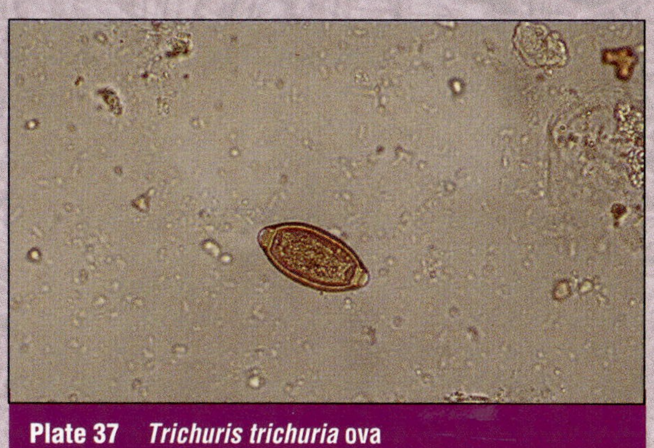

Plate 37 *Trichuris trichuria* ova

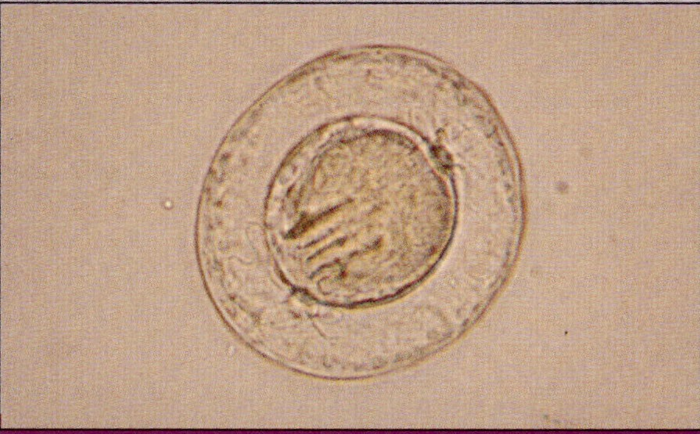

Plate 38 *Hymenolepsis nana* ova

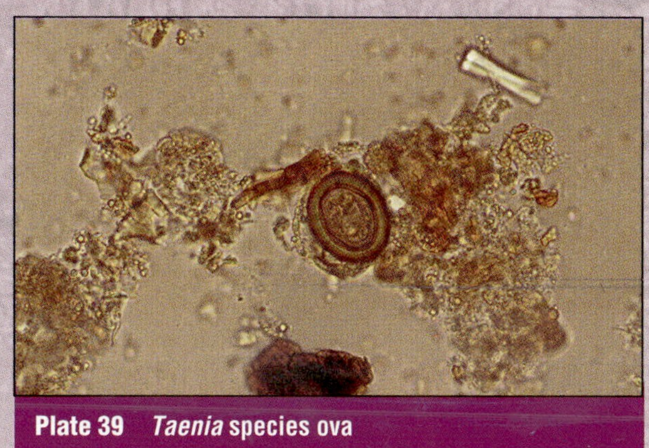

Plate 39 *Taenia* species ova

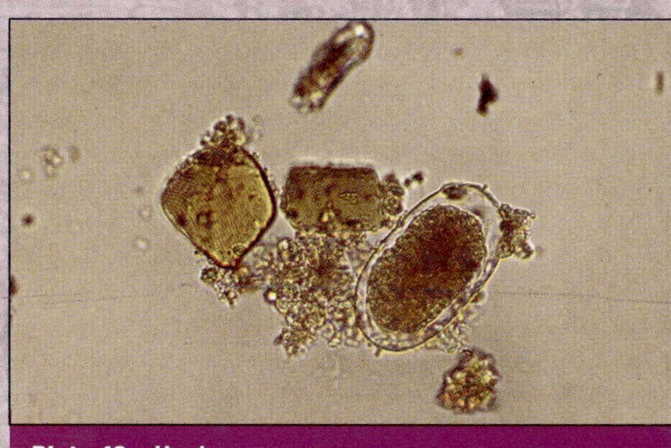

Plate 40 Hookworm ova

Plate 41 *Clonorchis sinensis* adult worm

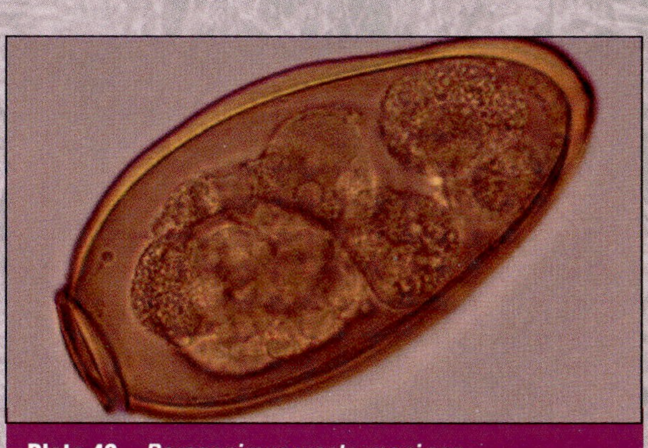

Plate 42 *Paragonimus westermani* egg

PARASITES (continued)

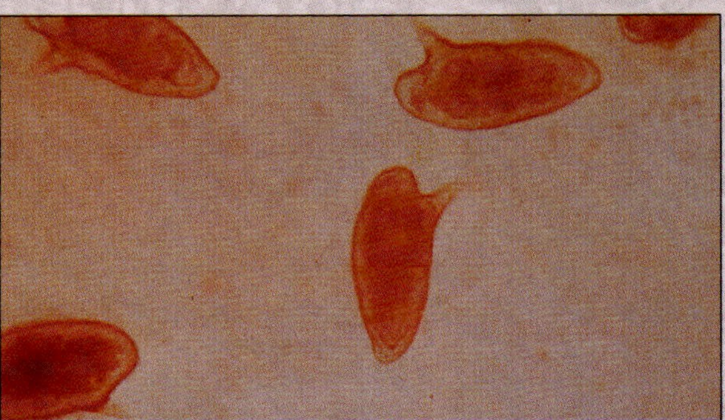

Plate 43 *Schistosoma mansoni* eggs showing lateral spines (Courtesy of the Armed Forces Institute of Pathology [AFIP]).

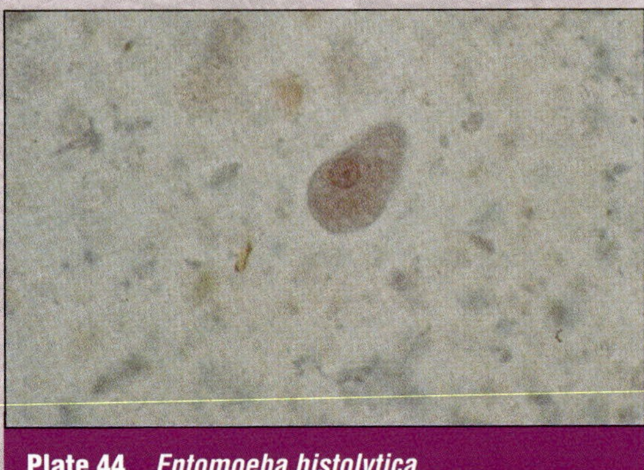

Plate 44 *Entomoeba histolytica.*

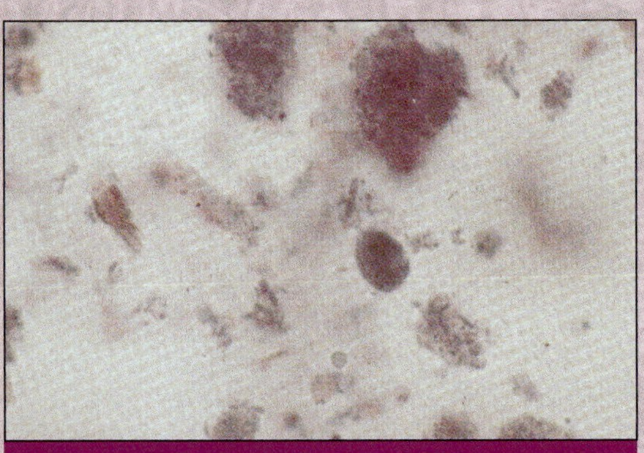

Plate 45 *Giardia lamblia.*

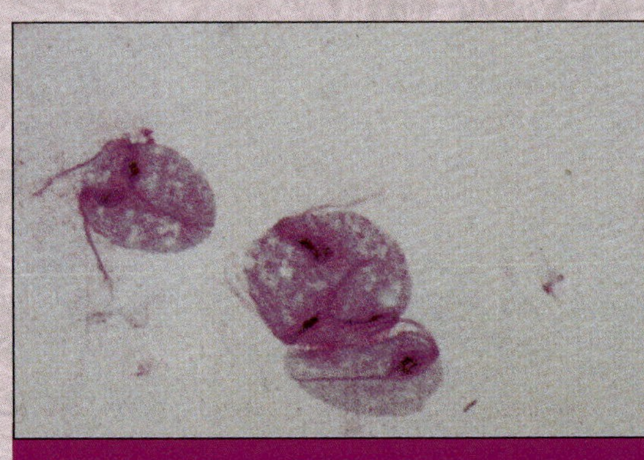

Plate 46 *Trichomonas vaginalis.*

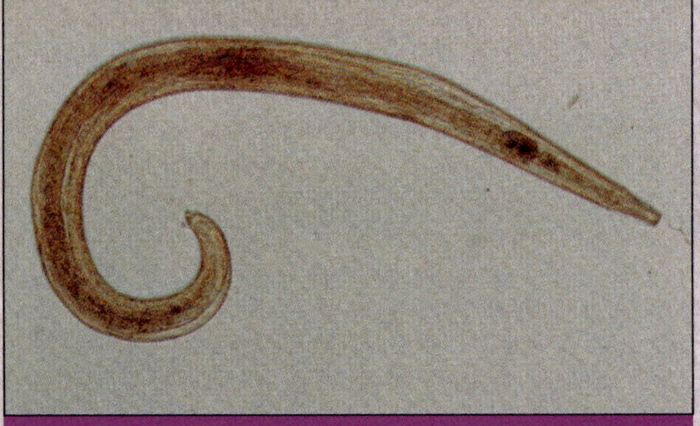

Plate 47 *Enterobius vermicularis* (pinworm).

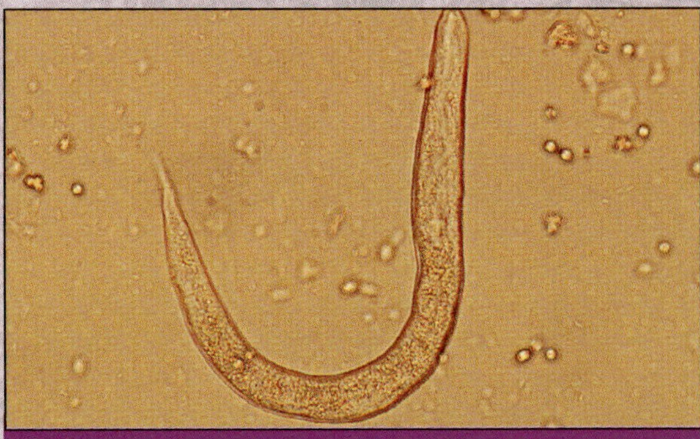

Plate 48 *Strongyloides stercoralis.*

DNA and phage protein coats, or **capsids.** For the first 10 to 15 minutes after the infection of the bacterial cell, no phages are detected. This phase is called the **eclipse period.**

Maturation. Over the next 10 to 15 minutes, actual phages start to appear very quickly. The phage DNA and phage protein coat are being packaged to form the mature infective phages.

Release. Soon after the initial phage infection, the bacterial cell bursts open, or **lyses,** to release new phages in search of other cells to infect. This process occurs as a result of a phage enzyme lysozyme, which is secreted near the end of the maturation stage to digest the bacterial host's cell wall. When this happens, the bacterial cell lyses and releases all the newly formed phages. These phages in turn infect other susceptible bacterial cells. This process of viral or phage infection and replication is repeated.

This activity may cause a variety of cellular changes, depending on the characteristics of the virus and the susceptibility of the host cell. It may cause no observable change or damage to the host. In this case the virus infection is termed **latent.** Conversely, such cell damage can result in disease. For example, HIV attaches to the CD4 receptor on T4 lymphocytes and monocytes, and the cell damage or destruction can result in disease.

A chemical substance called **interferon** is produced by cells after they become infected or parasitized with a virus. Interferon has been found to prevent replication of viruses in other cells of the same kind. It appears to be an important factor in the recovery from viral infections. Interferon has also been shown to prevent cancer cells from reproducing. The major drawback to the use of interferon for cancer treatment was once the cost. Six pints of human blood yield barely enough white blood corpuscles to produce a single day's supply of interferon for just one patient. This makes the price of one millionth of an ounce $1500; a pound of interferon would cost about $22 billion. However, the cost of making interferon is no longer a problem. A new technique of making interferon in the laboratory has made the production of interferon less costly and more efficient.

Some viruses, such as the influenza virus, are capable of rapid change in their genetic material. When this happens, a new viral strain is produced that can infect people who used to be immune to the virus.

Many different ways of classifying viruses have been tried, but no single way has proven entirely satisfactory. Listed are some of the groups of viruses that contain members pathogenic to humans. They are classified by the type of nucleic acid and by the size, shape, and substructure of the parasite (Figure 12–4).

- **Poxvirus group**—relatively large, brick-shaped viruses containing DNA, and chiefly pathogenic for the skin. Examples: smallpox, cowpox.
- **Herpesvirus group**—medium-sized, twenty-sided viruses containing DNA. Latent infections may occur and last the lifespan of the host. Examples: cold sores, shingles, chickenpox.
- **Adenovirus group**—medium-sized, cube-shaped viruses containing DNA. Examples: catarrhs, some types of conjunctivitis.
- **Papovavirus group**—small, cube-shaped viruses with circular DNA. Example: wart virus.
- **Myxovirus group**—medium-sized viruses of helical form containing RNA. Example: influenza viruses.

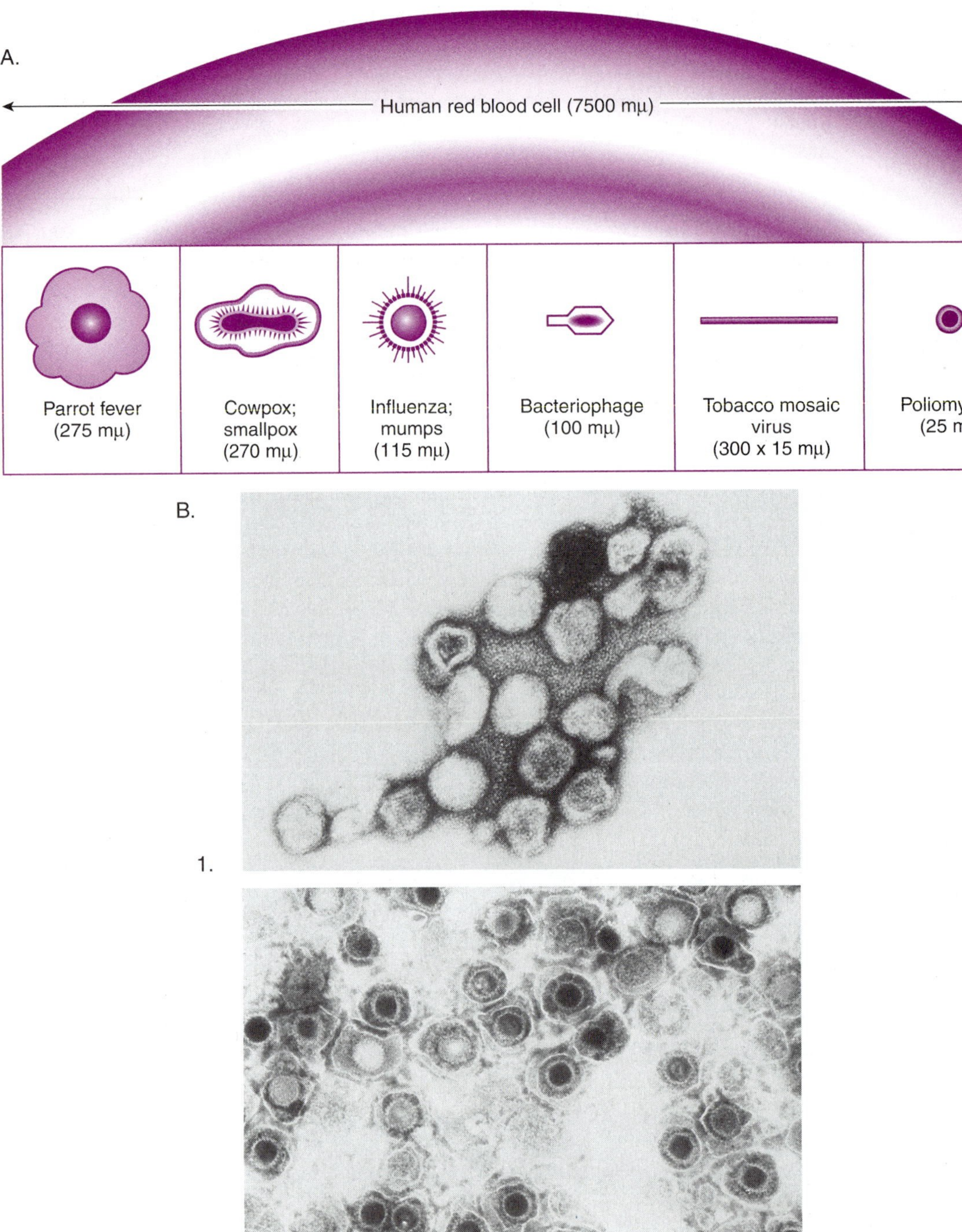

Figure 12–4 (A) Relative size and shape of various viruses as compared with that of a human red blood cell, (B) examples of viruses: (1) rubella and (2) herpes simplex (*Courtesy of Centers for Disease Control and Prevention, Atlanta, GA*)

- **Paramyxovirus group**—similar to but larger than the myxoviruses. Examples: measles, mumps.
- **Rhabdovirus group**—bullet-shaped viruses containing RNA. Example: rabies.
- **Arbovirus group**—arthropodborne viruses (carried by insects, ticks, or mites). Examples: yellow fever, equine encephalitis.
- **Picornavirus group**—small, cube-shaped viruses containing RNA and divided into two groups: enteroviruses (include poliovirus) and rhinoviruses (most common cause of colds in human beings).

VIRUS FACTS

We should be aware of these facts about viruses: (1) they are generally more resistant to some disinfectants than are most bacteria; (2) most of them have about the same susceptibility to heat, except the hepatitis viruses, which are very resistant; and (3) most viruses are not affected by sulfonamides or other antibiotics, so that giving penicillin for a common cold only adds to the resistance factor of penicillins and does nothing for the cold. Today the following facts are pertinent:

- You can get HIV if you have unprotected sex. Unprotected sex can increase the chances of getting any of the other sexually transmitted diseases including genital warts, chlamydia, herpes, gonorrhoea, syphilis, and hepatitis to name a few.
- Latex condoms are effective barriers.
- Mothers can transmit HIV to their unborn children.
- Women have a higher risk of getting infected during heterosexual sex.
- Not all who have HIV have AIDS. It is important to know that many diseases are caused by specific viruses, and that treatment is not the same for all.

VIRUS MYTHS

In addition to the above viral facts, it should be noted that several myths about viruses still exist today. The ideas that viral detection is of academic interest only, is of epidemiological interest only, and that viruses are too slow and difficult to grow are easily dispelled in that today there are much easier and faster detection methods. Viral cell culture media can be purchased commercially as may any bacteriological culture media. Although serological tests may be faster than culture, they are not necessarily easier or cheaper to perform. Today the following myths are pertinent: (1) Your partner may get offended if you ask him to use a condom; (2) you can get HIV if you use the same toilet seat that an HIV-infected person used; (3) you can get HIV from breathing the air around an HIV-infected person; (4) if you get an HIV test, others will know your test result too; and (5) using a condom will reduce the pleasure of having sex.

AIDS VIRUS

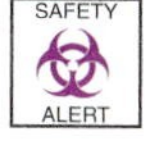

At this point, some very important and basic information about the virus that causes **acquired immunodeficiency syndrome,** commonly called **AIDS,** should be presented in a logical and forthright manner to the microbiology student and health care professional.

Acquired Immunodeficiency Syndrome

To date, much publicity and media attention still focuses on the gay population and intravenous (I.V.) drug users. Although it is true that these populations are at the greatest risk, today HIV infection (and then AIDS) is a disease that affects all walks of life just as any other sexually transmitted disease. In our world, one teenager is infected every day with the virus. Females and heterosexuals alike are contracting the disease. On a good note, however, since the blood supply has been tested universally the incidence of hemophiliacs' infections have decreased. Without a doubt, much controversy and emotionalism still surrounds AIDS.

The following information is intended to answer the various questions that a health care professional may have about AIDS, such as: What causes AIDS? What are its symptoms? What is the mode of transmission of AIDS? How infectious is it? What preventive measures should be taken to avoid its transmission or acquisition?

Discovery of AIDS

Between October 1980 and May 1981, five previously healthy young men were treated for a pneumonia caused by the parasite, *Pneumocystis carinii.* They were treated at three different hospitals in Los Angeles. Doctors and health care professionals took special note of this situation. Before this time, *P. carinii* pneumonia occurred only in patients who were **immunosuppressed** (suppression of the immune system, such that there is a decreased ability to fight disease and infections), especially those patients receiving cancer therapy. At the same time, a rare and unusual blood vessel malignancy called **Kaposi's sarcoma** was being diagnosed with increasing frequency in young males in California and New York. By July, 1981, twenty-six cases of Kaposi's sarcoma had been diagnosed in young previously healthy men. Seven of these men also had serious infections, and four of them had *P. carinii* pneumonia. In North America, male homosexuals, drug addicts, Haitians, and hemophiliacs were the first noted to be infected. Today, the disease has been found in all walks of life among male and female heterosexuals, homosexuals, intravenous (I.V.) drug users, babies who have been infected during fetal life or as nursing infants, and hemophiliacs. Certainly, the high-risk groups still include I.V. drug users and sexually promiscuous men and women.

These cases were an early indication that an epidemic of a previously unknown disease was on the horizon. Meanwhile, Robert Gallo, a physician from Connecticut, was studying **enzymes** that produced DNA in blood cells and looking for a **retrovirus** (an RNA virus that carries an enzyme capable of forming DNA from RNA) that could cause human leukemia. He happened upon a method to cultivate **T-lymphocyte** cells in tissue culture, which allowed him to grow one of his retroviruses, "human T-cell lymphoma virus," or HTLV. At first his discovery received little attention because there was no disease associated with HTLV, until Japanese researchers identified their "adult T-cell leukemia" (ATL) virus, a particularly aggressive leukemia the same as Gallo's HTLV virus. It soon became evident that this virus was found throughout most of the Caribbean, northern South America, and much of Africa, where it was endemic. Gallo hypothesized that it originated in Africa, where monkeys as well as people were infected, and it made its way to Japan and the Americas as a stowaway in slave ships. Now, reports were adrift linking a rare skin cancer, Kaposi's sarcoma, and a usually harmless parasite *Pneumocys-*

tis carinii with enlarged lymph nodes and a cancer called non-Hodgkin's lymphoma. These **afflictions** were seen mostly in young, white males (many of whom were homosexuals and I.V. drug users), who had frequent transfusions, and Haitians. In central Africa, people were dying of this disease, irrespective of gender. The disease was named the acquired immunodeficiency syndrome (AIDS). Dr. Gallo surmised that this syndrome might have been caused by a virus and quite naturally thought of his retrovirus.

Meanwhile, in Paris, Dr. Jacques Leibowich was doing similar work. He found his HTLV virus in a French AIDS patient who had received a blood transfusion while in the civil service in Haiti. Dr. Leibowich's sister provided him with blood from a leukemia patient in Zaire for the African connection. A third researcher, Luc Montagnier of the Pasteur Institute, was working with a retrovirus called "lymphadenopathy-associated virus" (LAV) that he thought was the cause of AIDS. His virus had been isolated from a Frenchman who had visited New York City in the 1970s.

Ultimately, professional discrepancies resulted, and in 1987 the U.S. team and the French group were given joint credit for discovering the HTLV-III/LAV as the cause of AIDS. As research progressed, the disease came to be known as AIDS. After nearly 20 years of living with this disease its incidence had grown from a mere few thousand cases in the United States to many millions of cases now found worldwide. Its origin is debatable, but it is generally thought that it originated in Africa as a mutant of a simian virus. It may have spread via migrant workers to Haiti, a popular resort area for American homosexual males who in turn spread the virus to the United States. The virus **human immunodeficiency virus** (HIV) (Figure 12–5), is carried in blood, semen, and body fluids, although urine has not been implicated to date. For people who have contracted AIDS, it is usually fatal. The virus is now known to be able to lie dormant for years, exhibiting no symptoms before its devastation strikes.

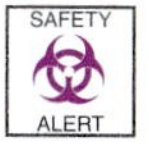

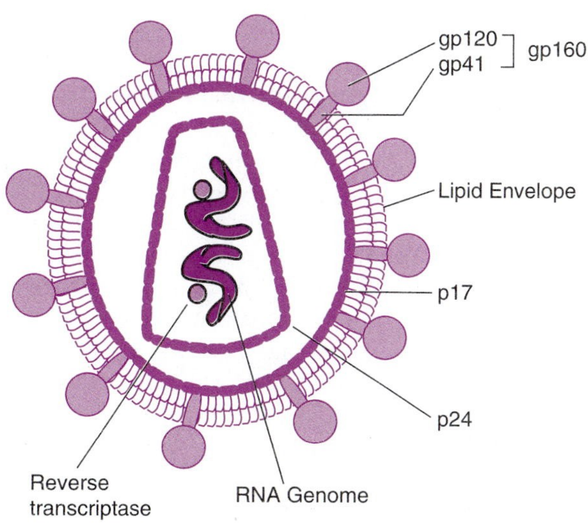

Figure 12–5 HIV virus

As research has progressed we are finding that certain drug combinations slow the rate of the invasive effects of the virus on white blood cell destruction, namely the T-lymphocytes, giving patients a longer life expectancy. A cure is not yet on the horizon, although scientists are working diligently to come up with an effective vaccine that will stop the virus's replication at various stages of its invasion into the white blood cells. The virus is affecting all populations and has moved beyond the large urban metropolitan areas to rural America. Infection among women is on the rise. It is now the fourth leading cause of death in young adults aged 25 to 44.

History and Causative Agent of AIDS

The causative agent of AIDS is a retrovirus (a virus, 90 to 120 nm in diameter, whose genetic material contains duplicate copies of high-molecular-weight, single-stranded RNA) (see Figure 12–5). In 1983, researchers working at the Pasteur Institute in Paris first isolated a new retrovirus from a patient with **lymphadenopathy** (an abnormal enlargement of the lymph glands such as seen in Hodgkin's disease, lymphatic leukemia, or infectious mononucleosis). It was called lymphadenopathy-associated virus (LAV). The following year, American researchers at the National Institutes of Health (NIH) isolated a similar retrovirus from an AIDS patient. They named their virus HTLV-3 for human T-cell lymphotropic virus, type III. Since the two viruses proved to be identical, and to avoid international tension in the scientific community, the organism is now called human immunodeficiency virus type 1 (HIV-I). A related strain (HIV-II) has subsequently been recovered from patients with AIDS in Africa.

Incubation period.

The **incubation period** (the period between becoming infected and the actual development of the disease symptoms) for AIDS is quite long, ranging from 6 months to 5 or more years. In some recent cases, doctors and health care professionals have discovered patients whose incubation period was up to 10 years.

After being infected with HIV, as with any infection, there is a lag period before antibodies are detected serologically. Sometimes a mild illness, not unlike flu symptoms, appears about 7 to 14 days after infection. This is often shrugged off as the flu when symptoms disappear. When these symptoms do not disappear as described previously, infection with HIV may be considered, especially if the patient acquires one of the alerting opportunistic infections. Sometimes no symptoms occur for years. Unless there is concern, one is not routinely tested for the presence of HIV. However, today it is accepted that once infected with the virus, AIDS will develop at some time in the future in all cases. In one study, however, only one-third of the patients infected actually had developed AIDS within a period of 3 years. It is projected that the remaining two-thirds will develop the disease by the tenth year. For a complete list of AIDS indicator diseases, see Table 12–1.

At present, there is no cure for AIDS; however, the opportunistic infections associated with AIDS can be treated. Several experimental drugs are being developed and tested on AIDS patients in the United States and Europe, particularly at the Pasteur Institute in Paris. Other doctors and health care professionals are treating patients with only minimal symptoms early in the onset of their disease to see if more serious symptoms can be prevented. The development of various vaccines has been reported in the media, but these findings must be taken with precaution. Researchers are working fervently to develop an AIDS vaccine and hopefully we will see one on the market soon.

Table 12–1 Some Common Infectious Agents and Syndromes Associated with AIDS

Infection	Cause	Organism Type
Thrush or moniliasis Pneumonia	*Candida albicans* Herpes simplex I Oran hairy leukoplakia *Pneumocystis carinii*	Yeast Virus Unknown Parasite
	Cryptococcus neoformans *Mycobacterium avium* *Streptococcus pneumoniae* *Mycobacterium tuberculosis* *Aspergillis* sp.	Yeast Bacteria Bacteria Bacteria Fungus
Toxoplasmosis Chronic diarrhea	*Toxoplasma* *Cryptosporidia* *Isospora belli*	Parasite Parasite Parasite
Malignancies	*Giardia lamblia* *Salmonella* *Shigella* Lymphoma Kaposi's sarcoma	Parasite Bacteria Bacteria Cancer Cancer
	B-cell lymphoma	Cancer
Other	Cytomegalovirus (CMV)	Virus

AIDS has been brought to prominence through the passage of the Ryan White Care Act of 1990, which provided disaster relief for cities hardest hit by the HIV epidemic. In 1991 when a famous basketball personality announced his positive results, thousands began to get tested for HIV. That same year a young dental patient, Kimberly Bergalis, was believed to have contracted the virus from her dentist. This incident was the catalyst to have all health care providers tested for the virus. New drugs came into play. By 1992 AIDS diagnosis was further defined by recognizing cervical cancers, pulmonary tuberculosis, and recurrent pneumonia as commonplace with the disease and announcing that a positive HIV test and a CD4 T-lymphocyte cell count of less than 200 was diagnostic for AIDS. Combination drug treatments were reported to be successful. Arthur Ashe, the U.S. Wimbledon champion tennis player, contracted HIV through tainted blood following surgery. As 1993 rolled in, research for a cure pressed on with no real headway, but great strides were made in public awareness of the disease as Congress found funds to increase education and prevention. The backbone of treatment before symptoms occur is zidovudine (AZT), which is shown to have little effect at this point but is better suited to combination therapy and to reducing risk of transmission from infected mothers to their newborn infants. By 1995 President Clinton recognized the need for more AIDS education and research by holding the first-ever White House AIDS Summit. Combination drug therapies are having success, as more are continuously being developed. The year 1995 marked the date that cryptosporidiosis became a serious health issue for HIV-infected patients wherever water treatment processes were not sufficient to kill this tiny, normally nonpathogenic parasite. By 1996 two new protease-inhibiting drugs, ritonavir and indinavir, were introduced with the high hope of controlling the disease. They have shown success in combination with other regimes. A herpes virus was found to be the causative agent for Kaposi's sarcoma. For the past 2 years, the CDC has been announcing a dramatic decrease in deaths due to AIDS, which indicates that more people with the virus are living with the disease much longer thanks to the successful regimes of combination therapies. Regimes are necessary because these drugs must be taken faithfully on time every day without fail. For the first time in the history of tracking the epidemic, the number of newly diagnosed AIDS patients has decreased thanks to the successful education and prevention measures taken in this country.

Signs and Symptoms of AIDS

AIDS is a disease that suppresses the body's natural immune system. Thus, a patient with AIDS cannot fight off cancers and most ordinary infections. Because they are immunocompromised, these patients are open to severe infections caused by organisms that are considered normal inhabitants of the atmosphere or body for healthy individuals. These infections are often referred to as **opportunistic** infections because they can take over the body the moment one's immune system is unable to fight them off. The term AIDS stands for:

A (acquired)—The disease is not inherited or caused by any form of medication;
I (immuno)—Refers to the body's natural defenses against cancers, disease, and infections;
D (deficiency)—Lacking in cellular immunity;
S (syndrome)—The set of diseases or conditions that are present to signal the diagnosis.

The first signs of HIV infection can be seen in 1 to 4 weeks with mononucleosislike symptoms that may include swelling of the lymph nodes, headache, fever, loss of appetite, and sore throat. These are symptoms commonly mistaken for the flu or other viral infection. Sometimes people develop skin rashes on the chest, abdomen, or back (but the symptoms are not to be confused with Kaposi's sarcoma). At this time it is usually too early to have formed detectable antibodies. All too often, though, no symptoms are detected for years as the immune system is still intact and able to fight off any minor symptoms such as those mentioned.

Eventually the body will **seroconvert,** that is, develop detectable antibodies. At this point the HIV test will be positive. The white blood cells, specifically the CD4 T-helper lymphocytes, will now be infected with the virus. The **CD4 cells** are special helper cells to the immune system that help fight the virus. Although one may remain healthy for years, there are often psychological symptoms of depression and anxiety about the future. It may be 5 years before any physical signs are seen. As long as the CD4 cells are producing, symptoms will be postponed. An afflicted person's general health and age also factor into the equation of how long he or she will remain healthy.

Next, as the immune system becomes compromised due to the destruction of the CD4 cells, infections that are normally easily overcome occur more frequently. The most common of these include thrush, caused by a yeast *Candida albicans;* shingles, caused by *Herpes zoster;* pneumonia, caused by *Streptococcus pneumoniae,* **oral hairy leukoplakia,** an infection resembling thrush of unknown origin; and idiopathic thrombocytopenia purpura, a condition that occurs when a person develops antibodies that attack the platelet cells in the blood, causing excessive bruising and bleeding. Additional generalized symptoms such as diarrhea, weight loss, fever, and fatigue become persistent.

Acquired Immunodeficiency Syndrome (AIDS)

As the immune system becomes increasingly compromised, the body is not able to fight off more serious infections that the normal immune system could suppress. Life-threatening infections develop that eventually result in the death of the AIDS patient.

HIV is carried in blood and semen. It can penetrate mucosal surfaces, as some cases of AIDS have developed following artificial insemination. It can be transmitted through blood and blood products, thus accounting for infection among hemophiliacs.

AIDS is the most severe type of HIV infection. When a patient has AIDS, the immune system is severely suppressed. Thus, the person becomes highly susceptible to certain cancers and opportunistic infections, including:

- Cancers, especially Kaposi's sarcoma and at times primary **lymphoma** (tumors) of the brain.
- Parasitic infections such as *Pneumocystis carinii* pneumonia and toxoplasmosis. (Toxoplasmosis is a disease caused by a sporozoan protozoa called *Toxoplasma gondii.* Human toxoplasmosis is acquired either orally or congenitally through the placenta from an infected mother. Oral transmission has a source either in cat feces or in inadequately prepared meat of infected animals. Orally acquired toxoplasmosis seldom causes illness and may often go undetected, marked only by fatigue and muscle pains. Acute toxoplasmosis is rare. Symptoms range from fever, lymphadenopathy, muscle fatigue, and pain to cerebral infection. Its symptoms can mimic aseptic meningitis, hepatitis, myocarditis, or pneumonia, depending on the site of the parasite.)
- Fungal infections such as candidiasis and histoplasmosis. (Histoplasmosis is an infection caused by the fungus, *Histoplasma capsulatum.* The symptoms range from a mild respiratory infection to more severe ones such as fever, anemia, **hepatomegaly** [liver enlargement], **splenomegaly** [spleen enlargement], **leukopenia** [reduction of the number of white blood cells in the peripheral blood], pulmonary lesions, gastrointestinal ulcerations, and suprarenal necrosis.)
- Viral infections such as cytomegalovirus disease, herpes simplex, hepatitis B, and non-A, non-B hepatitis. (Cytomegalovirus [CMV] disease is a particularly severe one in immunosuppressed persons, especially those with AIDS. Symptoms range from hepatitis and mononucleosis to pneumonia.)

The symptoms of AIDS are often nonspecific. These symptoms are often similar to such illnesses as the common cold or the flu. When they persist, one may become suspicious of a more serious malady. Some of these suspicious symptoms may include:

- Prolonged fatigue and/or malaise that is not due to physical exertion or other disorders
- Persistent fevers or night sweats
- A persistent, unexplained cough
- A thick, whitish hairlike coating in the throat or on the tongue
- Easy bruising or unexplained bleeding

- Recent appearance of discolored or purplish lesions of the mucous membranes or skin that do not go away and slowly increase in size
- Chronic diarrhea
- Shortness of breath
- Unexplained lymphadenopathy (swollen glands) that has persisted over 3 months
- Unexplained weight loss of 10 or more pounds in less than 2 months

Symptoms and treatment of the secondary infectious agents that ultimately lead to the demise of the AIDS patient are described in Table 12–2.

Table 12–2 Some Common Opportunistic Infections Found in AIDS Patients

Disease & Description	Symptoms	Treatment
Thrush This is the most common infection among HIV-positive people. It is a condition that is located in the mouth and is caused by a fungus, *Candida albicans.*	White patches on the walls of the mouth, gums, and tongue are good indications of infection. May experience a burning sensation and altered sense of taste. It is irritating more than anything else.	Clotrimazole, troches, and nystatin
Herpes zoster (shingles) A virus that causes chicken pox in children. Anyone who has had chicken pox has the virus for *Herpes zoster* in the nerves of their body. Immune deficiencies and stress are the two main factors that cause reactivation of this virus as shingles in adults.	Shingles looks like a red rash that normally appears in a specific area, and may look like a band around the body. It is very itchy and painful. Headaches, fever, and fatigue may accompany the rash.	Analgesics are used to control the pain. Oral acyclovir works best when started as early as possible to decrease the severity of the symptoms.
Herpes simplex It is a common sexually transmitted disease. In HIV/AIDS patients it may become a chronic condition. As the immune function decreases, the frequency of herpes simplex and the severity increases.	Herpes simplex affects the rectal, genital, and esophageal regions. Painful lesions are observed that can erupt into ulcerations of the area.	Oral Acyclovir 200 mg four times a day for 2 weeks or longer, or until the lesions disappear. New forms of this type of drug are being developed that have an increased effect on the disease.
Oral hairy leukoplakia This infection of the mouth resembles thrush. The cause is unknown.	White patches in the mouth	None

Table 12–2 Continued

Disease & Description	Symptoms	Treatment
Idiopathic thrombocytopenia purpura When a person develops antibodies that attack the platelets, which are responsible for the clotting of blood. This condition can go undetected.	Excessive bleeding and bruising	Use of zidovudine (AZT), prednisone, I.V. gamma globulin, a splenectomy, danazol, or no treatment at all.
Pneumococcal pneumonia This infection of the lungs is one of the most common causes of pneumonia in people with AIDS.	Lung congestion, difficulty breathing. A pneumococcal vaccine may be appropriate for prevention and treatment.	Antibiotics, penicillin derivatives
HIV-related lymphoma Tumors of the lymph glands	Very large lymph glands in the neck, groin, or under the arms	Radiation and chemotherapy
Toxoplasmosis encephalitis Caused by the parasite *Toxoplasmosis gondii,* found in the stools of cats and uncooked meats. It can cause a brain infection leading to neurological impairment and seizures.	Headaches, fevers, lethargy, confusion, and seizures; uncoordinated walking and loss of balance also occur.	Sulfadiazine and/or pyrimethamine. Clindamycin may be used for those with sulfa drug allergies. Folinic acid is administered. Also AZT may be helpful. Treatment continues for life, once diagnosed.
Cytomegalovirus infection About 90% of AIDS patients develop CMV. It presents as a monolike illness. The virus is similar to that of toxoplasma and pneumocystis.	It is located in the blood and distributed to all parts of the body, causing infections in many different organs. Eye infections and lung infections are common.	Ganciclovir and foscarnet
Cryptococcus neoformans The fungus *Cryptococcus neoformans* is found in the soil and pigeon droppings. The brain is the most serious site of infection.	Fatigue, fever, nausea, vomiting. Accompanying headaches are not always specific to one region of the head. Encephalitis, inflammation of the brain, along with altered mental states, memory loss, confusion, and behavioral changes, may also be present.	Amphotericin B, with or without flucytostine (5FU). Once stable the patient is treated with fluconazole for life.

Table 12–2 Concluded

Disease & Description	Symptoms	Treatment
Pneumocystis pneumonia A parasite, *Pneumocystis carinii,* is the cause. PCP is the most common opportunistic infection, therefore **prophylaxis** (i.e., use of drugs to prevent infection) is important.	Usually seen in patients with CD4 counts under 200. Early medical intervention is important. Symptoms include fever, respiratory problems, and other pneumonia-like indications.	Trimethoprim/sulfamethoxazole bactrim or septra, dapsone, or pentamidine
Cryptosporidium Drinking water is the most common route for this parasitic infection.	Diarrhea and weight loss	No effective treatments at this time
Kaposi's sarcoma A condition in which tumors of the blood vessels develop. Cause is unknown, but recently a suspect virus has been isolated. This malignancy originates in the endothelial or lymphatic cells.	Small, nonpainful reddish, purple, or black tumors or lesions arise anywhere on the skin, in the GI tract, mouth, lungs, groin, liver, and lymph glands. Even though treated, recurrences are common.	Local lesions are treated only if painful or interfering with cosmetic problems. Radiotherapy, cryotherapy, or intralesional injections with vinblastine are also used.
Mycobacterium tuberculosis MTB can occur at any stage of AIDS. The immune system need not be compromised to get this disease.	Night sweats, cough, fever, and weight loss. The problem with treatment involves the multidrug resistant strains, and noncompliance to the rigorous treatment required.	Isoniazid (INH), along with pyridoxine (vitamin B_6.) Other combinations with INH include ethambutol, rifampin, or streptomycin.
Mycobacterium avium complex MAC generally occurs during the later stages of the disease in patients with CD4 counts below 100. It is common to find MAC in 50% of patients at autopsy.	Fatigue, chills, night sweats, fever, weight loss, diarrhea, and abdominal pain. Such common symptoms make it difficult to diagnose.	Drug combinations are used, including clarithomycin and one or two others such as ethambutol and/or clofazamin. Other drugs include amikacin, azithromycin, ciprofloxin, and rifampin. Once on treatment, it is continued for life.

AIDS-Related Complex (ARC)

AIDS-related complex (ARC) was previously identified as the precursor to the disease AIDS. Once infected with HIV, a series of symptoms may ensue, including diarrhea, weight loss, fatigue, fever, night sweats, lymphadenopathy, **lymphopenia** (lowered lymphocyte count), and **hypergammaglobulinemia** (excess gamma globulin proteins in the blood). These symptoms may last a long time before developing into full-blown AIDS, and their onset may be delayed long after initial infection. AIDS is diagnosed when at least two additional markers for the disease develop, such as *Pneumocystis carinii,* Kaposi's sarcoma, candidiasis or thrush, cryptosporidiosis, atypical mycobacteria, toxoplasmosis, cryptococcosis, lymphomas (tumors of lymphoid tissue), parasitic infections, life-threatening opportunistic infections, or a significantly lowered T-cell lymphocyte count. Although the actual term ARC is seldom used today, it serves to identify the various periods that a patient will experience during the course of the disease.

Effective January 1993 the Centers for Disease Control and Prevention (CDC) published a new classification system for HIV infection. This classification system first assumes the patient has tested positive for the HIV virus. The basis of this new classification system is designed to assist health care providers in monitoring the progress of the patient by regular T4-cell counts. Research has shown that HIV will attack only those white blood cells that contain one particular type of marker site on the surfaces of the cells. The markers through which the HIV gains entry to a cell are known as the CD4 marker sites. Of the two types of lymphocytes, only the T4 cells have CD4 marker sites. T cells that have CD4 marker sites are the helper cells; thus, the term *T4 helper cell* was coined. Other T cells, called the "suppressor cells," have only CD8 marker sites, and therefore cannot be penetrated by the virus. Additionally, **histiocytes** and **macrophages** have the same CD4 marker sites and therefore are also susceptible to the virus.

Clinical categories for the classification of HIV infections are now designated as A for asymptomatic, acute onset (primary), or persistent generalized lymphadenopathy (PGL); B for symptomatic conditions, but no A conditions (The B symptoms may include wasting, chronic diarrhea, recurrent skin rashes, and yeast infections. This designation was formally recognized as ARC.); and C for AIDS indicator conditions, which include any of the following diseases: extrapulmonary *Cryptococcus neoformans* (which may be disseminated throughout the body), cytomegalovirus (CMV); *Mycobacterium avium–intracellulariae* (MAI), *Pneumocystis carinii* pneumonia (PCP), Kaposi's sarcoma, and disseminated *Toxoplasmosis gondii.*

The key to the prognosis of each of these categories is further subdivided, based on the T-helper cell counts. Normal T4 cell counts are 500 to approximately 800 per microliter. Level 1 counts are equal to or above 500 per microliter. Level 2 counts will be between 200 and 499 per microliter. Level 3 counts are equal to or less than 200 per microliter. In any of the three categories, a count this low indicates the presence of AIDS and must be treated immediately with azathioprine (AZT) (Table 12–3).

All patients who fall into categories A3, B3, C1, C2, and C3 should be treated immediately for HIV infection (Table 12–3). Patients who fall into the A1 and B1 categories need not be started on prophylactic treatment for PCP. Patients in categories B2 and B3 are required to be treated prophylactically for PCP, with the drug of choice being an aerosol pentamidine. Patients who fall into the A2 and A3 categories may be

Table 12–3 Revised Classification System for HIV Infection and Expanded AIDS Surveillance Case Definition for Adolescents and Adults

	CLINICAL CATEGORIES		
CD4+ T-CELL CATEGORIES	(A) ASYMPTOMATIC, ACUTE (PRIMARY) HIV OR PGL	(B) SYMPTOMATIC, NOT (A) OR (B) CONDITIONS	(C) AIDS-INDICATOR CONDITIONS
(1) >500/μl	A1	B1	C1
(2) 200–499/μl	A2	B2	C2
(3) <200/μl	A3	B3	C3

started on trimethylprim-sulfamethoxazole as prophylactic treatment. Under this new system, patient prognosis and early antibiotic therapy can be monitored, with strong efforts to maintain T4 cell counts of above 500 per microliter.

Asymptomatic Infection (Categories A1 and A2)

Today it is known that people who have been infected with HIV will probably go on to develop symptoms of the disease; but there are some HIV-seropositive people that to date have not developed symptoms of AIDS. Continued monitoring and research will determine the statistical reality of such persons remaining **asymptomatic** yet infectious carriers. It is known that any person infected with the virus can pass it on to others. It is important to be knowledgeable about this disease, practice safe sex, and if testing positive for HIV to follow the prophylactic therapy precisely as directed by a physician.

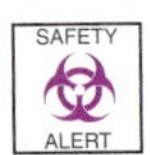

High-Risk Groups for AIDS

Although the high-risk groups remain essentially the same, we should not forget that this disease is no longer confined to these groups. Heterosexual females have risen high on the list of infected patients. Too many young people say, "This can't happen to me." First ask yourself if you know of anyone that has had a sexually transmitted disease, and chances are very good you will know someone who has been infected with HIV. Individuals at the highest risk of contacting AIDS are

- Homosexual and bisexual men with multiple sexual partners
- Male and female intravenous drug users who share needles and syringes
- Heterosexual males and females who have multiple partners
- Any person not practicing safe sex procedures
- Female sexual partners of males in the high-risk group
- Infants born to parents who are at risk for AIDS

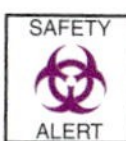

Transmission of AIDS

The transmission of HIV occurs in three ways:

- Sexual intercourse during which semen enters the body (about 75% of the adults in the United States who have AIDS contracted it through sexual intercourse)
- Sharing of hypodermic needles among I.V. drug users, when infected blood is injected into the body (accounts for 17% to 25% of the AIDS cases in the United States)
- In utero or at birth from an infected mother to her unborn or newborn infant

Transmission of HIV through transfusion of blood or blood products has been all but eliminated, possibly because blood banks and plasma centers test all blood donors to determine whether they have been exposed to HIV. Also, federal guidelines require that individuals in high-risk groups do not donate blood or blood products.

The virus cannot be contracted through air, feces, food, urine, or water. Even close nonsexual contact such as coughing, sneezing, embracing, shaking hands, and sharing eating utensils cannot spread the virus.

New York, New Jersey, Washington D.C., Florida, and California still have the highest incidence of AIDS in the United States. Males outnumber females and CDC is reporting a significant rise in numbers of cases in women ages 25 to 44 attributed to only heterosexual exposure. In Africa it has long been a heterosexually transmitted disease. In Romania many orphaned children became infected due to the extremely poor state of hygiene and sanitary precautions taken by overworked staff and an undersupply of sterile utensils not limited to but including syringes, needles, and catheters. HIV is a worldwide infectious disease. Asia and eastern Europe are now beginning to see the explosion of the disease. In 1994 only 30,000 cases of AIDS were identified in all of eastern Europe. Today (1998) the figures have jumped to over 200,000, a sixfold increase in only 4 years. Former Soviet bloc countries have been hardest hit: For example, in the Ukraine, which has the highest HIV rates (approximately 110,000 compared with only 44 reported in 1994), there are almost four times as many cases of HIV infection as found in all of eastern Europe only 3 years ago.

Measures to Prevent Transmission and Acquisition

People who have AIDS must take precautions to reduce the chances of giving the virus to others. Also, those in the risk groups must take measures to reduce their chances of contracting AIDS. Thus, these measures should be followed by all persons.

- Limit the number of sexual contacts, as each new sexual partner increases the chance of infection.
- Do not donate blood, blood products, sperm, or any other parts of the body if you are in the high-risk group.
- Abstain from sexual acts during which blood or semen is exchanged, as in anal, oral, and vaginal intercourse. At the very least, never have unprotected sex.
- Do not share hypodermic needles or syringes.

- Make sure that soiled articles, materials, and surfaces are thoroughly cleaned with soap and hot water after incidents involving bleeding. Also, bleach is an excellent disinfectant.
- Cover an open cut, sore, or wound with a bandage.

Recommendations for health care personnel to prevent the acquisition of AIDS include the practice of universal precautions:

- Use the same precautions when caring for AIDS patients as for those patients with hepatitis B virus.
- Avoid direct contact of skin and mucous membranes with blood, blood products, excretions, secretions, and tissues of people with AIDS or people who are likely to have it.

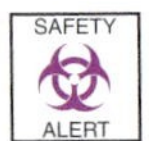

Standard Precautions and the Health Care Worker

With the inception of the concept of standard precautions, whereby all patients and samples are treated as though they are infectious, the techniques for isolation procedures have become more standardized without compromising a patient's right to privacy. These precautions, if followed consistently by all health care personnel, will prevent accidental exposure to HIV as well as to hepatitis B virus. The precautions include wearing gloves when handling body fluids or materials contaminated with body fluids; wearing impermeable protective gowns, masks, or shields when the chance of spattering exists; using disposable mouthpieces for cardiopulmonary resuscitation (CPR); cleaning spills immediately with 10% bleach; not leaving bodily fluids exposed to the air; using disposable personal hygiene utensils for patients; properly disposing of contaminated materials into biohazard containers; disposing of needles and sharps in a hard-wall container; and not resheathing or breaking needles. Laboratory personnel and nurses, especially those working in the emergency room and surgery have the greatest risk for accidental exposure, so it is important to follow the guidelines even as severe traumas or life-threatening emergencies occur.

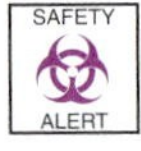

Laboratory Diagnosis of HIV

HIV has been grown in tissue culture from peripheral blood, and on occasion saliva, of patients with ARC. Recently another retrovirus, HIV-II, has been shown to cause AIDS, but the prevalence of this virus is very low in the United States. Today, all donor blood is screened for both types of AIDS as well as hepatitis and a number of other potential bloodborne pathogens. Common are the enzyme-linked immunosorbent assay (ELISA) and Western blot procedures for the detection of the HIV **antibody** (a protein substance produced by the immune system to fight off the presence of a foreign antigen). These tests are highly sensitive and specific but do miss people who have been infected recently and who have not yet had time to make detectable antibodies (lag phase). The ELISA test procedures are the first screening test of choice for HIV antibodies. These tests demonstrate less than 1% false negative results but may show a much higher rate of false positive results. The Western blot confirmation test will weed out most of the false positives. To date there has been no real gold standard test developed, and more research efforts are directed at developing a vaccine than at developing more antibody-detection tests. Laboratories in California use an immunofluorescent assay (IFA) as a supplement to the ELISA with great reliability. Radioactive methods of antibody detection are being fielded with much promise.

These antibody-detection tests detect antibodies produced by the virus, and do not diagnose the disease AIDS. The applicable symptoms are diagnostic of the disease. The presence of antibody does not mean that one has AIDS. It merely means that one has been infected with the virus. Whether the disease will develop in that individual is not determined by the screening tests.

Laboratory Diagnosis of Infections Associated with AIDS

Patients who are infected with HIV will, as statistics are demonstrating, develop full-blown AIDS at some time in the future. For some it may be only a few months to the first symptoms; for others it may be years. Early symptoms include an ordinary cold or virus infection that does not go away, fatigue, weakness, and general malaise. As the disease progresses a number of infections may befall the patient. Along with the infection, immunological studies will bear out a drastic decrease in the number of T-helper lymphocytes—white blood cells important to the immune system that are specifically attacked by the virus. Positive serological tests are confirmed with a Western blot test. Some of the infections that befall the AIDS patient were listed in Table 12–1.

Historical background of hepatitis. Outbreaks of yellow jaundice took a high toll on military personnel during World War II, until the surgeon general ordered the withdrawal of the then recently mass-produced Rockefeller yellow fever vaccine. The vaccine was great in preventing yellow fever but some 200,000 people contracted hepatitis between 1942 and 1945. At that time no one was aware that serum or blood could be a reservoir for another disease. In 1956, Saul Krugman, a young professor of pediatrics at New York University Medical School, was asked to assist at a state school for retarded children where hepatitis was rampant. Overcrowding and poor sanitary conditions guaranteed a haven for the virus. His goal was to rid the school of hepatitis by preventing the disease. To prevent the disease, a vaccine was needed. His controversial methods of inducing the disease in the children (who were bound to get it anyway) brought much concern. Nevertheless, he proceeded by giving shots of **gamma globulin** (the part of the plasma rich in antibodies) to children, with parental consent. He gave the children doses of diluted serum from children who had already contracted hepatitis. Then, after they had recovered from the induced disease, he fed them another dose of infected serum. This time his children remained healthy; but then problems arose as almost one in every twelve of these children suffered another bout of hepatitis within a year. He remembered the Rockefeller yellow fever vaccine problems. Perhaps there were two hepatitis diseases. Further studies with the children through 1967 finally revealed two distinct types of hepatitis, one a highly contagious variety transmitted by direct exposure (type A) and another, equally infective but transmitted by blood (type B).

Meanwhile another researcher, Barry Blumburg, a **geneticist** (one who studies genetic defects) working at one of the cancer institutes, was looking for proteins in **recipients** (people who receive a blood transfusion) of blood that may not have been part of their own gene pool to see if they made antibodies (protein substance produced by the immune system in response to a foreign protein) to these antigen markers. He found a new antibody in hemophiliac patients that reacted with the blood of an Australian aborigine. This Australian antigen was found in leukemia patients and also in those with Down's syndrome. Dr. Blumburg tested his antigen against Dr. Krugman's type A and type B hepatitis-infected blood. The testing revealed the Australian antigen to be indeed present, but only in the type B samples. The Australian antigen is definitely a marker for the hepatitis B strain. The hepatitis B virus became known as the hepatitis B surface antigen. In 1976, Blumburg won the Nobel Prize for physiology or medicine in recognition of his discovery of the hepatitis B surface antigen.

An explosion of research followed this discovery, and in 1970 the first widespread testing of donor blood for the Australian antigen began. Maurice Hilleman, a virologist with Merck Sharp & Dohme Laboratories, is credited with developing the first hepatitis B vaccine. Interestingly, it is prepared with the serum of hepatitis carriers and recovering hepatitis patients. When the virus could not be grown in tissue culture to make a vaccine, Hilleman turned to the infected serum laden with the hepatitis antigen particles to prepare a safe vaccine. Between 1978 and 1980 a massive vaccination trial was carried out on over 1000 volunteers solicited from high-risk groups located in New York City. The results were astounding. In a double-blind study only 3% of those receiving the vaccine contracted hepatitis; 27% of those receiving the placebo contracted hepatitis after 18 months. Merck Sharp & Dohme was then licensed to market the vaccine on November 17, 1981.

Today, all health care workers are urged to receive the hepatitis B vaccination series as a precautionary measure. But let us not forget that researchers are now working on the latest of the hepatitis viruses. Hepatitis C virus (HCV), formerly referred to as non-A, non-B, awaits vaccine development.

HEPATITIS

Viral hepatitis is the most common liver disease, and it is found worldwide. The viral agents of hepatitis include hepatitis A, hepatitis B, hepatitis C (non-A, non-B), and hepatitis D. Other agents causing a secondary hepatitis include the Epstein-Barr virus, cytomegalovirus, and herpesvirus.

Hepatitis A, also known as infectious hepatitis, is caused by a small RNA virus belonging to the picornavirus class. The virus has a 2- to 6-week incubation period before symptoms appear. Although the illness may last up to 6 months, the virus is no longer found in the feces once the patient becomes jaundiced. This form of hepatitis is transmitted in sewage-contaminated water and in areas where personal hygiene is poor. Immune globulin injections may prevent the onset of this disease.

Hepatitis B (HBV) (formally referred to as the Australia or hepatitis-associated antigen) was discovered in 1966. HBV is a complex DNA virus belonging to the class hepadna. The virus has an outer surface structure called the "hepatitis B surface antigen"

(HBsAg) and an inner core component called the "hepatitis B inner core antigen" (HBcAg). It is inside the core that a single molecule of the double-stranded DNA particle is found. This means that there are two antigens associated with this virus, both of which are coded for on the DNA strand. It is no wonder researchers had a difficult challenge preparing a suitable vaccine for this elusive virus. Hepatitis B (formerly called serum hepatitis) has a long incubation period, up to 6 months, and is transmitted through blood contact. It has the same modes of transmission as HIV. Often, infected persons will have no outward symptoms; but make no mistake, hepatitis B is a very serious illness, and one that health care workers have feared most. Many have died from this disease, and until the advent of the hepatitis B vaccination series it killed many health care workers infected via needle sticks or direct contact with contaminated blood. The vaccine, first made available in 1982, has been refined to such a point that today a series of three immunizations are given on day 0, days 25 to 30, and again on day 180. Should there be accidental exposure, starting the series within 24 hours affords excellent protection.

Hepatitis C, once referred to as non-A, non-B hepatitis, is now included as a bloodborne pathogen. It is also found in water, like hepatitis A virus (HAV) (see Figure 12–6). Many infected with this virus will become carriers as do those with hepatitis B. Diagnosis of this virus is based on nonreactions to HBV and HAV testing and elevated alanine aminotransferase (ALT/SGPT) (an enzyme associated with liver function) levels, because at present the serological test for this virus antibody has not been perfected. As research progresses it has been suggested that more than one viral agent may be responsible for non-A, non-B hepatitis.

Hepatitis D is a pathogen that superinfects some patients already infected with hepatitis B. It appears that HBV is required as a helper to initiate a delta infection. This virus is also a bloodborne agent that apparently is a defective or incomplete RNA virus incapable of causing disease except in the presence of hepatitis B virus. Serological testing confirms the presence of this virus.

Modern medical authorities recognize not only hepatitis A, B, and C, but also the fact that it has become the alphabet soup disease with hepatitis D, E, F, and G, identifiable.

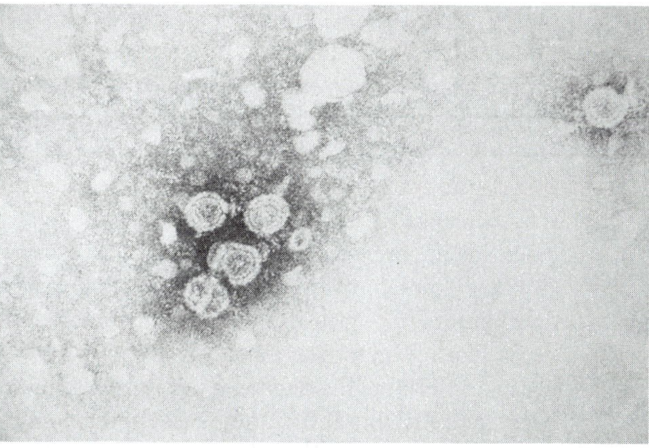

Figure 12–6 Hepatitis B (*Courtesy of Centers for Disease Control and Prevention, Atlanta, GA*)

Cures are not evident in the near future, but with good hygiene, no needle sharing, education, testing of the blood, and vaccines, hepatitis can be controlled. Children at the elementary and middle school levels are now being vaccinated against hepatitis B. Hepatitis C, D, E, F, and G are now in the forefront of researchers' activities, with hepatitis C being of the most concern, for it is known to be transmitted by blood-to-blood contact. Often referred to as the stealth disease, it comes on without any warning. There is no cure at this time, but researchers have found that combination therapy with ribaviron, which seems to interfere with the virus's ability to replicate, and interferon alpha-2b, which can then boost the immune system's ability to fight the disease, has shown to be more effective than with interferon alone.

Today's health care professionals must be wary of not just one virus capable of causing serum or bloodborne hepatitis but at least three or four varieties. As we move into the twenty-first century so too will research in developing vaccines for all forms of bloodborne pathogens. Regardless of the availability of vaccines, we must take proper precautions at all times to protect ourselves and our patients from other unknown or as yet undetected potentially harmful agents.

Prions

A new infectious agent may be on the forefront of our future. **Prions** (also known as rogue proteins) describe particles known as **proteinaceous infectious particles.** They were first described in 1984 by Dr. Stanley Prusiner as potential disease-causing agents. Unlike virus particles that exist in a single form, prions can exist in multiple molecular forms. Also, the presence of prions are nonimmunogenic (i.e., they do not result in the formation of antibodies), whereas viruses result in an immune response to form antibodies. These particles or prions contained nothing but protein—no RNA, DNA, or nucleic acids. Lastly, prions contain only one component, prion protein designated as the scrapie form (PrPSc) which is encoded by a chromosomal gene. Viruses consist of nucleic acid, protein, and often other constituents. Dr. Prusiner suggested that these prions might be responsible for causing certain degenerative disorders of the central nervous system and that they could be the cause of both inherited and communicable diseases. Dr. Prusiner also suggested that prions could multiply in an incredible way, by converting normal protein molecules into dangerous ones simply by inducing the benign molecules to change their shape. Fifteen years later the scientific community has finally recognized the truth to his suggestions. Prions are responsible for transmissible and inherited disorders. They also cause sporadic disease which is neither communicable nor inherited. Additionally, modern-day evidence supports the theory that prions of entirely different proteins may contribute to other **neurodegenerative** diseases that are prevalent in humans.

The known prion diseases, all fatal, are sometimes referred to as **spongiform encephalopathies** because they frequently cause the brain to become riddled with holes, much like a sponge. The most common form of a spongiform encephalopathy is found in sheep and goats. This disease, a prion disease, is known as **scrapie,** because infected sheep become so irritable and in some cases develop an intense itch that they scrape off their wool or hair. Bovine spongiform encephalopathy (BSE) is known as mad cow disease. This disease was identified in Great Britain first in 1986 when it struck cows, thus causing them to be very uncoordinated and apprehensive. In the course of the emerging epidemic it was discovered that a food supplement given to cows included a meat and bone supplement from dead sheep. A change in the processing procedures of sheep carcasses in the late 1970s resulted in a processing method that did not eliminate the scrapie agent. In 1988 the British government banned the use of animal-derived feed supplements, which then ended the epidemic until 1996 when mad cow disease reemerged for a short period.

Human prion diseases are more obscure. One called kuru has been seen only among the Fore Highlanders of Papua New Guinea. They call it the "laughing death." As early as 1957 National Institute of Health (NIH) researchers described a strange fatal disease marked by loss of coordination (**ataxia**), and later dementia among the highlanders who probably acquired the disease through ritual cannibalism. The Fore tribe honored their dead by eating their brains. Since this practice has stopped, kuru has disappeared.

Creutzfeld-Jacob disease (CJD), in contrast, is well known and occurs worldwide. It is of concern to health care providers because the disease can be transmitted through a needle stick injury or any other blood-to-blood contact. CJD becomes evident when dementia sets in. It appears sporadically, striking one in a million around the age of 60. About 10% to 15% of the cases are inherited, but many are inadvertently spread by attempts to treat other medical problems. For example, CJD has been diagnosed after corneal transplants, implantation of dura matter or electrodes in the brain, use of contaminated surgical instruments, or an injection of growth hormone derived from human pituitary glands.

The remaining human prion disorders Gerstann-Straussler-Scheinker (GSS) syndrome and fatal familial insomnia (FFI) are also characterized by loss of motor control, dementia, paralysis, wasting, and death. The prion protein has been isolated from a man's mutated gene in the case of Gerstann-Straussler-Scheinker syndrome in which he and his family were dying of the disease. FFI is also an inherited disease in which dementia follows difficulty in sleeping.

SUMMARY

The study of viruses is an interesting subject, because research is on the forefront of the new millennium and new viruses and treatments are on the horizon. Viruses act by penetrating cells and releasing their DNA or RNA into the nucleus of the cells. Rapid replication takes place and the virus moves on to do its damage. Today one of the most prominent viruses is HIV. Although no cure is available, clinical trials are starting with 1000 volunteers. Super cocktails of drugs in combination have shown great promise in the treatment of the symptoms of this hideous disease. Previously we knew only about hepatitis A and hepatitis B. There was some discussion of a non-A, non-B hepatitis, which we recognize now as hepatitis C. Additionally hepatitis D, E, F, and G are now recognized. Immunizations for hepatitis B, once only given to health care workers, now is given routinely to all infants. There is now even a vaccination for the *Varicella* virus (chicken pox) on the market.

HIV, once a sure death sentence, is responding to drugs that, however toxic, are adding many years to their victims' lifespan. There are numerous side effects to this disease, in the form of opportunistic infection. Many are harmless saprophytes to the healthy individual but, in a patient with full-blown AIDS, can be the actual cause of death. Death rates from AIDS may be decreasing in the United States, but just the opposite is happening in Asian and eastern European countries. Table 12–1 explains the effects of some of the opportunistic infections found. Health care professionals need to be aware of and practice standard precautions at all times to lower their risk of contamination.

Now that a successful vaccine protocol is available for hepatitis B, researchers can begin to concentrate on the newer hepatitis strains, namely hepatitis C, D, E, F, and G. Hepatitis C is as infective as hepatitis B and is transmitted in the same manner. Soon a vaccine will be available for routine use against this virus.

Prion diseases, once unknown, have opened a new avenue to infectious diseases. Scientists were always aware of the possibility of a bloodborne connection with Creutzfeld-Jacob disease, but were unable to associate a known disease particle as the cause. We now know about prion infectious agents, which are proteinlike infectious particles. They can exhibit multiple molecular forms and contain only protein—no DNA or RNA is present. Most prion diseases cause neurogenic diseases. Most are fatal, as they attack brain tissue. Unfortunately no symptoms occur before the dementia sets in and by then it is too late.

REVIEW QUESTIONS

A. General Questions: Provide complete answers to each of the following.

1. What is a host?

2. Name some localized infections and systemic diseases caused by viruses.

3. Why must an electron microscope be used to see a virus?

4. What is interferon, and why is it so important? What is the major drawback to its use?

5. What are some of the characteristics of viruses of which the health care professional must be aware?

6. What causes AIDS?

7. What do the initials A-I-D-S signify?

8. What are the three possible outcomes from infection by the causative agent for AIDS?

9. Describe three of the possible opportunistic infections that can trouble an AIDS patient.

10. What are the symptoms of AIDS, and what is its incubation period?

11. Who are the people at risk of contracting AIDS?

12. What are the three ways of transmitting the causative agent of AIDS?

13. What are some preventive measures a health care professional should use to avoid the acquisition of AIDS?

14. What is the one useful benefit of the HIV antibody test?

B. Multiple-Choice Questions: Select the letter of the choice that best answers the question.

1. Viruses contain which of the following components?
   a. cell wall, DNA, core, protein coat
   b. cell wall, RNA, core, protein coat
   c. a nucleic acid, core, protein coat
   d. a nucleic acid, protein coat
2. Viruses reproduce by a process known as ________.
   a. uncoating c. release
   b. adsorption d. replication
3. Large brick-shaped viruses, pathogenic to the skin, are the ________ group.
   a. papovavirus c. poxvirus
   b. arbovirus d. adenovirus
4. Parasitic infections associated with AIDS infections include which of the following organisms?
   a. *Giardia lamblia, Candida albicans, Isospora belli*
   b. *Giardia lamblia, Enterobius vermicularis, Isospora belli*
   c. *Isospora belli, Giardia lamblia, Cryptosporidia*
   d. *Toxoplasma, Cryptosporidia, Entomoeba histolytica*
5. The AIDS virus has been known by other names in the past, and they are ______.
   a. LAV, HTLV-3, ARC c. HIV-I, HIV-II, HIV-III
   b. HIV-I, HIV-II d. LAV, HTLV-3
6. HIV infection can be acquired by ________.
   a. anyone who uses I.V. drugs and shares needles
   b. teenagers who practice unprotected sex
   c. adults who have multiple partners
   d. all of the above

7. Standard precautions include the wearing of ________ when the chance of spills or spatters may occur.
   a. gloves, gown, and mask
   b. impermeable protective clothing, gloves
   c. impermeable protective clothing, mask
   d. impermeable protective clothing, gloves, shield
8. Serum hepatitis, known as ________ , is of most concern to health care workers.
   a. hepatitis A
   b. hepatitis B
   c. hepatitis C
   d. hepatitis D
9. Infectious hepatitis is caused by ________.
   a. unsanitary conditions
   b. eating contaminated food
   c. a needlestick injury
   d. contaminated blood

C. Completion Questions: From the following list of terms fill in the blands with the correct choice.

rickettsia	phage	T-lymphocyte
louse	maturation	trimethylprimsulfamethoxazole
flea	hepatitis D	interferon
replication	*Rickettsia prowazekii*	uncoating
hepatitis C	*Mycoplasma pneumoniae*	lysozyme
aerosol pentamidine	*Chlamydia trachomatis*	hepatitis B
Weil-Felix	hepatitis A	CD4 receptor
proteus		

1. A virus that attacks bacteria is referred to as a ___________.

2. The substance ___________ prevents ___________ of the virus and is also helpful in the treatment of cancers.

3. ___________ is the only one of the four kinds of hepatitis that is not transmitted by blood.

4. Presently a vaccine is available only for the ___________ virus.

5. AIDS-related complex has been recategorized into groups that use the ___________ count as an indicator of progress of the disease.

6. Patients testing positive for the HIV virus, with a T-cell count 450/μl and no other symptoms, should begin prophylactic treatment with ___________.

7. Patients testing positive for the HIV virus, with a T-cell count 410/μl and respiratory symptoms, should begin prophylactic treatment with ___________.

D. Matching Questions: Match the terms in Column I with their corresponding terms in Column II.

Column I		Column II
_______	1. arbovirus	a. common cold
_______	2. enterovirus	b. rabies
_______	3. herpesvirus	c. HBsAg & HBcAg
_______	4. rhabdovirus	d. non A non B
_______	5. rhinovirus	e. yellow fever
_______	6. adenovirus	f. superinfects HBV
_______	7. hepatitis A	g. RNA virus
_______	8. hepatitis B	h. poliomyelitis
_______	9. myxovirus	i. warts
_______	10. paramyxovirus	j. shingles
_______	11. hepatitis C	k. conjunctivitis
_______	12. hepatitis D	l. mumps
_______	13. papovavirus	m. influenza

CHAPTER

13 Microbiological Techniques

OBJECTIVES

After completing this chapter, you will be able to:

- differentiate between the hanging-drop and wet-mount techniques.
- perform the technique involved in the preparation of a smear from a bacterial culture and one from pus material.
- explain the importance of the fixation step in slide preparation.
- differentiate between simple staining and differential staining.
- list three examples of a simple stain and three examples of a differential stain.
- perform a Gram stain.
- list five relative differences between a gram-negative and gram-positive cell wall.
- perform an acid-fast stain.
- explain what stain is used for the demonstration of rickettsias.
- explain the value of the use of the negative staining technique.

KEY WORDS

Brownian movement
coagulate
counterstain
differential staining
fixing
gram variable
inoculating loop
morphology
precipitate
reagent
simple staining
"vital" stain

Light microscopy is a most important technique. It allows the microbiologist and health care professional to examine and study bacterial structure or **morphology.** However, before one can examine microbes under the microscope, certain procedures must be used to prepare the specimens for light microscopy. These techniques are needed because microbes would otherwise appear "featureless," and transparent and motile bacteria would have to be made motionless. Two basic techniques are used to prepare specimens for light microscopy. One technique involves the examination of living bacteria or other microbes by suspending them in water or other suitable fluid. The second uses smeared, dried, fixed, and stained specimens on a glass slide.

THE HANGING-DROP AND WET-MOUNT TECHNIQUES

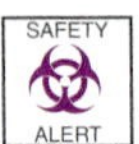

Bacteria and other microbes can be examined in a normal living state by suspending them in a fluid. Live microbial examination helps a health care professional to discover such characteristics as bacterial group arrangements, shape, size, and motility. There are two wet preparations used for live microbial study. One is the hanging-drop technique, which is performed using a coverslip, petrolatum or petroleum jelly, and a special slide with a concave depression in the center (Figure 13–1); the other preparation is the wet-mount technique. Instead of the concave slide a regular glass slide is used. The procedures for the hanging-drop and wet-mount techniques follow.

A wet-mount slide is made by first applying a rim of petrolatum or petroleum jelly around the edges of the coverslip. Using a sterile dropper or inoculating loop containing the microbe, transfer a drop of the liquid suspension to the center of the coverslip. Carefully lay the glass slide over the coverslip, making sure the petrolatum has contact with the glass slide on all four sides; press very gently. Now invert the glass slide so that the coverslip is uppermost. The jelly prevents the inexperienced eye from interpreting the effects of air current as movement of the bacteria. It also prevents rapid evaporation of the material. The hanging-drop slide is prepared using the concave slide instead of the regular glass slide. The hanging-drop technique tends to be the choice when examining suspended material for motility, whereas the wet-mount preparation is used more frequently when looking at larger microbes such as fungi, protozoans, and yeasts. Using a microscope with excellent resolution and the 100X and 450X magnifications, these larger microbes can be seen very clearly. Even without staining, their internal structures can be seen. However, to see the internal structures more clearly, a **"vital" stain** is used. A "vital"stain is one that can be taken up by an organism without distorting or destroying the organism or its internal structures. Examples of such a stain are weak solutions of iodine, methylene blue, and janus green B. Smaller microbes such as bacteria are too small and transparent to be seen with good resolution in wet preparation, even using the oil-immersion objective. However, their motility, their natural groupings into chains, clusters, or packets, and their reactions to certain chemical substances can be seen.

In all wet preparations, all small particles, including both motile and nonmotile bacteria, show **Brownian movement.** Brownian movement is a rapid motion caused by the continuous movement of liquid molecules that constantly bombard the suspended microbes.

When a motile microbe is suspended in a wet preparation, the organism changes position in relation to the other organisms and also may have a characteristic pattern. Movement of motile bacteria can be dashing, spinning, sluggish, or undulant. The

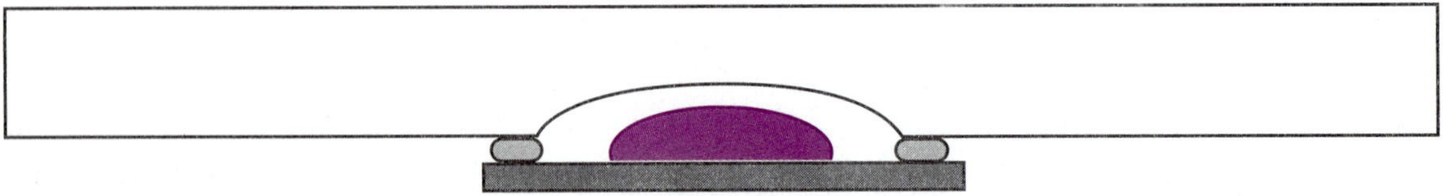

Figure 13–1 Hanging-drop preparation viewed from the side and showing the drop hanging into the depression of the concave slide from the coverslip, which has been rimmed with petrolatum

following are situations in which the hanging-drop and/or wet-mount preparations are used:

1. to observe the morphology of spiral bacteria
2. to observe motile bacteria in a liquid medium that allows them to move freely
3. to observe cell inclusion bodies such as vacuoles and fatty material
4. to observe cellular changes during cell division and to determine how fast this division occurs

The most appropriate types of microscopy for unstained wet preparations are darkfield and phase-contrast microscopy, because the illumination provides more contrast for visualization of organisms than brightfield microscopy.

FIXED, STAINED SMEARS

Fixed, dried, and stained smears are often used in light microscopy to provide for greater resolution of bacteria and of internal structures in larger organisms. Such treatment results in the whole or part of the organism achieving a dramatic contrast to the unstained background.

Preparation of Bacterial Smears to be Stained

The most typical way of examining bacteria is to first make a thin film of the bacteria on a clean slide. The material is allowed to air-dry before it is fixed and stained. Smears are prepared in the following way:

Procedure 13–1 Preparing a Slide for Staining

Steps

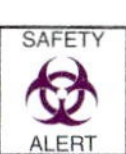

1. Secure a disposable, precleaned slide.

2a. Prepare a smear from a bacterial colony culture or a plate.

   i. Holding the culture plate in the left hand and the **inoculating loop** or needle in the right, sterilize the needle by holding it perpendicular in the Bunsen burner flame until it is red hot, then let the loop cool. (Using a hot loop may cause the bacteria-laden material to spatter, causing contamination of yourself and the surroundings. Additionally, hot looping will kill the bacteria taken onto the loop.)

   ii. With a twisting motion, remove the cotton plug or cap by grasping it between the little finger and the palm of the right hand. The part of the plug or cap protruding outward from the hand should not touch the fingers or other surfaces. When the culture tube is open, it is held nearly horizontal, so that dust particles laden with bacteria cannot drop directly into it (Figure 13–2).

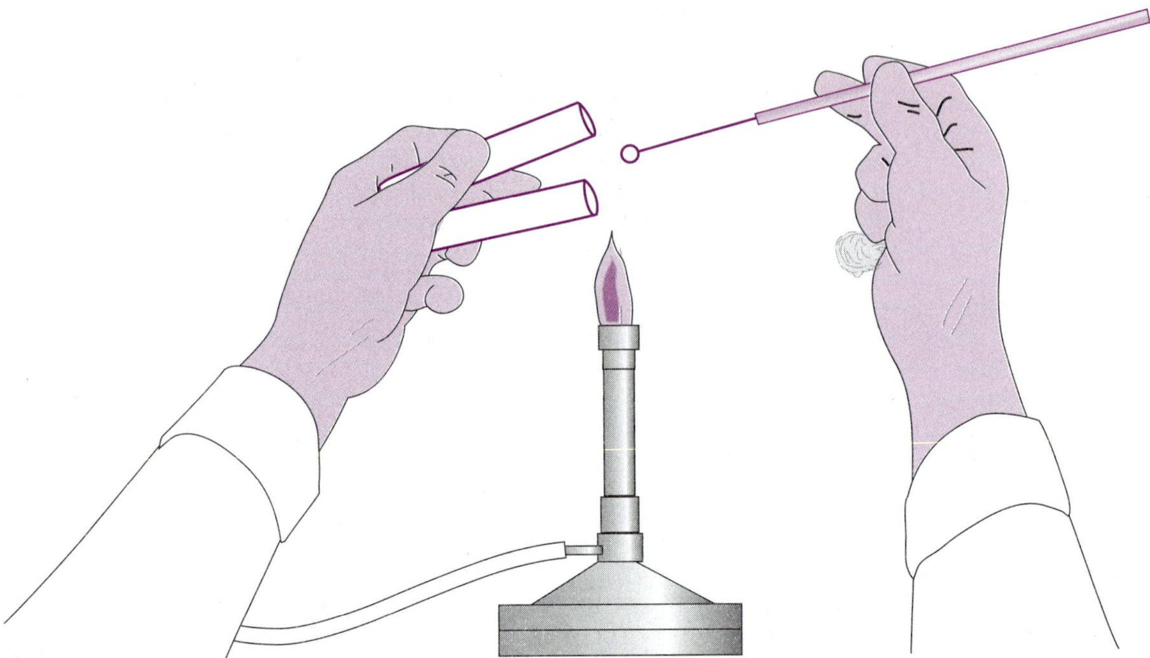

Figure 13–2 Handling test-tube cultures (The cotton plugs have just been removed from the two culture test tubes, prior to making a transfer. The plugs are held by the fingers of the right hand, which holds the inoculating loop, and cannot be seen. The test tubes are held nearly horizontal and close to the flame.)

iii. Whenever a tube is opened, the exposed lip of the tube is quickly passed through a hot Bunsen burner flame. Flaming the open lip will prevent bacteria in the air from entering the tube and contaminating the bacterial suspension.

iv. Carefully insert the cooled sterilized loop into the culture tube and remove a small quantity of the culture with the inoculating loop. Then spread the drop to make a thin smear.

v. The bacteria can be spread over the glass slide by the following method. The drop can be spread out slowly with the inoculating loop by making several circular paths through it, each time carrying the mixture farther away. This way, the smear will have the required thinness in the outer portions of the smear as well. Figure 13–3 shows this technique.

vi. Pass the mouth of the culture tube through the flame again and replace the cotton plug.

vii. Flame-sterilize the inoculating loop and lay it aside. (*Note:* When flame-sterilizing an inoculating loop contaminated by small drops of fluid laden with microbes, pass it gently and slowly into the cooler part of the Bunsen burner flame and slowly heat to redness. This prevents spattering of live microbes into the air.)

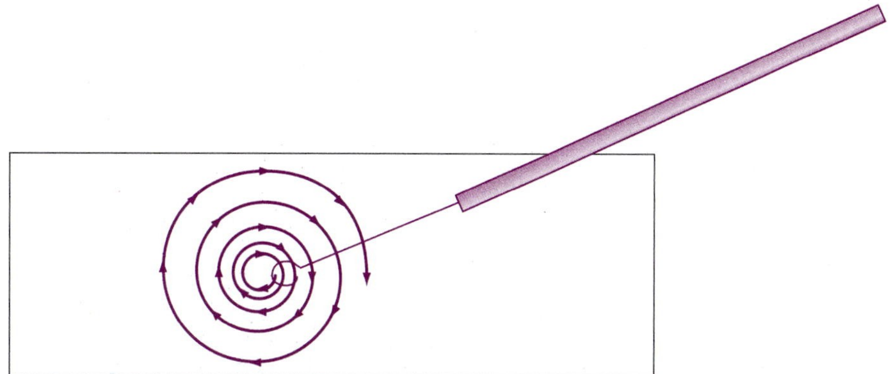

Figure 13–3 Circular path of the inoculating loop in the preparation of a thin smear

2b. Prepare a smear from pus or other material.
   i. Sterile cotton swabs are used to transfer larger amounts of material onto a slide. Roll the cotton swab along a clean glass slide to make a thin, even film. Generally, water is not needed for a smear of this kind. Dispose of cotton swab immediately into a container designated for biohazard waste.
3. Let the smear air-dry.
4. After the smear is completely dry, pass the slide, smear side up, through the Bunsen burner or Bacticinerator flame three times. (Slides may also be heat-fixed by placing them on a smooth-surfaced hot plate for a few minutes.) This heating procedure is called **fixing** the slide. The heat **coagulates** (curdles or clots) the cell protein of the bacterium to the slide. The bacteria in a fixed state are not all dead. They are just affixed to the glass slide so that they will not fall off during further handling. However, too much heat fixation can burn or distort cells, and should be avoided. Smears are sometimes fixed by placing a few drops of methyl alcohol (CH_3OH) on the slide and allowing it to air-dry. This causes less distortion.
5. After fixation, the slide is ready for staining.

The actual staining method used depends on the type of structure or structures needed to be examined through the microscope. Some of the more widely used stains are discussed next.

Simple Staining

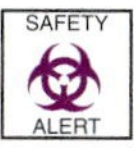

Only a single stain is added to the bacterial smear in **simple staining.** This procedure is used to stain the entire cell or specific structures in the cell. The fixed smear is covered with a stain for a certain time, according to the stain in use. Even the weakest dyes need no more than 3 minutes application time.

The smear is either air-dried or dried by pressing the slide gently between several layers of filter or bibulous paper. The cells should stain evenly with this technique. The stained smear is ready for microscopic examination.

Methylene blue is a common stain used in simple staining. It is often applied to a fixed bacterial suspension to stain whole cells a blue color without staining the background material. Methylene blue is classified as a basic dye, which means the charge carried by the dye ion is positive (+). Methylene blue binds mainly to the DNA and RNA of the cell.

Acidic dyes are dyes carrying a negative (−) charge on the dye ion. These include acid fuchsin, congo red, and safranin. They stain basic compounds in a cell, such as proteins carrying a basic charge. Sudan IV is a stain that is very soluble in fat. It is often used to identify the location and presence of fat droplets in bacteria.

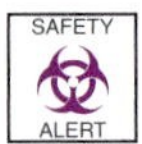

Differential Staining

Differential staining is a very detailed technique that helps to bring out differences between bacterial cells or parts of a bacterial cell. Differential staining is much more complex than simple staining because more than one stain is applied to the bacterial cells.

There are several widely used differential stain techniques, including the Gram stain, the acid-fast stain, and the Giemsa stain.

Gram staining.

The Gram stain is one of the most important and widely used differential stains in both bacteriology and microbiology. The Gram stain was developed by a Danish physician, Dr. Hans Christian Gram, in 1884. He developed this technique while working in a morgue in Berlin. This stain was developed to help him to distinguish pneumococcal bacteria from the cell nuclei in infected lung tissue. Dr. Gram was dissatisfied with his stain, because not all bacteria kept the stain. However, what Dr. Gram thought was a defect in his staining technique forms the basis for the most widely used stain to classify bacteria into one of two groups.

It is not known who first had the idea to use the Gram stain as a diagnostic method to separate bacteria into two groups. Many modifications to the original Gram stain method have occurred. One of the more widely used procedures is the one proposed by Kopeloff and Beerman. Gentian violet is used as the major stain. Other **reagents** used are an iodine solution, a decolorizing agent such as alcohol, acetone, or an alcohol-acetone mixture, and a **counterstain** such as Bismarck brown, dilute carbol fuchsin, or safranin. Color-blind people may find it helpful to use Bismarck brown as the counterstain.

The formula for the various stains mentioned in this chapter are found in the instructor's guide.

The basic Gram stain procedure is as follows:

Procedure 13–2 Gram Stain

Steps

1. Heat, fix the smear, then apply a basic purple stain, such as gentian violet or crystal violet to the fixed smear. Leave the stain on for 1 to 2 minutes. This will stain all bacteria purple.
2. Wash off the stain with water, using a wash bottle or an adapted hose connected to the faucet.

3. Rinse the stained smear with an iodine solution. Then add more iodine solution and let it set for 1 to 2 minutes. (The dilute iodine solution is made by dissolving 2 grams of iodine in 10 milliliters of normal NaOH solution and then adding water to bring it to a volume of 100 milliliters or, if available, use a commercial iodine solution.) The iodine solution or mordant decreases the solubility of the gentian violet stain within the bacterium by combining with the dye to form a dye–iodine complex. The dye is now "fixed" firmly in the bacterial cell.
4. Wash off the dilute iodine solution with water.
5. Drop by drop, apply acetone-alcohol decolorizing solution to the slide. Let the decolorizing solvent drain off, and watch the slide carefully. The acetone-alcohol will easily strip (decolorize) the purple–dye iodine complex from some but not all bacterial species. At the end of this step, gram-positive organisms will be purple. The gram-negative organisms will be colorless.
6. When no more purple color is seen in the acetone-alcohol drippings, wash the slide immediately with water. (Decolorization generally takes only 5 to 10 seconds.) Be careful to not over-decolorize.
7. Counterstain the smear for 1 minute with red safranin solution. The bacteria that were decolorized by the alcohol will absorb the safranin and appear either reddish or pink. The bacteria stained by the safranin are gram negative. Those that retain the gentian violet stain will appear purple and are said to be gram positive.

The Gram-stain reaction is characteristic for each different species of bacterium. The precise mechanism that causes bacteria to react differently to the Gram stain is not yet fully understood. The answer appears to be related to differences in the makeup and structure of the bacterial cell wall. Gram-negative bacteria have thinner cell walls containing a higher percentage of lipids than do gram-positive cell walls. Experimental data show that during decolorization the acetone-alcohol solvent extracts and dissolves the lipids from the gram-negative cell wall. This increases the permeability or porosity of the gram-negative cell wall, and the purple dye–iodine complex is extracted. Thus, the gram-negative bacteria is decolorized. The gram-positive cell walls with a lower lipid content become dehydrated during decolorization with the acetone-alcohol treatment. Thus, the pore size decreases, reducing the permeability of the cell wall and trapping the insoluble purple–dye iodine complex inside.

Although gram-negative organisms are constant in their reaction, gram-positive organisms occasionally show a borderline or **gram-variable** reaction. Sometimes, in old cultures, some gram-positive bacteria degenerate and lose their ability to retain the gentian violet stain. When this occurs, it will be stained by the safranin and show a gram-negative reaction. Also, gram-positive bacteria that have been exposed to an acid media or too much decolorizer will show the gram-negative reaction. It is very important, therefore, to follow the established procedures.

The Gram stain is an important diagnostic tool used to identify unknown organisms. Therefore, much reliance is placed upon the Gram stain in the diagnosis of gonorrhea, meningitis, and other diseases. Table 13–1 shows the reaction to the Gram stain of some major pathogenic bacteria.

The gram-negative and gram-positive bacteria have other differences besides their characteristic reaction to the Gram stain. Gram-negative bacteria are usually more sus-

Table 13–1 Some Important Pathogenic Bacteria and Their Reaction to the Gram Stain

Gram-Positive Reaction (+) (Reaction of the Purple Stain)		Gram-Negative Reaction (−) (Loss of the Purple Stain)		Gram-Variable Reaction (+/−)	
Bacterium	Disease It Causes	Bacterium	Disease It Causes	Bacterium	Disease It Causes
Bacillus anthracis	Anthrax	*Bordetella pertussis*	Whooping cough	*Mycobacterium leprae*	Leprosy
Clostridium botulinum	Botulism (food poisoning)	*Brucella abortus* (bovine strain)	Infectious abortion in cattle and undulant fever in humans	*Mycobacterium tuberculosis*	Tuberculosis
Clostridium perfringens	Gas gangrene, wound infection	*Brucella melitensis* (goat strain)			
Clostridium tetani	Tetanus (lockjaw)	*Brudella suis* (porcine strain)			
Corynebacterium diphtheriae	Diphtheria	*Escherichia coli*	Urinary infections, intestinal disorders		
Staphylococcus aureus	Carbuncles, furunculosis (boils), pneumonia, septicemia, toxic shock syndrome	*Haemophilus influenzae*	Meningitis, pneumonia		
Streptococcus pyogenes	Erysipelas, rheumatic fever, scarlet fever, septicemia, strep throat, tonsilitis	*Neisseria gonorrhoeae*	Gonorrhea		
Streptococcus pneumoniae	Pneumonia	*Neisseria meningitis*	Nasopharyngitis, meningitis		
		Pseudomonas aeruginosa	Respiratory and urogenital infections		
		Rickettsia rickettsii	Rocky Mountain spotted fever		
		Salmonella paratyphi	Food poisoning, paratyphoid fever		
		Salmonella typhi	Typhoid fever		
		Shigella dysenteriae	Dysentery		
		Vibrio cholerae	Cholera		
		Yersinia pestis	Plague		

Table 13–2 Some Basic Differences between Gram-Negative (−) and Gram-Positive (1) Bacteria

	Basic Differences	
Characteristic	**Gram Negative (−)**	**Gram Positive (+)**
Cell-wall composition	High lipid composition (11%–22%)	Low lipid composition (1%–4%)
Permeability of basic dyes like crystal violet	Less permeability	Marked permeability
Nutritional requirements	Relatively simple	Relatively complex for many species
Resistance to mechanical or physical treatment	Less resistant	More resistant
Sensitivity to penicillin	Less sensitive	More sensitive

ceptible to disintegration by physical treatment or exposure to some enzymes and less susceptible to penicillin than gram-positive bacteria. It has been discovered that gram-negative bacteria are very susceptible to streptomycin. Infection with gram-negative bacteria may result in an extreme condition called "endotoxin shock," and some gram-positive bacteria such as *Staphylococcus aureus,* which can cause toxic shock syndrome, can be quickly fatal. Table 13–2 shows some relative differences between gram-negative and gram-positive bacteria.

Acid-fast staining. There are some important bacteria that are distinguished from all others by the fact that they are stained with great difficulty. However, once they are stained with a powerful stain, they resist the decolorizing action of an acid-alcohol solvent. They are thus said to be "acid-fast" (alcohol to which has been added about 3% of concentrated acid). The tuberculosis bacterium and other members of the genus *Mycobacterium* are acid-fast, and this is one of their most outstanding characteristics. Thus, the acid-fast stain is invaluable as a diagnostic tool for examining specimens from patients suspected of having tuberculosis. It is also used as a stain for mycobacteria that have been grown in culture.

The procedure generally used to demonstrate the acid-fast staining properties of an organism is the Ziehl-Neelsen technique. The recommended steps are as follows.

Procedure 13-3 Acid-Fast Stain

Steps

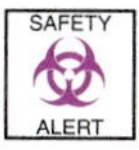

1. Place the slide on a ring stand, and stain the fixed smear with carbolfuchsin (Ziehl's formula). Apply a Bunsen burner flame under the slide for 3 to 5 seconds until the

stain steams. *Do not boil* the stain, and do not allow it to dry on the smear. (The heat from the Bunsen flame causes the stain to penetrate the lipid substances in the cell wall of certain bacteria.)

2. Wash off the carbolfuchsin with water.
3. Immerse the slide into an acid-alcohol solvent until the smear is decolorized; a very faint pink color remains. (The acid-alcohol solvent is 95% alcohol with 3% concentrated hydrochloric acid.) Decolorization causes the carbolfuchsin stain to be removed from everything in the smear except the acid-fast organisms. These organisms will retain the red carbolfuchsin color.
4. Wash off the acid-alcohol solvent with water.
5. Counterstain the smear with methylene blue or malachite green for about 30 seconds. This second stain serves as a contrast, dying everything in the smear except the acid-fast organisms. The organisms that absorb the blue or green counterstain are said to be non-acid-fast.
6. Wash off the counterstain with water and dry the smear.

Giemsa staining. The Giemsa staining technique is generally useful in locating rickettsias within host cells. (See Chapter 11 for more information on rickettsias). Rickettsias stain differentially and can be observed within the cytoplasm of the host cell. This stain is also used to stain blood films to examine protozoa, such as the malaria parasite.

Negative staining. The negative staining technique involves the staining of the background of a bacterial smear with an acidic black dye such as india ink or nigrosin. This procedure makes bacterial cells readily visible in an otherwise dark film, hence the term *negative staining*. This type of staining technique is comparable in appearance to a darkfield presentation. In practice, the microbial suspension is mixed with black india ink or nigrosine. The suspension is then spread in a thin film across a clean glass slide and allowed to dry. Upon microscopic examination, the microbes appear contrastingly colorless or transparent outlined against the dark background. This stain is traditionally used to help identify certain yeast cells that cause encephalitis. There is less vigorous chemical or physical treatment of microbes in negative staining, which is one advantage it has over the fixation, staining, and decolorization steps of other stains. Although these steps might cause some distortion in the cell, this is greatly lessened in negative staining. Negative staining is especially useful in staining capsulated organisms.

Other Stains

Capsule stain. Bacterial capsules are usually stained by the negative staining method or a variation of it. One capsule stain is the Welch method. The microbial smear is first treated with a hot crystal violet solution followed by a rinse with a copper sulfate solution. Copper sulfate ($CuSO_4$) is used to remove any excess stain, because the conventional water rinse would dissolve the bacterial capsule. The copper salt also colors the background. Thus, the bacterial cell and background appear dark blue and the capsule a much paler blue. One of the bacteria causing pneumonia, *Streptococcus pneumoniae*, is susceptible to the capsular stain.

Flagella stain. Flagella found on flagella-bearing bacteria are much too thin and fine [12 to 30 nanometers (nm) in diameter] to be visible in the light microscope. Prior to staining, the flagella are treated with a suspension of tannic acid salts. The tannic acid forms a heavy deposit or **precipitate** around the cell walls and flagella of the bacterium. This treatment helps to increase the apparent diameter of the flagella, so future staining with basic fuchsin makes the flagella quite visible in the light microscope.

In multitrichous bacteria, the flagella clumps into bundles during movement. These bundles may be thick enough to be observed on living cells by darkfield or phase-contrast microscopy.

Nucleic stain. Nuclei of cells can be stained with the Feulgen stain, which is specific for DNA, the genetic material.

Spore stain. In unstained cell suspension, spores can be seen as intracellular refractile bodies. However, in regularly stained cell preparations, they appear as colorless areas. The spore wall is relatively impermeable, but various stains, such as malachite green or carbolfuchsin, can be made to penetrate it by heating the bacterial preparation. The spore-wall impermeability prevents the spore from being decolorized by the alcohol treatment. The spores can be seen later counterstained with safranin.

A suggested procedure for the spore stain is as follows.

Procedure 13–4 Spore Stain

Steps

1. Prepare a smear of *Bacillus subtilis* from a 24-hour broth and fix over the Bunsen burner flame.
2. Flood the smear with 5% malachite green or carbolfuchsin. Then heat the smear over a steaming water bath for 2 to 3 minutes.
3. Wash with water.
4. Apply the safranin and counterstain for 30 seconds.
5. Wash, blot dry, and examine the slide using the oil-immersion objective lens.

SPECIMEN COLLECTION

Laboratory results are only as valid as the quality of specimen obtained. Therefore, it is essential that strict adherence to laboratory protocol must be followed when collecting microbiological specimens. The following are guidelines that all microbiological laboratories will, as a minimum, reject.

Specimen Source	Proper Specimen Collection	Unacceptable Specimens
Anatomical and surgical pathology	-Pathologist or physician will select suitable samples and put directly into a sterile container for prompt delivery to the lab. -Tissue abscesses from brain, lung, plural cavity, pelvis, liver, etc. must be cultured for anaerobic organisms. -Collect pus from the abscesses using a sterile needle and syringe, expelling all air from the syringe. Cork the needle to avoid oxygen contamination.	-any received in fixatives, formalin, alcohol, etc.
Blood cultures	-Select venipuncture site by palpation of the vein. -Using a circular motion, cleanse site with 70% isopropyl alcohol. -Let air-dry 1 minute. -Using the same circular motion, cleanse the site with povodone iodine, iodophor, or iodine. -Let air-dry 1 minute. -Do not palpate the site again unless the gloved finger has been cleansed in the same manner as the venipuncture site. -Collect 10–20 ml blood using a syringe and needle. -Immediately dispense the blood into the blood culture medium whose rubber top has been cleansed and dried according to the manufacturer's directions. -Usually blood culture bottles are inoculated in triplicate at timed intervals.	-samples collected in routine vacutainer tubes, red, lavender, etc.
Ear	-The physician will collect samples from the inner ear using sterile equipment and culturettes. -Carefully cleanse the external ear with detergent to remove the normal bacterial flora before the sample is taken.	-dry samples left out for long periods before being taken to the lab -any swab received dry
Eye	-Collect cultures before application of any antibiotics or irrigation procedures. -Use a sterile culturette to collect purulent material from the lower cul-de-sac and the inner canthus of the eye.	-samples taken after antibiotic drops have been added -any swab received dry

Specimen Source	Proper Specimen Collection	Unacceptable Specimens
Throat/nose	-Use a sterile culturette to collect tonsillar material by vigorously swabbing the areas of inflammation. -Using a tongue depressor will aid in the collection process. -Advise the patient to breathe regularly through the mouth to avoid gagging.	throat/nose swabs -any swab received dry
Sputum	-A first-morning deep-cough specimen is recommended. Advise patient to raise sputum and expectorate into a sterile container. -Patients suspected of having a tuberculosis or fungal infection must use appropriate safety containers for collection to avoid aerosol spread of germs. -For mycobacteria collect at least three daily specimens. -Deliver promptly to the lab to avoid overgrowth of normal respiratory flora.	-those consisting of saliva only (percentages of white blood cells and epithelial cells will be evaluated using Gram stain techniques) -any received in nonsterile containers
Bronchial washings	-The physician will collect the washings using a bronchoscope. -Place the washings in a sterile container and deliver promptly to the lab. -Bacterial, fungal, mycobacteria, and parasitology studies are usually ordered on these samples.	-bronchial washings received in nonsterile containers -any received in nonsterile containers
Transtracheal aspirations	-Patients with a trachaeotomy or those on a respirator may require transtracheal aspirations. -The area around the trachaeotomy is well disinfected before a catheter is inserted and sputum is suctioned from the trachea. The sample is put immediately into a sterile container and transported to the lab. -Transtracheal aspirations are usually incubated in an anaerobic atmosphere.	-transtrachial aspirations delivered in an aerobic environment unsuitable for anaerobic culture
Lung biopsy	-Physicians will perform this procedure, often at bedside. -Care must be taken to process these specimens with the utmost of care and very thoroughly as they are taken at great risk to the patient.	-any received in formalin

Specimen Source	Proper Specimen Collection	Unacceptable Specimens
Urine	**Clean Catch** -Cleanse the periurethral area (tip of penis, labial folds, vulva) with two separate soapings and rinse with sterile water. -Patient then urinates a portion of urine into the toilet and stops. The next portion is collected into a sterile container. The last portion of urine is voided into the toilet. -Deliver specimen immediately to the lab. Any delay requires refrigeration.	-any received in nonsterile containers -a delay or more than 1 hour between collection and delivery to the lab -specimens that have not been refrigerated while awaiting
	Catheter -For an in-place catheter, disinfect the wall of the catheter at the juncture with the drainage tube. -Using a syringe and 21-gauge needle puncture the cleansed area and aspirate the urine. -Transfer the urine to a sterile container and deliver immediately to the lab.	delivery to the lab
Genital	**Urethral** -In males the purulent discharge may be collected on a sterile swab and plated directly on the appropriate transport medium (Thayer Martin). A second swab is saved for a Gram stain smear. -*Neisseria gonorrhoeae* is very delicate and can die before the specimen reaches the lab. -A small calcium alginate swab may also be gently inserted several centimeters directly into the urethra to obtain a productive sample. **Vaginal/Cervical** -The cervix is the best site for female collections -The physician will use a sterile speculum moistened with warm water so as not to kill the gonococcus. -The cervical mucous plug is removed with a cotton ball and forceps. -A sterile swab is then inserted into the cervix, rotated, and allowed to remain for several seconds before removing. -Plate immediately to transport medium and send an additional swab to the laboratory.	-any received on a dry swab -any delayed more than 10 minutes unless in a transport media designed to hold or preserve organisms causing genital infections (esp. gonorrhoea, chlamydia, and herpes) -a delay of more than 30 minutes for delivery of Thayer Martin plates for gonorrhoea -dehydrating transport media

Specimen Source	Proper Specimen Collection	Unacceptable Specimens
Anal	Insert a cotton swab about 1 inch into the anal canal; move it from side to side to collect sample from the anal crypts. -If fecal material is observed, the swab should be discarded and the procedure performed again.	-any grossly contaminated with feces, annotate on the report
Stool	-Collect stool in a bedpan. -Select portions that have blood or mucus and transfer to a plastic stool container. -Deliver to laboratory immediately as pH changes when temperature of stool drops, decreasing recovery potential of pathogens. -Rectal swabs may also be collected by inserting a cotton swab beyond the rectal sphincter, rotating the swab, and withdrawing it carefully.	-enema-induced specimens -stools that have been refrigerated -prolonged delay in plating the specimen
CSF	-Usually three sterile tubes are collected by the physician using a needle and syringe. The first tube filled is labeled specimen 3 (as it was last to be withdrawn), the second tube filled is labeled specimen 2, and the last tube filled is labeled specimen 1. -The tubes are delivered first to the microbiology lab where cultures are taken off first using the tube that has been labeled specimen 3. -A portion is prepared for direct fungal and bacterial examination. -The CSF is then delivered to other laboratory departments for cell counts and chemistry studies.	-NEVER rejected -note time received and condition of specimen on the final report
Body fluid aspirations (joint, pleura, etc.)	-The skin areas around the aspiration site must be well disinfected so as not to introduce bacteria into the site or contaminate the specimen. -The aspirate is collected by a physician, the needle is corked, and the sample is promptly delivered to the lab. -If the syringe was washed with sterile heparin before the aspiration, the fluid will not clot.	-NEVER rejected -note time received and condition of specimen on the final report
Wounds	-Aerobic and anaerobic cultures should be taken. Follow the anaerobic collection procedures described on the culturette package. -Care must be taken to not contaminate the specimen with skin flora or airborne organisms. -If material is aspiratable this technique is preferred so as to avoid cross contamination.	-dry swabs left out for a long period.

SUMMARY

In this chapter procedures for examining bacteria are described. A hanging-drop preparation examines the motility of an organism. Staining a bacterial culture or a sample of body material requires preparation of the material on a slide, spread thinly, and then adhered by heat-fixing to ensure that the material does not wash off the slide during staining. The Gram stain procedure is an important staining procedure in the microbiology laboratory, for it is with this stain that the identification process begins. Other stains include the acid-fast stain (Ziehl-Neelson technique) for tuberculosis, the Giemsa stain for finding parasites in blood, and the negative stain (often called the india ink stain) for watching yeast cells in such fluids as spinal fluid. Capsular stains enhance capsules of *Streptococcus pneumoniae* as they are easily dissolved by the Gram stain technique. Because flagella on bacteria do not stain routinely, special stains employing tannic acid can enhance these fine appendages to allow their observation in the microscope. Spore stains enable us to better see the spores. In routine Gram stains they appear only as colorless bodies, but with a malachite green stain the stain actually penetrates the spore wall to prevent it from being decolorized by the alcohol treatment. An important section on specimen collection concludes this chapter. A specimen identification is only as good as the technique by which it was collected. Samples left sitting exposed to the air, urines not transported immediately, and spinal fluid samples not delivered directly to the microbiology lab can all result in misdiagnosis.

STUDY AND DISCUSSION

- Individually, or in small groups, prepare a report on Dr. Hans Christian Gram to find out more information about the development of the now famous Gram stain.
- Discuss with your instructor and become familiar with the safety procedures and precautions that must be strictly followed in a microbiology laboratory.

REVIEW QUESTIONS

A. General Questions: Provide complete answers to each of the following.

1. What is the difference between a simple stain technique and the differential stain technique?

2. Describe a situation in which it would be preferable to use a simple stain rather than a differential stain.

3. Briefly describe the Gram stain. Why is it a differential stain?

4. What are the basic differences between gram-negative and gram-positive bacteria?

5. Why is the Gram stain one of the most important and widely used microbial stains?

6. Briefly describe the acid-fast stain. When is it used?

7. What staining procedure is used for the observation of rickettsias?

B. Multiple-Choice Questions: Select the letter of the choice that best answers the question.

1. The stain of choice for differentiation of bacteria is the ________ stain.
   a. Wright's
   b. Giemsa
   c. Gram
   d. Ziehl-Neelsen
2. Vital stains ________ .
   a. distort internal structures
   b. stain living cells
   c. include crystal violet
   d. kill bacteria
3. Hanging-drop preparations will ________ Brownian movement.
   a. maximize
   b. minimize
4. Brownian movement is caused by ________ .
   a. air currents
   b. bacterial motility
   c. molecular collisions
   d. shaking the broth suspension
5. Gram-positive bacteria stain ________ .
   a. blue
   b. purple
   c. red
   d. golden

6. Hot looping will ________ .
   a. kill the bacteria
   b. spatter
   c. burn the media
   d. all of the above
7. Flaming the open lip of a culture tube is done to ________ .
   a. prevent bacteria in the air from entering the tube.
   b. prevent bacteria in the tube from escaping.
   c. prevent contamination of the air
   d. none of the above
8. In the Gram stain the mordant is ________ .
   a. crystal violet
   b. acetone-alcohol
   c. iodine
   d. safranin
9. The acid-fast stain is a stain for ________ .
   a. tuberculosis
   b. athletes' foot
   c. yeast infections
   d. intestinal bacteria
10. India ink stains are traditionally used to identify ________ .
   a. tuberculosis
   b. athletes' foot
   c. yeast infections
   d. intestinal bacteria

C. Completion Questions: From the following list of terms fill in the blanks with the correct choice.

a. Safranin **b. Crystal violet**

1. ________ stains red
2. ________ stains purple
3. ________ counterstain
4. ________ primary stain
5. ________ gram negative
6. ________ gram positive
7. ________ teicholic acid
8. ________ lipoprotein
9. ________ *Staphyloccus*
10. ________ penicillin sensitive

D. Matching Questions: Match the terms in Column I with their corresponding terms in Column II.

Column I		Column II
________	1. bacteria	a. nucleic stain
________	2. acid-fast bacilli	b. Giemsa stain
________	3. motile bacteria	c. capsule stain
________	4. *Bacillis subtilis*	d. spore stain
________	5. yeast	e. flagella stain
________	6. *Streptococcus pneumoniae*	f. Gram stain
________	7. nuclei	g. Ziehl-Neelsen
________	8. malaria parasites	h. india ink
________	9. gram positive	i. safranin
________	10. gram negative	j. crystal violet

SECTION 2

ACHIEVEMENT REVIEW

A. **The three main classifications of bacteria are shown. Identify each type in the space provided.**

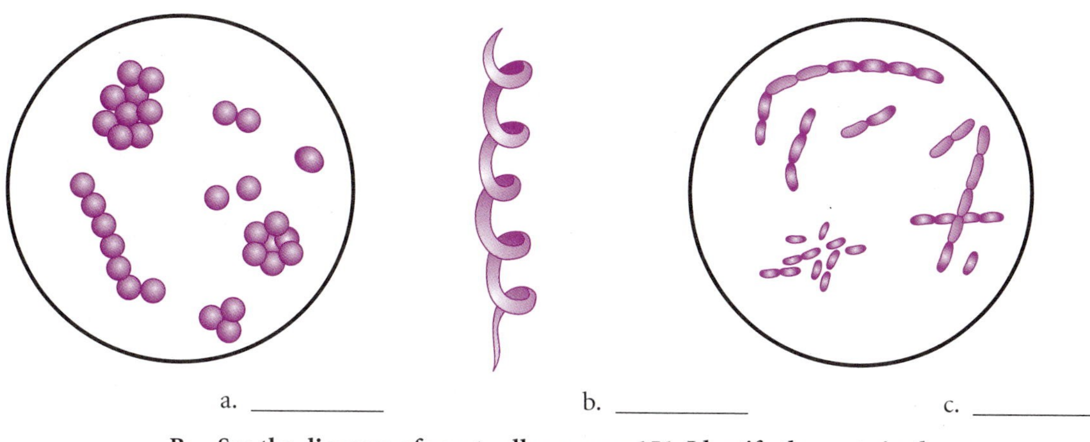

a. __________ b. __________ c. __________

B. **See the diagram of yeast cells on page 151. Identify the parts in the spaces provided, and complete statements 1 to 5.**

1. The reproductive process shown is called __________ .
2. The change process that yeasts produce in food is called __________ .
3. A disease caused by a form of yeast is __________ .
4. Yeasts may be killed by __________ .

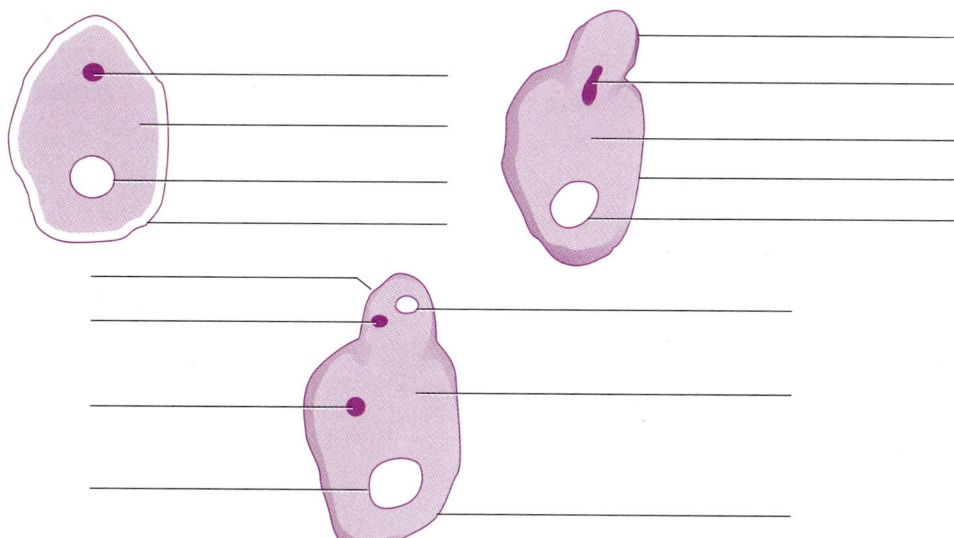

5. __________ is the gas given off during the action of yeasts on sugar in solution.

C. **Match each word or term in Column I with the statement in Column II that is most closely associated with it.**

Column I		Column II
______	1. fermentation	a. filterable virus
______	2. spores	b. protozoa
______	3. Ziehl Neelson	c. bacteria
______	4. one-celled animals	d. enterioorganisms
______	5. india ink	e. mold
______	6. germsa stain	f. clostridium
______	7. athlete's foot	g. bacteria
______	8. flagella	h. tuberculosis
______	9. one-celled plants	i. parasites
______	10. measles	j. capsular stains
		k. yeast

D. **In the spaces provided, identify the parts of each protozoan shown on pages 170 and 174. Complete statements 1 to 5.**

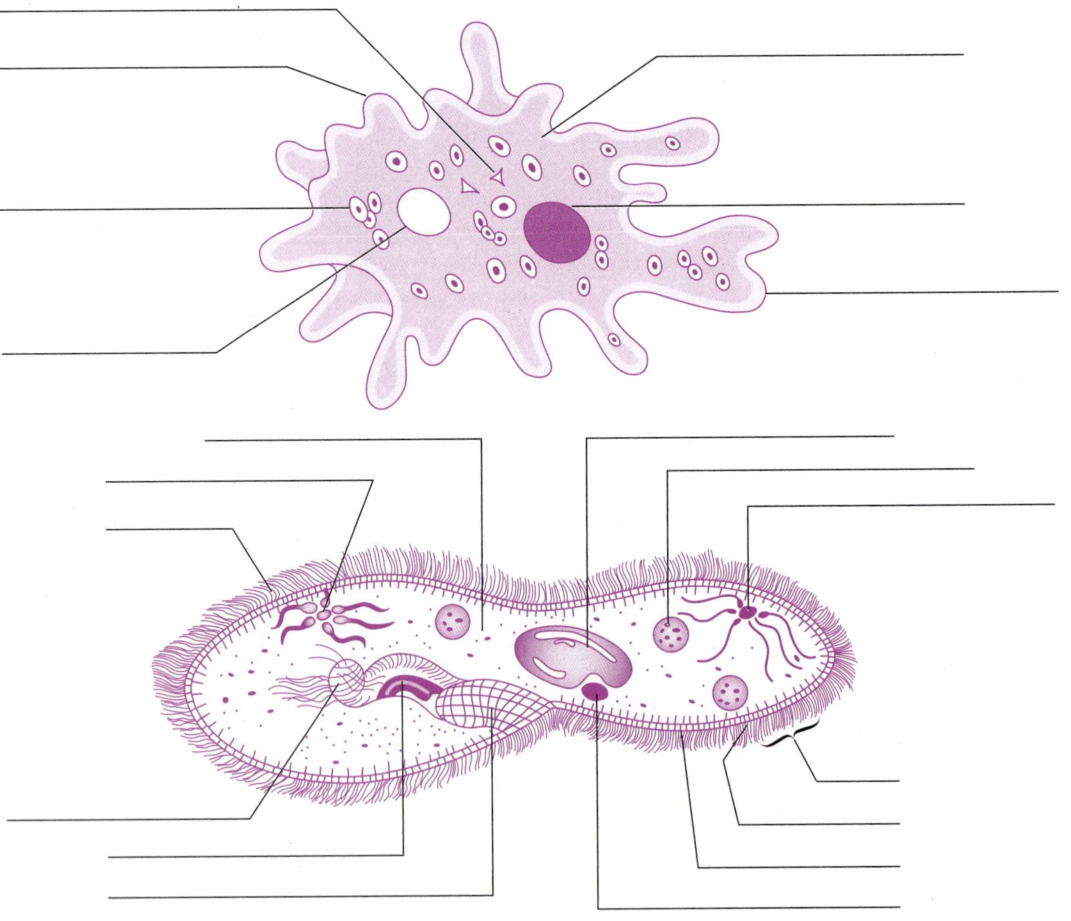

1. Three diseases caused by protozoa are ___________ , ___________ ___________ , and ___________ .

2. The process by which protozoa feed is called ___________ .

3. Two harmless protozoa found in stagnant water are ___________ and ___________ .

4. A protozoan transmitted to people through the bite of the *Anopheles* mosquito causes ___________ .

5. In human beings, protozoa are likely to be found in several locations. Two such locations are the ___________ and ___________ .

E. Illustrated are two molds as seen under the microscope. Identify the parts in the spaces provided, and complete statements 1 to 5.

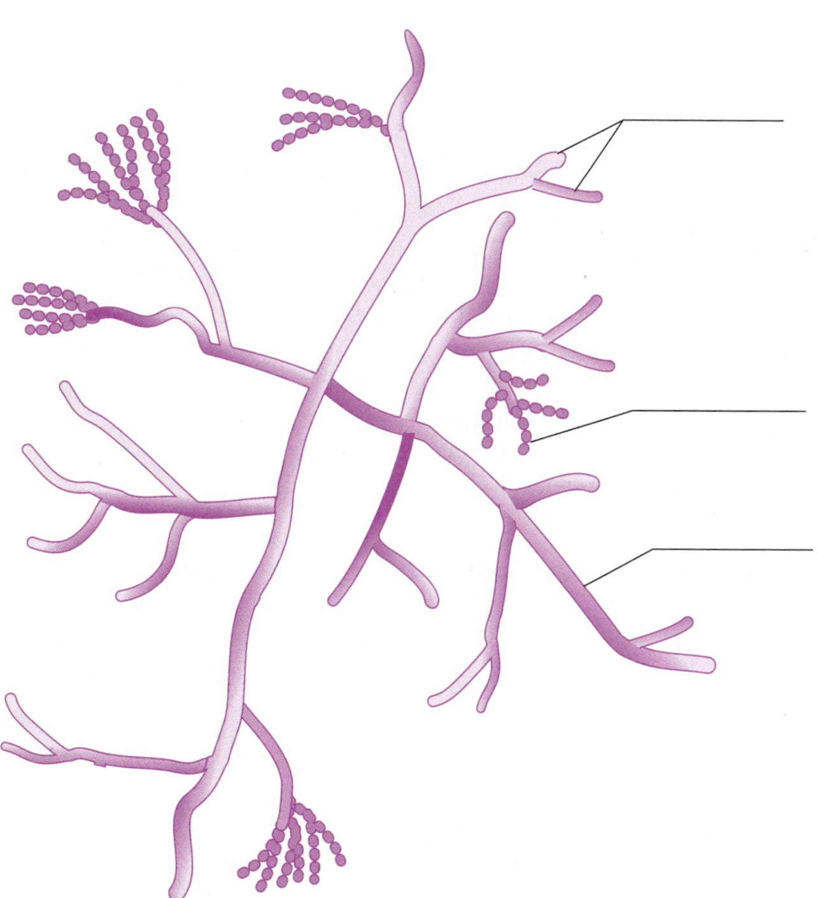

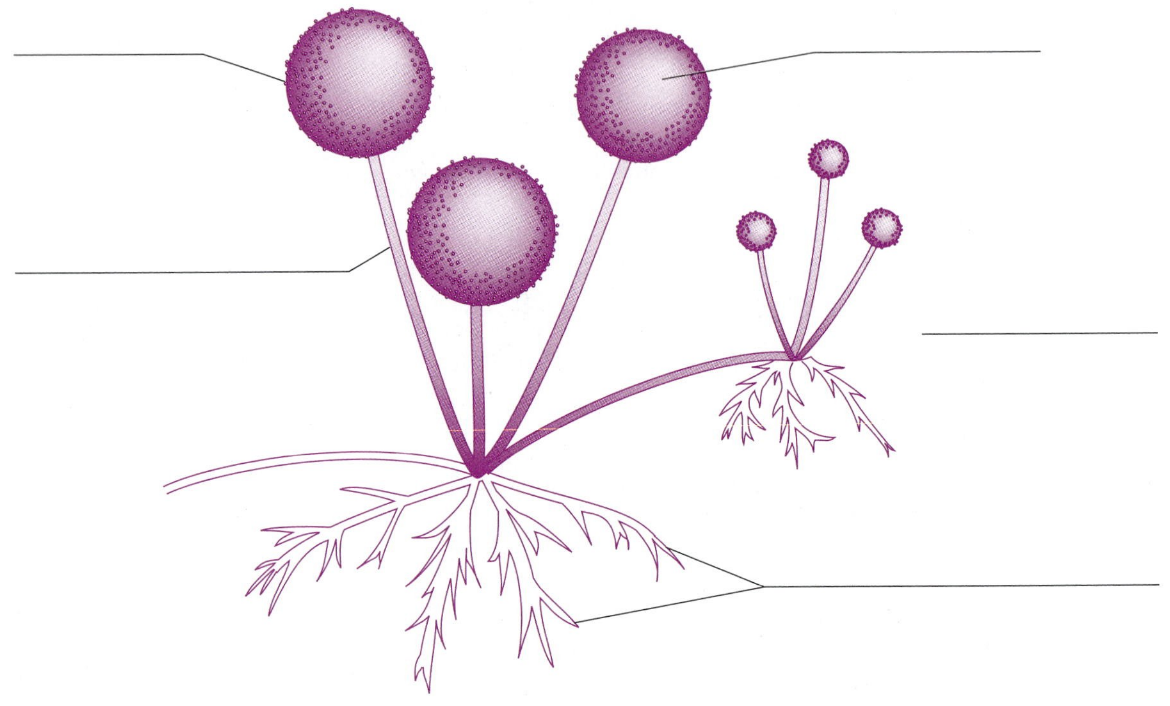

1. Three conditions favorable for the growth of molds are ___________ , ___________ , and ___________ .

2. Two diseases caused by molds are ___________ and ___________ .

3. A useful antibiotic obtained from bread mold is ___________ .

4. Molds release into the air thousands of ___________ , which start new mold growths when they contact substances that can nourish them.

5. One way to prevent mold growth is to ___________ .

F. Insert the word or phrase that best completes the following sentences.

1. Molds belong to a group of plants called ___________ .

2. Bacteria may be classified according to their degree of harmlessness as ___________ and ___________ .

3. Of the above two types of bacteria, the ___________ type is of more concern to the health care professional.

4. The unit of measurement for bacteria is called the ___________ .

5. Three beneficial activities of microorganisms are ___________ , ___________ , and ___________ .

6. A form of microorganism so small that it passes through a porcelain filter is called a ___________ .

7. Three diseases caused by viruses are ___________ , ___________ , and ___________ .

8. A health professional flames the loop of an inoculating needle in order to ___________ .

9. A bacterial population consisting of millions of bacteria is called a ___________ .

10. An animal or plant that supports a parasite is called a ___________ .

11. A permanent preparation made by spreading a drop of culture on a glass slide is called a ___________ .

12. Two culture mediums used to grow bacteria in the laboratory are ___________ ___________ and ___________ .

13. Bacteria are everywhere except in a ___________ environment.

14. A form of microorganism that causes typhus is ___________ .

15. Most diseases are caused by ___________ and ___________ ___________ .

16. Poliomyelitis is caused by a ___________ .

17. The term *pathogenic* means ___________ , or ___________ .

18. AIDS is caused by the ___________ virus.

19. One symptom produced by the causative agent of AIDS is swollen glands or ___________ .

G. Insert the word or expression that best completes each statement. Some words may be used more than once.

90 minutes	*Stapyhlococcus*	water	kill
45 minutes	neutral	contamination	temperature
Streptococcus	acidic	moisture	yeasts & molds
60 minutes	disinfectant	darkness	yeast & protozoa
sterile	25,000	*Estomoeba coli*	unfavorable
16×10^6	molds	syphilis	20 to 30
Balantidium coli	yeasts	gonorrhoea	40 to 45
stationary	250,000	coldness	protozoa
	food		

1. A nonmotile bacterium is one that is ___________ .

2. An example of spherical bacteria found in pairs is the one that causes ___________ .

3. An example of a spirillum is one that causes ___________ .

4. An example of a spherical form that produces boils is ___________ .
5. It is possible for a bacterium to divide after ___________ minutes.
6. Most bacteria prefer a ___________ medium.
7. All methods of preserving foods depend upon producing ___________ conditions for the growth of bacteria.
8. The effect of direct sunlight on bacteria is to ___________ them.
9. Under favorable conditions, a single bacterial cell may produce ___________ ___________ of bacteria in twelve hours.
10. Four conditions needed by bacteria for growth are ___________ , ___________ , ___________ , and ___________ ___________ .
11. The medium agar, provides bacteria with both ___________ and ___________ .
12. Refrigeration retards the growth of bacteria because it produces the unfavorable environmental condition of ___________ .
13. Something free from bacteria is referred to as ___________ .
14. All health care professionals should wash their hands thoroughly with disinfectant soap and water after tending patients to prevent ___________ .
15. The fungi may be divided into the ___________ and ___________ groups.
16. Of these groups, only ___________ consists of more than one cell.

H. From the list of terms below fill in the blanks with the correct choice.

mitochondria	plasmid	Pili	vacuole
prokaryote	cytoplasm	solvent	solute
ribosomes	nucleus	lysosome	isotonic
phagocytosis	hypertonic	cell wall	cytologist

1. Tiny grainy structures attached to the endoplasmic reticulum called ___________ are protein factories of the cell.
2. The ___________ is the control center for all cell activity.
3. The ___________ produces most of the cell's energy.
4. The cell material outside the nucleus is called the ___________ .
5. Fine hair-like structures found protruding from the cytoplasmic membrane of bacterial cells are called ___________ .
6. A ___________ is a space or cavity found in the protoplasm of a cell.
7. The substance that is being dissolved is called the ___________ .
8. The substance doing the dissolving is called the ___________ .

9. A section of DNA taken from a donor and inserted into recipient DNA is called a ___________ .
10. A unicellular organism lacking a true nucleus is called a ___________ .
11. The ability of some white blook cells to engulf bacteria is known as ___________ .
12. The cell organelle that aids in digestion is the ___________ .
13. A solution whose salt concentration is the same as the body's fluids concentration is called a(n) ___________ solution.
14. A solution with a salt concentration greater than that of body fluids is said to be ___________ .
15. The outer rigid structure of plant cells is the ___________ .
16. A ___________ studies the structure and pathology of cells.

I. Matching Questions: Match the terms in Colum I with their corresponding terms in Column II.

	Column I	Column II
________	1. Complex cells	a. vacuole
________	2. 2N chromosomes	b. micron
________	3. Micrometer	c. lipoprotein layer
________	4. sex cells	d. RNA
________	5. simple cells	e. Meiosis
________	6. N chromosomes	f. prokaryotes
________	7. Ribosomes	g. Mitosis
________	8. Pinocytosis	h. haploid
________	9. gram-negative bacteria	i. osmosis
________	10. diffusion of water	j. eukaryotes
________	11. respiratory enzymes	k. teichoic acid layer
________	12. Flagella	l. cytochromes
________	13. pili	m. fimbriae
________	14. gram positive	n. scientific names
________	15. binomial nomenclature	o. locomotion

J. Select the word or expression that best completes each statement.

1. Biologists refer to rod-shaped bacteria as
   a. bacilli.
   b. cocci.
   c. spirilla.
   d. streptococci.
2 Properly canned foods will not spoil because they have been
   a. homogenized.
   b. pasteurized.
   c. stabilized.
   d. sterilized.
3. The classification of bacteria that does form spores is
   a. bacilli.
   b. spirilla.
   c. cocci.
   d. viruses.

4. If the name of a kind of bacterium ends in *coccus*, then the shape of the individual bacterium is
   a. elongated.
   b. rectangular.
   c. spherical.
5. Spiralla are types of
   a. bacteria.
   b. molecules.
   c. protozoa.
   d. virusues.
6. The hairlike projections found in some bacteria are the
   a. cilia.
   b. villi.
   c. flagella.
   d. pseudopods.
7. A string of spherical bacteria make up a group called
   a. *Diplococcus.*
   b. *Streptococcus.*
   c. *Staphylococcus.*
   d. *Bacillus.*
8. A bacterium that forms spores is the
   a. *Streptococcus.*
   b. *Staphylococcus.*
   c. *Diplococcus.*
   d. tetanus organism.
9. The purpose of a Ziehl-Neelsen is to determine ______ .
   a. acid-fast properties.
   b. capsules.
   c. gram properties.
   d. fungal properties.
10. Sputum specimens consist of ______ .
    a. mucus.
    b. saliva.
    c. white blood cells.
    d. mucus and white blood cells.

K. True/False

1. Specimens that cannot be processed immediately may be refrigerated for up to 2 hours ____ .
2. The best urine sample for processing is one that is collected using the clean catch midstream method and brought to the lab immediately ____ .
3. Wound cultures require aerobic and anaerobic culturing ____ .
4. Genital specimens are cultured only on blood agar ____ .
5. When spinal fluid is collected it must be delivered to the lab for cell counts before culture material is removed ____ .
6. In collecting blood cultures the area must be prepped with alcohol and iodine to prevent skin contamination ____ .
7. Syringes used to collect fluid aspirations should be washed with an anticoagulant such as heparin before the aspiration to prevent clotting ____ .
8. If a patient is constipated and cannot produce a stool specimen as needed for culture, it is best to give a fleet enema to loosen the bowels ______ .
9. CSP samples collected in open test tubes or regular blood-collecting tubes will not be processed for culturing ____ .
10. Tissue samples or lung biopsies for culture from an AIDS patient must be submitted in formalin as a safety measure to protect the laboratory worker ______ .

SECTION

3 INFECTION AND IMMUNITY

CHAPTER

14 How Microorganisms Cause Infection

OBJECTIVES

After completing this chapter, you will be able to:

- name four ways in which microorganisms may be transmitted.
- list four sources of entry into the body.
- identify bodily secretions and excretions that contain bacteria.

KEY WORDS

biohazard	commensal	fomites
carrier	droplet infection	standard precautions

TRANSMISSION OF MICROORGANISMS

Microorganisms may be transmitted from an infected individual to a susceptible person in the following ways:

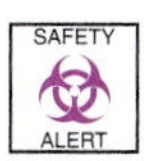

- Contact with an infected person
  - A. Direct contact: This method involves handling, touching, coughing, sneezing, and blood-to-blood and secretions-to-secretions contact.

1. Handling/touching: Many bacteria are readily transmitted one to another by touching an infected area. Boils involving staphylococcal infections can be transmitted by not cleaning the infected site properly, then by touching something else without proper handwashing techniques. Hospital staphylococcal infections in newborn nurseries are one of the most dreaded instances of touching contact.
2. Coughing/sneezing: Viral infections such as the flu and the common cold are readily passed on by not covering the mouth when coughing and the nose when sneezing, thus allowing the air droplets containing these viruses to be inhaled by others.
3. Secretions-to-secretions contact: This method would include kissing and sexual intercourse to transmit STDs such as gonorrhea, syphilis, genital warts (human papalloma virus), herpes, chlamydia, and HIV.
4. Blood-to-blood contact: Blood transfusions with tainted blood can readily pass on hepatitis A, B, and C and HIV.

B. Indirect contact: This method implies that the infected person has not been in contact with the host or carrier, but rather the host or carrier has contaminated something (most often food) with which the infected person later comes in contact.
   1. Handling articles: A good example would be the laundering of contaminated bedding of someone with dysentery, salmonella, or hepatitis A without using proper handwashing techniques.
   2. Touching contaminated substances: Poor personal hygiene and handling substances contaminated by a patient in isolation could result in the passage of infectious materials.
   3. Eating food prepared by an infected person: This method has been known to transmit typhoid fever, intestinal diarrhea (*E. coli*), hepatitis A, and dysentery. See the list of standard precautions on page 272 (as well as in Appendix C) for preventive measures in transmitting diseases.

- Contact with human carriers

A **carrier** is someone who harbors a pathogen (a disease-causing microorganism) with or without developing any symptoms from the pathogen. Even so, the pathogen can be transmitted to a susceptible individual, who may develop the disease. Respiratory secretions given off when coughing or sneezing and human fecal material from carriers can contaminate food and water, thus providing an avenue of infection to others. Such was the case of the infamous "Typhoid Mary," perhaps the best-known carrier of all times.

During the early twentieth century, Mary worked as a cook in a well-known restaurant in New York City. A large outbreak of typhoid fever alarmed health officials who, upon investigation, traced the source to a salad served by the restaurant as its trademark. Upon bacteriological testing of stool samples taken from the staff, the culprit was found to be harbored by "Mary," a cook who frequently failed to wash her hands when returning to work. Mary, of course, was a classic carrier and had never had any symptoms of the disease herself.

More recently, a particularly virulent strain of a common bowel **commensal** *Escherichia coli* was found to have caused a serious food poisoning outbreak in children who had eaten hamburgers at a fast-food restaurant. Several deaths were even reported from this strain of *E. coli.* It is particularly important to note that good handwashing techniques must be strictly adhered to by all who work in restaurants.

In Milwaukee, Wisconsin, the city water supply was found to have become contaminated with *Cryptosporidium,* a rare protozoan parasite generally found in cow dung. It was thought that it got into the city water supply by runoff from farms. This disease produced flulike symptoms, stomach cramps, and diarrhea for up to 2 weeks in the epidemic proportions of residents who fell victim.

- Contact with animal or insect carriers

This category includes any type of animal (cattle, domestic animals, wildlife, horses, and pigs) or insect (flies, mosquitoes, ticks, and mites) capable of transmitting a disease to a human. People can contract certain diseases from the bite of or direct contact with an animal. Eating meat and other products from a diseased animal can also be a cause of disease to humans. Some diseases transmitted to people by animal or insect carriers are described in Table 14–1.

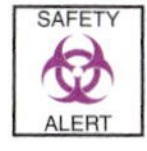

- Contact with inanimate or airborne carriers

This category includes air, dust, food, soil, water, instruments, and fomites.

MICROORGANISM INVASION

Microorganisms entering the body may or may not cause infection. The invasion of bacteria is similar to an enemy army invading a country. If the defenses of the country are good, the invasion fails; if the defenses of the body are strong and numerous, the bacteria are killed and no infection results. On the other hand, weak defenses may allow for a successful invasion of bacteria.

The effectiveness of an invasion of bacteria will depend upon:

- the kind of organism and its virulence
- the number of organisms
- the resistance or body defenses
- the location of the invasion

Pathogenic organisms may enter the body through several routes: the respiratory tract, the alimentary canal, the genitourinary tract, abrasions in the skin, and mucous membranes of the eye.

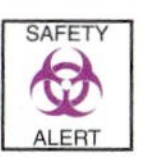

Respiratory Tract

Many diseases, especially respiratory infections, are spread through the air by **droplet infection.** This fine spray of mist is discharged by sneezing and coughing. If this spray

Table 14–1 Some Microorganisms Transmitted to Humans by Animal Carriers

Disease	Microorganism	Symptoms in Humans	Animal Carrier(s)	Method of Transmission
Anthrax	Gram-positive bacillus: *Bacillus anthracis*	Skin develops pustules (small boils), area surrounding pustules becomes hard and edematous	Cattle, birds, pigs, goats, horses, sheep	Contaminated hair, hide, wood
Plague	Gram-negative bacillus: *Yersinia pestis*	Extremely high fever, inflammation of lymph glands, pneumonia, severe internal and external bleeding	Rodents	Flea bites rodent, which in turn bites person
Q fever	Rickettsia: *Coxiella burnetti*	Acute infection, characterized by pneumonia, fever, nausea, and vomiting	Birds, rats, domestic animals	Tick bite and inhalation of the airborne microorganism
Rocky Mountain spotted fever	Rickettsia: *Rickettsia rickettsii*	Fever characterized by a rash	Wild rodents	Tick bites wild rodent, which in turn bites person
Rabies	Virus: Rabies virus	Severe headache, high fever, alternation between depression and excitement, difficulty in swallowing characterized by spasms in the throat and chest	Skunks, bats, cats, dogs	Bite from an animal carrying the infected saliva
Malaria	Protozoan: *Plasmodium vivax*	Alternation between high fever and chills, profuse sweating and anemia	Monkeys	Mosquito bite
Ringworm	Fungus: Several species of microorganisms causing fungal skin infections—dermatophytes	Skin infection characterized by raised, circular, reddish swellings	Cats, dogs, domestic animals	Direct contact
Lyme disease	Spirochete bacterium: *Borrelia burgdorferi*	Erythema migrans at tick bite site. Later muscle, joint pain, malaise. Still later, arthritis, neurologic disorders	Deer, rodents	Human tick
Hemorrhagic fever	Dengue virus	Sudden fever lasting 2–7 days, skin hemorrhages, circulatory failure, bleeding gums, A-I hemmorhage and hematuria	Aedes mosquito	Mosquito bite to humans—never person to person

comes from a person with a cold, influenza, tuberculosis, or any other respiratory ailment, it contains pathogens. Another person may get the disease by inhaling the droplets if his or her resistance is low.

Dust may also potentially spread infection. Tiny dried particles of animal and human wastes can be borne through the air by dust. This is also true of pathogenic bacterial spores. In this manner, infected waste particles and pathogens may be carried into a person's warm and moist respiratory tract, where they breed and multiply.

Gastrointestinal Tract

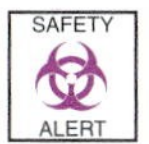

Contaminated or infected food and drink can spread disease. Organisms that live in our intestines will be spread through contaminated food objects. Some diseases spread by food and drink are typhoid fever, dysentery, undulant fever, and food poisoning.

The health care provider should know how to handle contaminated, disposable materials and how to sterilize dishes and other articles used by patients.

Genitourinary Tract

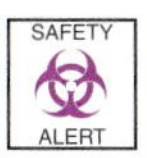

Bladder infections, syphilis, and gonorrhea are examples of diseases caused by organisms that infect the genitourinary tract. It is extremely important that all health care professionals observe **precautions** when working with patients and handling any body fluids. Gloves must be worn at all times when giving genitourinary care.

Abrasions in the Skin

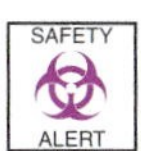

We are all familiar with an infected finger resulting from an unsterilized cut in the skin. Lockjaw or tetanus bacteria may enter a very deep puncture in the skin.

Insect and vermin bites can also transmit infection. Mosquitoes carry the microorganisms that cause malaria and yellow fever. The tsetse fly carries the organisms that cause African sleeping sickness; flies carry the bacteria of typhoid fever, tuberculosis, and dysentery. Animals may transmit rabies; body lice may transmit typhus fever; and bubonic plague is sometimes spread by fleas.

HEALTH CARE PROCEDURES

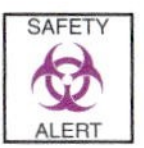

Microorganisms leave the body through secretions and excretions such as saliva, urine, sputum, feces, blood, and nasal discharges. Disposable, soiled tissues should be bagged and discarded; any equipment that has come in contact with body discharges should be made aseptic.

Health care personnel must also be aware of the dangers in transmission of pathogens through **fomites.** Fomites are inanimate objects that can carry pathogens and thus serve as disease carriers. For instance, pathogens from the respiratory, gastrointestinal, and genitourinary tracts, as well as from the skin of a patient, can contaminate bedding, clothing, drinking and eating utensils, bedpans and urinals, and medical equipment. Of course, a health care provider must properly dispose of or sterilize such articles. Refer to Chapter 18 for more on destruction of microorganisms.

STANDARD PRECAUTIONS

With the passage of the OSHA final rule in Health Care Workers Protection from Potential Blood Borne Pathogens in June 1992, employers and employees have a shared responsibility to inform and educate and to comply with the guidelines. Simply stated, all **biohazardous** and potentially biohazardous materials must be treated as though they are infectious. Similarly, all patients and their body fluids will be treated in the same manner.

1. Gloves must be worn at all times when handling all body fluid material.
2. Sharps as well as broken glass must be disposed of in a hard-walled sharps container. Such containers will be strategically placed and readily available for use.
3. Employers must provide nonpermeable protective clothing for those at risk of contamination by potentially hazardous body fluids.
4. Employers must make available, at no cost to the employee, hepatitis B vaccinations. Employees may decline but are required to sign a waiver of liability. Employees do have the right to request the vaccinations at a later date without cost to them.
5. Employers must provide education and training for their employees.
6. To clean a biohazardous spill, a 3% to 10% bleach solution is poured over the site, allowed to sit, then wiped up with disposable towels.
7. Spills in instrumentation will also be cleaned with bleach. Equipment sent for repair will be sprayed with a disinfectant bleach before being serviced.
8. Biohazardous trash will be properly disposed of according to weight and volume generated by a facility. Generally, less than 50 pounds of biohazardous waste is exempt from removal by a biohazardous waste management company.
9. Clothing worn on duty by health care personnel will not be worn outside the workplace, even to and from work.

SUMMARY

Microorganisms can be spread by direct contact, touching, sneezing, coughing, kissing, sexual intercourse, needle sharing, or indirect contact such as handling contaminated articles of an infected person or eating food prepared by an infected person. Coming in contact with a carrier can cause a person to become ill even when the carrier has no sign of illness.

The severity of an infection may depend on the organism's virulence, the type of organism, the body's resistance capabilities, and the location of the invasion.

Organisms may enter via the respiratory tract through sneezing or coughing tiny droplets into the air. They can enter the gastrointestinal tract by eating contaminated food and drink. They can also enter via the genitourinary tract as bladder or urethral infections. Abrasions to the skin can easily be an entry port for tetanus bacteria. Some mosquitoes can infect you with their bite by leaving the virus or parasite in your blood stream.

Standard precautions, common sense, and good handwashing techniques can prevent the microorganisms from gaining entry to cause infections.

STUDY AND DISCUSSION

- Prepare a report on the famous Typhoid Mary case.
- Explain the difference between direct and indirect contact.
- Explain what fomites are; list ten examples.
- Prepare a report on how the U.S. government controlled mosquitoes when building the Panama Canal. Why was this necessary?
- Discuss how a health care professional would administer first aid treatment for a skin wound.
- A health care professional is caring for a patient with typhoid fever. Explain how he or she would sterilize thermometers, bedpans, and dishes, and dispose of particles of uneaten food, as well as urine and feces.
- Discuss droplet infection. List precautions that will help prevent the spread of disease by this method.

REVIEW QUESTIONS

A. General Questions: Provide complete answers to each of the following.

1. List four different ways that microorganisms can enter the body.

2. What are disease carriers? Do they show disease symptoms? Name three types of disease carriers.

3. Name two diseases that can be spread through contaminated food and drink.

4. Identify two diseases that can be spread through the genitourinary tract.

5. Name one microorganism that can enter the body through a deep wound.

6. Name a disease transmitted by the saliva of an animal. List its symptoms.

7. List three diseases transmitted by insect bites. What are the microorganisms that cause these diseases?

8. Explain droplet infection. Which disease can be spread in this manner?

9. Explain how a health care provider would prevent a cough from spreading through droplet infection.

10. After bacteria enter the body, what determines whether a person does or does not get the disease?

11. Make a list of some of the careless practices by which microorganisms can be passed from diseased persons to persons who are well.

12. List four ways in which a health care professional can prevent transmission of pathogens to healthy persons.

B. Multiple-Choice Questions: Select the letter of the choice that best answers the question.

1. The spread of microorganisms by direct contact includes all of the following except _____ .
   a. touching an infected person's skin
   b. touching contaminated clothing
   c. coming in contact with respiratory secretions
   d. blood transfusions
2. Carriers of infectious agents _____ .
   a. do not become ill with the disease
   b. carry a less virulent stain of the pathogen
   c. carry only nonpathogenic organisms
   d. can spread their microorganisms to others who may become very ill with the disease
3. Respiratory infections are easily spread by _____ .
   a. droplet infections, sneezing, and coughing
   b. droplet infections and contaminated urine
   c. cow dung and droplet infection
   d. contaminated food, coughing, and sneezing
4. Fomites are _____ .
   a. bacterial infections originating on the farm
   b. dead decayed matter
   c. inanimate objects such as bedding
   d. normal flora of the upper respiratory tract
5. Standard precautions state that_____ when handling body fluids.
   a. gloves will be worn at all times
   b. gloves are optional
   c. gloves are recommended to be worn
   d. gloves are not necessary, except when the potential for contamination may be present

C. Completion Questions: From the following list of terms fill in the blanks with the correct choice.

saprophytes	fleas	mites	respiratory	gastrointestinal
commensals	ticks	lice	urinary	

1. Bacteria that are considered to be normal flora are also known as ___________ .
2. Lyme disease, carried by deer and rodents, is transmitted to humans via ___________ .
3. Undulant fever attacks the ___________tract.
4. Tuberculosis enters the body through the ___________ tract.
5. Bubonic plague is spread by ___________ .

D. Matching Questions: Match the terms in Column I with their corresponding terms in Column II.

Column I		Column II
_______	1. malaria	a. birds
_______	2. rabies	b. cattle
_______	3. Q fever	c. household pets
_______	4. plague	d. *Cryptosporidium*
_______	5. anthrax	e. mosquito
_______	6. Lyme disease	f. *Escherichia coli*
_______	7. ringworm	g. deer
_______	8. Milwaukee water supply	h. dogs, rodents
_______	9. fast-food restaurant	i. wild rodents
_______	10. Rocky Mountain spotted fever	j. flea bites

CHAPTER

15 Body Defenses

OBJECTIVES

After completing this chapter, you will be able to:

- provide a detailed explanation of the ways in which the human body protects itself from disease.
- describe the first line of defense.
- describe the second line of defense.
- explain how the third line of defense produces antibodies.
- describe how phagocytosis aids in the body's defense.

KEY WORDS

agglutinins
antibodies
antigens
antigen-antibody response
antitoxins
Candida albicans
Clostridium botulinum
Clostridium tetani
complement
Corynebacterium diphtheriae
degranulation
Enterobacter aerogenes
erythrocytes
exotoxin
Escherichia coli
fever
fixed phagocytes
general infection
hemolysin
incubation period
inflammation
leukocidin
leukocytes
local infection
lockjaw
lyse
lysins
lysosome
mobile phagocytes
opsonins
phagocytosis
phagolysosome
phagosome
precipitins
Pseudomonas aeruginosa
pus
pyogenic bacteria
reticuloendothelial system (RES)
Staphylococcus aureus
wandering phagocytes

BODY DEFENSES

We have focused upon some of the more harmful effects of an invasion by bacteria. The human body, however, is neither helpless nor completely vulnerable to these threats. In fact, the body is equipped with three main lines of defense against such unwelcome invasion: (1) the skin and mucous membrane; (2) circulatory defenses; and (3) antibodies (immune response).

Skin and Mucous Membrane

The first line of defense against invading pathogens is the external barrier of the unbroken skin and mucous membranes. Only when the skin is damaged, such as by burns, cuts, or scratches, are pathogens able to penetrate.

The skin kills or inhibits bacterial growth through its secretions. Lactic acid from the sweat glands and fatty acids from the sebaceous (fat) glands and the low pH environment that they produce fight off many pathogens.

Respiratory tract.

The mucous membranes and the cilia (tiny hairlike projections) lining the nose and nasal passages filter and trap inhaled dust and pathogens. Cilia lining the posterior nasal passages, bronchi, and trachea then sweep the entrapped dust and pathogens toward the throat. From there they are removed from the body by coughing, sneezing, and even swallowing. In addition, the lysozyme enzyme found in nasal secretions, saliva, and tears **lyses,** or kills, certain gram-positive bacteria.

Digestive tract.

Harmful pathogens in the digestive tract are destroyed by powerful digestive juices, the acidity of the stomach, and the alkalinity of the intestines. Mucous secretions from the digestive tract will entrap many pathogens, where they await destruction by bactericidal enzymes or phagocytes. The normal actions of peristalsis (muscular intestinal contractions) and defecation also remove pathogens from the intestine.

Of course, not all enteric (intestinal) bacteria are harmful. Some, such as ***Escherichia coli*** and ***Enterobacter aerogenes,*** are quite useful. They help to keep a normal balance in the digestive tract, and aid in getting rid of wastes. *E. coli* also helps in the production of vitamin K.

Genitourinary tract.

The genitourinary tract has its harmful pathogens flushed out by frequent urination and vaginal mucosal secretions. The occurrence of bladder infections is usually due to infrequent urination, especially after intercourse. In females, vaginal infections are common when oral contraceptives are taken because they reduce the acidity of the vagina. Also, after extensive antibiotic treatment the yeast ***Candida albicans*** may grow freely in the vagina, causing candidiasis or moniliasis. Because the normal protective vaginal flora is destroyed by prolonged antibiotic use, pathogens are allowed to flourish unchecked.

Circulatory Defenses

Often, if pathogens break through the first line of defense, other defenses (elements found in the circulatory system) move in to destroy them. These include the phagocytes, antibodies, and interferon.

Phagocytes.

Phagocytes are cells—specifically the monocytes, neutrophils, macrophages, and cells of the reticuloendothelial system—that are capable of engulfing bacteria. The process of **phagocytosis** can be described as the ameboidlike movement of these white blood cells to approach, surround, and engulf foreign material. Phagocytosis is necessary to remove dead blood cells, pathogens, and unused cellular secretions, as well as dust and dust particles that may find their way past first-line defenses. There are two types of phagocytes: fixed and mobile.

Fixed phagocytes are cells firmly attached to the tissue of the liver, spleen, bone marrow, and lymph nodes, and to intestinal and blood vessel linings. These tissues make up the **reticuloendothelial system (RES).** The lymph nodes remove bacteria from the lymph before they reach the large ducts leading to the bloodstream. If bacteria have gotten past the body defenses and entered the blood, phagocytes of the liver, spleen, and bone marrow will filter out the invading bacteria.

The **mobile phagocytes** (also known as **wandering phagocytes**) are in fact white blood cells, or leukocytes. When the body is invaded they increase in number and migrate to the injured site (Figure 15–1). There they will destroy the invading pathogens by phagocytosis.

The process of phagocytosis is started by a leukocyte as soon as a bacterium approaches it (Figure 15–2). When the bacterium sticks to the leukocyte, two pseudopods extend from the leukocyte to surround the bacterium. The two pseudopods fuse and form a vacuole called a **phagosome,** which entraps the bacterium.

Then a **lysosome,** the organelle that contains digestive enzymes, fuses with the phagosome. They form a **phagolysosome.** Within the phagolysosome the bacterium is killed in minutes. This digestive process is called **degranulation,** because the granules in the granulocytes are used up and therefore decrease in number. Additionally, the neutrophils die and are themselves phagocytized by the macrophages. Bacteria that survive the phagocytic process can break out of the cell and even establish themselves in secondary sites within the body. Additional inflammatory reactions can occur in these secondary sites, particularly if the patient's resistance has been lowered. The macrophages can also dispose of damaged or dying cells, remove old red blood cells from the spleen, and remove debris. The monocyte phagocyte may also be involved in removing cancer cells. It is thought that these phagocytes can suppress the growth of spontaneously arising tumors and be involved in tissue rejection.

Antibodies

When pathogens cannot be destroyed by the first or second lines of defense, the third line of defense, the **antibodies,** take over. Antibodies are produced and released in response to the presence of a foreign substance or pathogen to produce immunity. Antibodies can be thought of as the body's protective soldiers coming to the defense of their territory, the human body, in response to the invasion of a foreign army or foreign antigen in the form of bacteria, viruses, parasites, and fungi.

Initiating this battle is the breaking of the skin or outer barrier that allows the foreign antigen entry into the body. An inflammatory reaction caused by the rushing of phagocytes forms the second line of defense. Finally, after a time (days or hours depending on the nature of the foreign invader), formation of antibodies completes the third line of defense—and destruction of the foreign antigen by the phagocytosis process. This period, between the time of the foreign antigen invading the body and the onset of the disease, is known as the **incubation period.** For some infections or diseases, this incubation or lag period can be a matter of a few hours or days. In some, the incubation period can be 7 to 14 days (typical for childhood communicable diseases) to months (hepatitis B) to years (human immunodeficiency virus).

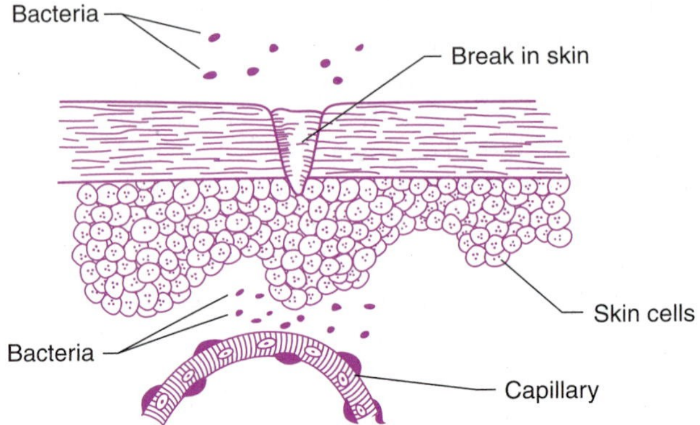

Break in skin permits entrance of bacteria

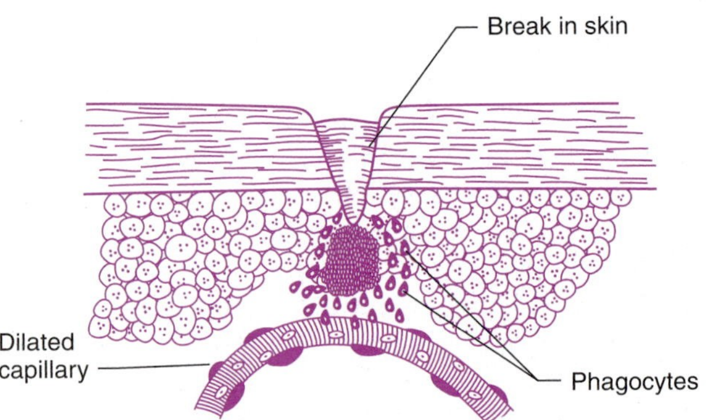

Phagocytes moving out of the dilated capillary to the point of injury

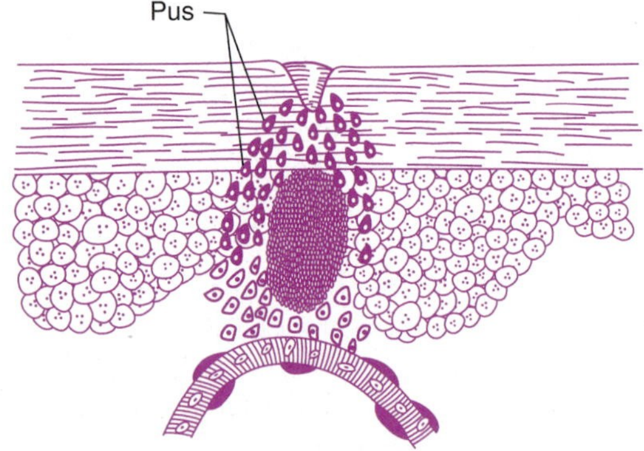

Accumulation of pus in the invaded area

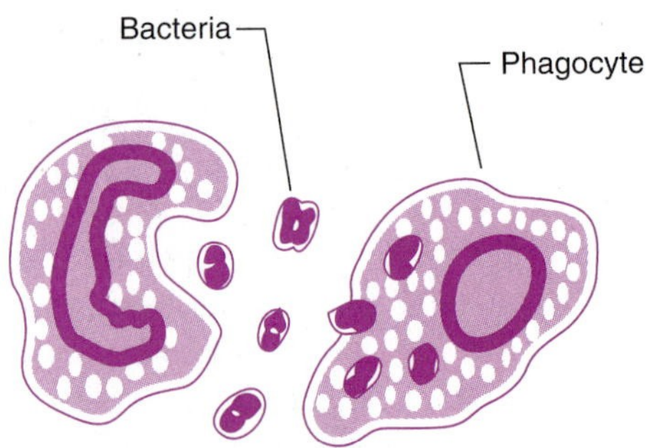

Phagocytes ingesting bacteria

Figure 15–1 Mobile phagocytes

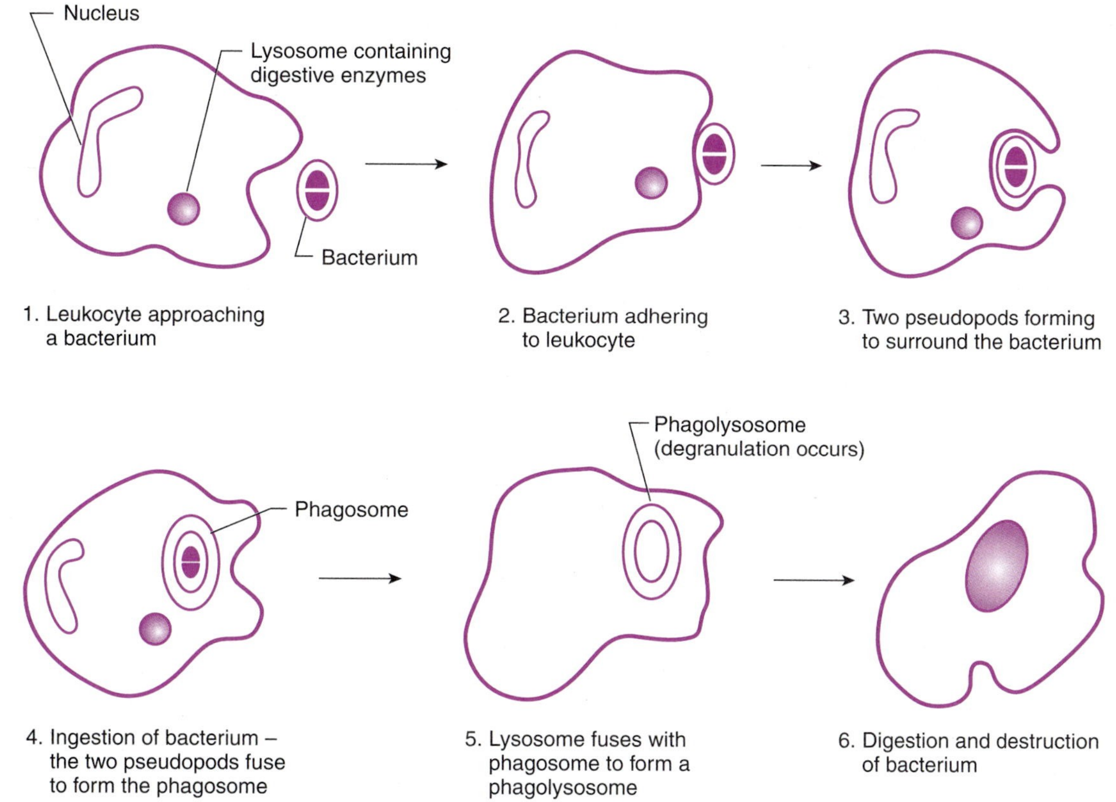

Figure 15–2 Process of phagocytosis

Pathogens tend to stimulate the production of antibodies in the blood and the lymph. These pathogens are called **antigens.** A specific microorganism or antigen will stimulate the production of a specific antibody. In turn, this specific antibody will destroy its specific antigen. This reaction is known as the **antigen-antibody response.** Carrying this process a step further, antitoxins are produced to neutralize specific bacterial toxins.

Complement

Additionally, some antibodies require the addition of special proteins called **complement** that circulate in the liquid portion of the blood in an inactive form until needed for assistance in the body's defense mechanism as part of the third line of defense. Complement can bind directly to an antibody to assist its destruction of a foreign antigen or it can set in motion a sequence of events, or a ripple effect of several complements (C1 through C4) that, when combined, either destroy the foreign antigen or prevent it from further destruction. People who have recurring infections, particularly those of the upper respiratory tract, ear infections, staphylococci, and gram-negative urinary infections, may have a deficiency in one of the four or more complements involved in the cascading or ripple effect that renders the complement active. Lack of pus formation at the site of a bacterial infection may also have a deficiency in one of the complements needed to complete the chain reaction necessary to activate the complement in an antigen-antibody response.

There are several different classes of antibodies of which every health care professional should be aware. A patient under your care may need an injection of one of the following substances at any time.

- **Antitoxins** neutralize and render harmless the toxins given off by bacteria.
- **Agglutinins** cause bacteria to clump together, thus making it easier for the white corpuscles to find and devour the bacteria.
- **Lysins** cause the bacteria to dissolve.
- **Opsonins** act on bacteria and make them more readily prey to be ingested by phagocytes.
- **Precipitins** cause bacteria to settle out of the bloodstream so that they can be filtered out and destroyed.

IMMUNE RESPONSE AND HIV (AIDS, THE DISEASE)

The human immunodeficiency virus enters the blood stream and rests in any of numerous sites within the body while the immune system silently begins its job to make specific antibodies to the HIV antigen, to increase the level of macrophages (phagocytes) to eat up the foreign invaders, and to release the killer T-helper cell lymphocytes that seek out and destroy any cells that are already infected with the virus. The problem is that HIV uses its own strategy and destroys the T-helper lymphocytes, which cripple the body's defense mechanism. HIV is outfitted with a special-shaped protein, called CD4, on the surface that just fits perfectly into receptors located on the T cells. The virus can now enter and infect the T-helper lymphocytes. Here the damage begins. The genetic information of the virus, which is RNA, is now transcribed into an identical form of the cell's DNA genetic information. Here the virus hides as DNA inside the T-helper cell's nucleus, eluding all body defenses.

At some point—months or even years later—HIV comes out of its hiding place in the T-helper cell nucleus and begins to reproduce many copies of the RNA, which are capable of producing proteins for the new viruses. These proteins are then packaged with the viral RNA and bud from the T cell. Each of these buds can then move on to infect and destroy other T cells. As the T-cell count drops lower and lower, resistance to outside infections becomes more frequent and more intense. Once the T-cell count drops to less than 200, a person is said to have full-blown AIDS and is prone to many opportunistic infections that usually result in death of the patient. Although many drugs are currently in use to stop the virus at various stages of its development, no real cure or vaccine is imminent or even on the horizon.

INFECTION

Internal defense structures function only after pathogenic bacteria have gained entrance into the body. Often these invasions are fought off so fast there is little evidence that the invaders were ever present at all. However, they sometimes result in local or general infections.

A **local infection** is one that is restricted to one area. A **general infection** is one that has spread to many parts of the body; it is recognized by finding bacteria in the bloodstream. The incubation period is the interval between the time bacteria enter the body until the first signs of disease appear.

When infections occur in the body, large numbers of white cells appear in the blood; thus, a high white cell count usually indicates that an infection is present.

Listed in Table 15–1 are some of the routinely encountered microorganisms found in the body that cause infections. Most of the listed organisms are indicative of localized infections. Keep in mind that when infections become generalized or disseminated throughout the body, such as in an immunocompromised patient, any microbe can be found anywhere in the body.

Table 15–1 Some of the Microorganisms Commonly Found in the Body

Site	Flora*	Pathogens
Throat	*Branhamella catarrhalis* Diphtheroids *Staphylococcus epidermidis* *Streptococcus viridans*	*Streptococcus pyogenes* (group A) *Staphylococcus aureus* *Neisseria gonorrhoege* *Haemophilus influenzae*
Nose	Diphtheroids *Staphylococcus epidermidis* *Streptococcus viridans*	*Branhamella catarrhalis* *Streptococcus pyogenes* (group A) *Staphylococcus aureus*
Ear (middle)	None	*Streptococcus pyogenes* (group A) *Staphylococcus aureus* *Haemophilus influenzae* *Pseudomonas aeruginosa*
Eye	None	*Streptococcus pyogenes* (group A) *Staphylococcus aureus* *Pseudomonas aeruginosa* *Haemophilus influenzae*
Sputum	Diphtheroids *Staphylococcus epidermidis* *Streptococcus viridans*	*Streptococcus pyogenes* (group A) *Staphylococcus aureus* *Klebsiella pneumoniae* *Streptococcus pneumoniae* *Candida albicans* *Myobacterium tuberculosis* *Pseudomonas aeruginosa* *Haemophilus influenzae* *Branhamella catarrhalis*
Urine	F. *Staphylococcus epidermidis* Diphtheroids M. None	*Escherichia coli* *Proteus* species *Pseudomonas aeruginosa* *Enterococcus* species *Staphylococcus saprophyticus*

continued

Table 15–1 Continued

Site	Flora*	Pathogens
Stool	*Escherichia coli* *Proteus* sp. *Klebsiella* sp. *Enterobacter* sp.	*Campylobacter* species *Salmonella* species *Shigella* species *Aeromonas* species *Escherichia coli* (some serotypes) *Giardia lamblia* *Entamoeba histolytica*
Genital	F. Lactobacilli *Staphylococcus epidermidis* M. None	*Neisseria gonorrhoeae* *Bacteroides* species *Streptococcus* (group B) *Trichomonas vaginalis*‡ *Candida albicans*†
Blood	None	All, especially: *Streptococcus viridans* *Staphylococcus aureus* *Escherichia coli*
Wounds and abscesses	None	*Staphylococcus aureus* *Escherichia coli* *Pseudomonas aeruginosa* *Clostridium* species *Streptococcus pyogenes* (group A)
Cerebrospinal fluid	None	*Neisseria meningitidis* *Haemophilus influenzae* *Streptococcus pneumoniae* *Cryptococcus neoformans*‡

*Normal flora found anywhere in pure culture should be considered to be potential pathogens.
†Parasites.
‡Fungi.
F Female.
M Male.

Fever and **inflammation** are two common responses to invasion by microorganisms. A high fever may be very destructive to the human host, but a moderate fever (102° to 104°F; 39° to 40°C) is a desirable response, because few bacteria can survive this temperature for long. Inflammation is characterized by four signs: redness, edema (swelling), heat, and pain. A dilation in the blood vessels brings more blood-carrying protective substances to the injured area, causing redness and heat. The walls enlarge, allowing the antibodies and white blood cells to come to the area, causing painful swelling and pressure on nerve endings. Should the struggle result in the death of many cells, a creamy white mixture of cell fluid containing living and dead leukocytes, bacteria, and damaged body cells appears at the site of infection. This mixture is known as **pus.** Sometimes the pus appears very thick and yellow; this is a purulent pus. Pathogens causing pus formation are called **pyogenic bacteria,** such as staphylococci and streptococci. The bacterium ***Pseudomonas aeruginosa*** is identified by formation of a blue pus.

FORMATION OF FOOD TOXINS OR POISONS

The pathogen ***Clostridium botulinum*** excretes a poisonous toxin that can cause botulism. Botulism is a very severe form of food poisoning; it is characterized by nerve destruction, which often proves fatal. Improper canning or smoking of foods that fails to kill all of the botulinum spores may cause them to grow and give off their deadly toxins.

The **exotoxin** given off by ***Staphylococcus aureus*** is a cause of diarrhea, nausea, and vomiting. These symptoms typically appear from 2 to 6 hours after the eating of contaminated food.

TISSUE DESTRUCTION

A classic example of tissue destruction is the tuberculosis bacteria, which invades and destroys living tissue. Another pathogen, streptococcus, gives off a **hemolysin** (*hemo* meaning "blood," *lysis* meaning "breakdown or destruction") capable of destroying **erythrocytes** (red blood cells). Some staphylococci and streptococci give off a **leukocidin,** which destroys **leukocytes** (white blood cells).

PRODUCTION OF TOXINS

Some pathogenic organisms give off toxins that destroy body tissue. These include the pathogens that cause diphtheria, scarlet fever, and tetanus (lockjaw). The exotoxin given off by ***Clostridium tetani*** leads to painful muscular contractions of the neck and jaw. This limits mouth movement (hence the term **lockjaw**), followed by thoracic, or chest, muscle paralysis. The usual result is death.

Diphtheria is caused by the pathogen ***Corynebacterium diphtheriae.*** This pathogen lodges in the nose, throat, and tonsils. Once established, it gives off a poisonous exotoxin that is circulated throughout the body until the entire bloodstream is poisoned. If diphtheria remains untreated, the lungs are likely to become clogged, leading possibly to death by suffocation.

SUMMARY

This chapter introduces the methods by which the body reacts to foreign invaders such as microorganisms to protect and help us recover from infection and disease. There are three recognized levels of body defenses. The first is the barrier of the skin, mucous membranes, and hair or cilia that help prevent foreign invaders from entering the body. The second line of defense involves the white blood cells of the circulatory system. Some white blood cells, specifically the neutrophils and monocytes, have the capability of actually circulating and then eating or engulfing the foreign organisms. Other substances in the blood include antibodies received from previous immunizations or infections, and a substance known as interferon. Both aid in ridding the body of foreign material. The third line of defense takes over when the foreign agent gets past the first two lines of defense. At this time the body has recognized the invader as foreign, so the immune system will activate to make specific antibodies (or soldiers) to that particular invader, whose job it is then to destroy the foreign material such as the bacteria. This process does not happen immediately but over a period of several days or weeks. An antigen- (the foreign invader) antibody complex is formed, sometimes with the help of a protein complement to destroy the invader or antigen.

STUDY AND DISCUSSION

- Demonstrate a prepared, stained slide under the microscope, showing a phagocyte-ingesting bacteria.
- A patient is complaining of a severe pain in his or her right side. The blood count shows a marked increase in the number of white corpuscles. Discuss the meaning of a high count.
- Explain how the skin protects our bodies against germs.
- Explain how a moderate fever is a reaction to bacterial invasion.
- How should a skin wound be treated?
- Tell what happens when there is a break in the skin.
- Give examples of how our body protects us when we inhale dust or other foreign particles.
- Name the three chief avenues of body defense.

REVIEW QUESTIONS

A. General Questions: Provide complete answers to each of the following.

1. Name six ways in which the body can protect itself against infection.

2. How does the skin protect the body against disease?

3. When is it possible for bacteria to gain entrance into the body through the skin?

4. Through what openings is it possible for bacteria to gain entrance into the body?

5. How does the body protect itself at these openings?

6. Which tubelike structure is a favorable place for the growth of bacteria?

7. What part do white blood cells play in protecting the body?

8. How do the blood and lymph act as body defenses?

9. What is a local infection?

10. What is a general infection?

11. Which type of infection is the harder to combat and why?

12. What are symptoms?

13. List some common symptoms of infection.

14. What is an incubation period?

15. Why must persons who have been exposed to disease-causing microbes be watched very carefully during the incubation period?

16. What is pus?

17. Explain what happens when there is a break in the skin.

18. Give a definition of *antibody.*

19. Give five different examples of antibodies.

20. Name two diseases that would call for the injection of an antitoxin if a person were seriously ill.

21. Explain why inflammation produces redness, swelling, heat, and pain.

22. Identify two foreign substances, besides disease bacteria, that will stimulate antibody production.

23. Describe how a white blood cell destroys bacteria.

B. Multiple-Choice Questions: Select the letter of the choice that best answers the question.

1. A hemolysin destroys _____ cells.
   a. epithelial
   b. blood
   c. nerve
   d. muscle
2. The first line of defense includes _____.
   a. formation of antibodies
   b. phagocytic activities of white blood cells
   c. natural resistance to infections
   d. skin, mucous membranes, and cilia
3. Microorganisms that invade the body are called _____.
   a. antigens
   b. antibodies
   c. complement
   d. agglutinins
4. An immediate response to the penetration of bacteria through the first line of defense may be _____ .
   a. fever
   b. inflammation
   c. phagocytosis
   d. antibody formation

5. _____ causes the bacteria to settle out of the bloodstream so they can be filtered and washed away.
   a. Antibodies
   b. Lysins
   c. Opsonins
   d. Precipitins

C. Completion Questions: From the following list of terms fill in the blanks with the correct choice.

nerves	toxins	endotoxins	exotoxins
antigens	antibodies	phagolysosome	lysosome
lysins	opsonins	antitoxins	muscles

1. Chemical poisons produced by some bacteria are called ____________.

2. The ____________ of *Clostridium tetani* destroys ____________of the neck and jaw.

3. ____________ act on bacteria and make them more ready prey for phagocytosis.

4. ____________ may be thought of as the soldiers fighting the enemy invaders, the ____________ in the body's defense mechanism.

5. An organelle that assists in the process of phagocytosis is the ____________ .

D. Matching Questions: Match the terms in Column I with their corresponding terms in Column II.

Column I		Column II
_______	1. *Clostridium tetani*	a. diarrhea/vomiting
_______	2. *Corynebacterium diphtheriae*	b. stool
_______	3. *Staphylococcus aureus*	c. nerve destruction
_______	4. *Clostridium botulinum*	d. sputum
_______	5. *Entamoeba histolytica*	e. hemolysin
_______	6. *Escherichia coli*	f. spinal fluid
_______	7. *Streptococcus*	g. lock jaw
_______	8. *Neisseria meningitidis*	h. vitamin K
_______	9. *Mycobacterium tuberculosis*	i. genital
_______	10. *Trichomonas vaginalis*	j. diphtheria

CHAPTER

16 Immunity

OBJECTIVES

After completing this chapter, you will be able to:

- explain what is meant by immunity and the different types of immunity.
- define antigen, autoimmunity, hypersensitivity, toxin, and toxoid.

KEY WORDS

acquired immunity
active acquired immunity
adaptive immunity
allergen
anaphylactic shock
anaphylaxis
antibodies
antigen
artificial acquired immunity
autoimmune disorder
autoimmunity
colostrum
hypersensitive
hypersensitivity
immunity
immunization
immunoglobulin
natural acquired immunity
natural passive acquired immunity
natural immunity
passive acquired immunity
rheumatic fever
thyroiditis
toxoid

When pathogens and foreign materials succeed in penetrating a person's first line of defense, the unbroken skin, the body's ability to resist these invaders and the diseases they cause is called **immunity.** Individuals differ in their ability to resist infection. In addition, an individual's resistance can vary at different times.

NATURAL AND ACQUIRED IMMUNITIES

Immunity is resistance to infections after a foreign antigen has penetrated the first line of defense. **Natural acquired immunity** occurs when a person has been infected with a microorganism and recovers from the disease, has had a subclinical or very mild infection, and/or is a carrier of the microorganism (yet shows no clinical symptoms). **Artificial acquired immunity** results from having been immunized, or vaccinated, with a killed or attenuated microorganism. Immunity received in these instances produces **active acquired immunity.** Sometimes immunity can also be acquired passively. **Natural passive acquired immunity** is passed from mother to child across the placenta. Artificially acquired passive immunity occurs when one receives gamma globulin, an antitoxin, or an immune serum (Table 16–1).

Natural immunity is inherited and is permanent. This inborn immunity consists of anatomical barriers such as the unbroken skin and cellular secretions such as mucus and tears. Phagocytes, along with T cells and B cells, are major cellular components of the immune response and a protein called complement, a major part of the humoral immunity component along with lysozymes and interferon, completes the list of contributors to natural immunity.

When the body encounters an invader, it tries to kill it by creating a specific substance to combat it. The body also tries to make itself permanently resistant to these intruders. **Acquired** or **adaptive immunity** is the reaction that occurs as a result of exposure to these invaders. Adaptive or acquired immunity allows the body to remember the invaders; thus, if the body is reinfected this immunity causes the T and B cells to respond more effectively to that microorganism. This is the immunity developed during an individual's lifetime. It may be passive or active.

Passive acquired immunity is borrowed immunity. It is acquired artificially by injecting antibodies from the blood of other individuals or animals into a person's body to protect him or her from a specific disease. The immunity produced is immediate in its effect. However, it lasts only from 3 to 5 weeks. After this period the antibodies will be killed by the individual's own reticuloendothelial system.

Because it is immediate, passive immunity is used in the treatment of virulent diseases. This is particularly true in treating diphtheria, measles, tetanus, and infectious hepatitis, in which there is hardly any time for a strong active immunity to develop.

A baby has temporary passive immunity from the mother's antibodies. These antibodies pass through the placenta to enter the baby's blood. In addition, the mother's milk and **colostrum** also offer the baby some passive immunity. Thus, a newborn infant may be protected against poliomyelitis, measles, and mumps. It should be noted that this passive immunity against poliomyelitis lasts for only about 6 weeks after birth. For measles and mumps it may last for nearly a year. Then the child must develop his or her own active immunity.

Table 16–1 Methods of Acquiring Immunity

	Natural	Artificial
Active	Have disease Be a carrier Have a subclinical case Recovered from disease	Vaccine (killed or attenuated microorganism)
Passive	Congenital, from mother to fetus	Gamma globulin Antitoxin Immune serum

Active acquired immunity is preferable to passive immunity because it lasts longer. The two types of active acquired immunity are natural acquired immunity and artificial acquired immunity:

- Natural acquired immunity is the result of having had and recovered from the disease. For example, a child who has had measles and has recovered will not ordinarily get it again, because the child's body has manufactured antibodies. This form of immunity is also acquired by having a series of unnoticed or mild infections. For example, a person who has had a mild form of a disease one or more times and has fought it off, sometimes unnoticed, is later immune to the disease.
- Artificial acquired immunity comes from being inoculated with a suitable vaccine, antigen, or toxoid. For example, a child vaccinated for smallpox has been given a very mild form of the disease; the child's body will thus be stimulated to manufacture its own antibodies.

Immunization is the process of increasing an individual's resistance to a particular infection by artificial means. It is an immunologic reaction or sensitization of the host in response to the presence of or exposure to a foreign substance. Immunization is produced by artificial means, usually by injection of a specific foreign **antigen** (protein substances such as bacteria, viruses, parasites, fungi, or any foreign substance that may cause disease) with the purpose of stimulating the production of **antibodies** (protein substance formed by the immune system in response to the presence of a foreign antigen to fight off the effects of the antigen). The building of sufficient antibodies to produce immunity or resistance may require several injections given over time. The antigen injected is usually a killed or attenuated version of the microorganism that would normally cause the disease. In this way the host does not become infected. Toxins or poisons produced by bacteria, dead or weakened bacteria, viruses, and foreign proteins are examples of antigens. Toxin stimulates the body to produce antibodies, while the antitoxin weakens or neutralizes the effect of the toxin.

A **toxoid** is a substance in which the toxin has been weakened by the addition of chemicals or heat, but not weakened enough to decrease the production of antibodies. Toxoids are used to protect individuals against diseases caused by toxins or toxin-producing bacteria, such as diphtheria and tetanus.

An **immunoglobulin** is a protein that functions specifically as an antibody. The five classes of immunoglobulins are immunoglobulin G (IgG), IgM, IgA, IgD, and IgE. IgG is the most abundant of the immunoglobulins. It is capable of crossing the placenta to provide temporary natural passive acquired immunity to an unborn baby. IgM is the largest of the antibodies, generally confined to the blood, and it functions in agglutination reactions. IgA is the predominant immunoglobulin found in tears, saliva, colostrum, and intestinal secretions. It is made by plasma cells and cells in the intestinal wall. IgD is found only in minute quantities and works with IgM. It may be found on the surface of B lymphocytes. IgE is found in trace amounts in plasma but is of major importance in desensitizing allergic reactions and in producing immunity to parasitic infections.

Autoimmunity

Autoimmunity is when an individual's immune system goes awry. It forms antibodies to its own tissues that destroy these tissues. This is also known as an **autoimmune disorder.**

Some autoimmune disorders are genetic (such as the "bubble" children) and sometimes diseases such as lupus can trigger an autoimmune response.

A well-known example of this disorder is **rheumatic fever.** A person may get a streptococcal infection, as in a strep throat, that slightly alters heart tissue. Later streptococcal infections can cause further heart damage, because the antibodies formed against the streptococci will also attack the altered heart tissue. This type of heart damage is known as rheumatic heart disease.

Other autoimmune disorders include **thyroiditis,** a severe inflammation of the thyroid gland, and most likely rheumatoid arthritis, an inflammatory joint disease.

Hypersensitivity

Hypersensitivity occurs when the body's immune system fails to protect itself against foreign material. Instead, the antibodies formed irritate certain body cells. A **hypersensitive** or allergic individual is generally more sensitive to certain allergens than most people.

An **allergen** is an antigen that causes allergic responses. Examples of allergens include grass, ragweed pollen, ingested food, penicillin and other antibiotics, and bee and wasp stings. Such allergens stimulate antibody formation, some of which are known as the IgE antibodies. An increase in IgE is found in individuals who are allergic, drug sensitive, or hypersensitive. The antibodies bind to certain cells in the body, causing a characteristic allergic reaction.

In asthma, the IgE antibodies bind to the bronchi and bronchioles; in allergic rhinitis or hayfever they bind to the mucous membranes of the respiratory tract and eyes, causing runny nose and itchy eyes. In hives and rashes they bind to the skin cells.

An even more severe and sometimes fatal allergic reaction is called **anaphylaxis** or **anaphylactic shock.** It is the result of an antigen-antibody reaction that stimulates a massive secretion of histamine. Anaphylaxis can be caused by insect stings and injected drugs such as penicillin. A person suffering from anaphylaxis experiences breathing problems, headache, facial swelling, falling blood pressure, stomach cramps, and vomiting. The antidote is an injection of either adrenaline or antihistamine. If proper care is not given immediately, death may occur in minutes.

Health care professionals should always ask patients whether they are sensitive to any allergens or drugs. This precaution is necessary to prevent negative and sometimes fatal allergic responses to injected drugs. People with such hypersensitivities should wear medical alert necklaces or bracelets to alert health professionals in the event of an emergency. Such tags have saved the lives of patients rendered unconscious or otherwise unable to communicate.

SUMMARY

In this chapter are two categories of immunity—natural and artificial—and within each category immunity can be actively or passively acquired. Much of our immunity comes by way of artificial active acquired immunity by receiving childhood immunizations against specific diseases. Artificial passive immunity includes the receiving of a nonspecific protein substance, such as gamma globulin, to boost the immune system into making antibodies. Natural active immunity involves actually contracting the disease (antigen) and allowing the body's third line of defense to make antibodies, which then are naturally acquired. Natural passive immunity is only transmitted by mother to child through the placenta or mother's milk.

Sometimes a person can develop an autoimmunity, in which case the body's immune system goes awry and the body develops antibodies to its own tissues. Some autoimmune disorders are genetic (such as the "bubble" children) and sometimes diseases such as lupus can trigger an autoimmune response. People with allergies often have excess of IgE antibodies which, in the case of respiratory allergies, will bind to the mucous membranes of the bronchi and bronchioles. This causes much discomfort and sometimes even anaphylactic shock when the allergy reaction is so severe that excesses of histamines are secreted causing severe breathing difficulties or heart failure. If antihistamines or adrenaline are not given quickly enough, death can result.

STUDY AND DISCUSSION

- Explain why antitoxin is administered to a child who is seriously ill with diphtheria, but a toxoid is prescribed for a child in whom the doctor wants to develop immunity to diphtheria.
- Explain why active immunity is better than passive immunity.
- Name three ways in which we may require active immunity.
- What is hypersensitivity?
- Discuss and outline the differences in the following terms:

a. antitoxin
b. toxin-antitoxin
c. toxoid
d. immunoglobulin

REVIEW QUESTIONS

A. General Questions: Provide complete answers to each of the following.

1. What is immunity?

2. What is natural immunity?

3. Name four sources of natural immunity.

4. What is acquired immunity?

5. Identify the two types of acquired immunity.

6. How is an individual's health related to immunity?

7. How is active acquired immunity obtained?

8. How long does active acquired immunity last?

9. How is passive acquired immunity attained?

10. How does an infant obtain passive acquired immunity?

11. How long does passive acquired immunity last?

12. What is the main difference between active and passive immunity?

13. When is passive immunization used?

14. What is an antigen?

15. What are antibodies?

16. What is hypersensitivity?

17. What are the common forms of hypersensitivity in humans?

18. What is anaphylaxis?

19. What are the symptoms of anaphylaxis?

20. How can anaphylaxis be effectively treated?

21. Name several diseases that produce long-term immunity in humans.

22. What is an allergy?

23. Give two common examples of allergies.

24. Name some common substances that cause people to be allergic.

B. Multiple-Choice Questions: Select the letter of the choice that best answers the question.

1. The most abundant immunoglobulin is ______ .
   a. IgG c. IgA e. IgE
   b. IgM d. IgD
2. The immunoglobulin responsible for desensitizing allergic reaction is ______ .
   a. IgG c. IgA e. IgE
   b. IgM d. IgD
3. Colostrum provides ______ immunity.
   a. active natural c. active artificial
   b. passive natural d. passive artificial
4. The purpose of being injected with antibodies from the blood of others is to ______ .
   a. produce an immediate long-lasting immunity
   b. produce a delayed long-lasting immunity
   c. produce an immediate but temporary immunity
   d. produce a delayed, temporary immunity
5. To offset a severe allergic reaction the person may receive ______ .
   a. adrenaline c. antitoxin
   b. histamine d. gamma globulin

C. Completion Questions: From the following list of terms fill in the blanks with the correct choice.

hives	hypersensitivity	anaphylaxis
allergen	autoimmune	immunoglobulin
immune	antigen	antibody

1. _______________ occurs when the body's immune system fails and severe allergies occur.

2. A severe allergic response may be _______________ while a much more mild response may be _______________ .

3. A bubble baby may be the victim of a/an _______________ disorder.

4. Rheumatic fever is an example of a/an _______________ disorder.

5. A protein substance formed in response to the presence of certain other proteins is called a/an _______________ .

D. Matching Questions: Match the situations in the statements listed below with their corresponding types of immunity. The types of immunity terms may be used more than once.

A. active natural
B. active artificial
C. passive natural
D. passive artificial

_____ 1. A child recovers from measles.

_____ 2. An adult has been vaccinated for smallpox.

_____ 3. Typhoid Mary

_____ 4. A traveller to a tropical country receives a gamma globulin shot.

_____ 5. Billy Jamison walks with a limp because he had infantile paralysis when he was 6 years old.

_____ 6. You have recently received a tetanus booster.

_____ 7. A new mother breast-feeds her baby.

_____ 8. A 12-year-old hemophiliac contracts AIDS.

_____ 9. A newborn baby has a demonstratable titer for rubella antibodies.

_____ 10. Your 3-month-old cousin has received his DPT immunizations for diphtheria, whooping cough, and tetanus.

_____ 11. The bacteriology staff have been given BCG vaccinations which result in positive skin tests for tuberculosis.

CHAPTER 17

Vaccines and Immune Serums

OBJECTIVES

After completing this chapter, you will be able to:

- provide a detailed explanation of vaccines and immune serums and how they protect us from disease.
- describe the schedule of childhood immunizations to parents.

KEY WORDS

antiserum
attenuated
booster
immune serum
vaccination
vaccine
vaccinia
variola

Vaccines and **immune serums** are used to produce immunity in a person. Vaccines are live, killed, or **attenuated** (thinned or weakened by chemical or physical means) microorganisms that are injected that will produce artificially induced active immunity. Naturally acquired active immunity results when one has been infected with the actual microorganism. Smallpox and polio vaccinations are examples of the use of vaccines to produce active immunity. Immune serums such as gamma globulin are antibodies injected to produce passive immunity. Before the development of the hepatitis B vaccine, gamma globulin was the health care worker's only chance at immunity from serum hepatitis (hepatitis B).

VACCINES

The first vaccine, a smallpox vaccine, was developed in 1796 by Dr. Edward Jenner, an English doctor. He observed that dairy workers who had contracted cowpox when milking cows never contracted smallpox, even when an epidemic raged. Dr. Jenner reasoned that if he transferred material from a pustule of cowpox to a healthy person, an immunity to smallpox would develop. This he proved experimentally. It is the basis of all vaccination. The word ***vaccination*** comes from the Latin word for "cow" (*vacca*) since a cow was first used for this purpose. Pasteur later used the principle for vaccination against rabies.

Vaccines are suspensions of pathogens that have been killed or weakened. These pathogens do not cause a disease, but they stimulate antibody formation. Vaccines are produced in a laboratory under exacting aseptic conditions. They can be made in the following ways.

Living Microorganisms Closely Related to the Pathogen

The smallpox virus, **variola,** is closely related to the cowpox virus, **vaccinia.** Thus, it was possible to develop a smallpox vaccine from a live cowpox virus. After receiving a cowpox vaccination the subject develops a mild, pustule infection while building antibodies to the cowpox virus. These antibodies can also combat the smallpox virus. At present, smallpox is no longer a major health problem, because it has been virtually eradicated.

Attenuated Live Pathogens

The vaccines used for vaccination against typhus, rabies, mumps, poliomyelitis, yellow fever, measles (rubeola), and German measles are made from attenuated, or weakened, live viruses. These viruses are attenuated by being grown in animal hosts, by means of cultivation in laboratory tissue cultures, or through the use of heat and chemicals. Attenuation weakens or thins out the virus but does not kill it. This protects the subject from contracting the disease although antibodies against the disease can still be produced.

The oral (Sabin) poliovirus vaccine is an attenuated mixture of three types of poliovirus. Its effectiveness is dependent on the virus remaining alive. Currently, only infants and children are being administered the vaccine, as there has been a very small chance (one case in a million for type I polio and one case in 5 million for type III polio) of a poliolike illness when used in adults. Today there is a new inactivated polio virus (IPV) vaccine being used to eliminate even the most remote possibility of developing the disease, from using the live oral polio vaccine (OPV). In addition, it has been reported that in rare cases, parents of children who received the vaccine have come down with poliolike infections.

Killed Pathogens

Certain vaccines come from pathogens that have been killed by heat or chemicals. Vaccines made this way are quickly and easily produced. Unfortunately, they are less effective than attenuated viruses because the immunity produced only lasts a short time. The Salk poliomyelitis vaccine (no longer used or manufactured in the United States), for instance, was made from three types of poliovirus. These viruses were grown in monkey-kidney tissue cultures and rendered inactive by formalin or ultraviolet light. The rabies vaccine is a killed vaccine prepared from infected embryonated duck eggs (DEV) or rabbit brain. Because the rabbit-brain preparations tend to have higher rates of neurological complications, the DEV vaccine is the preferred immunizing agent. Because the effects of rabies disease and the immunization process is so devastating, the vaccine series is preceded by the injection of an antirabies immune globulin serum with the purpose of establishing some immediate antibody protection to diminish the severe effects of the virus. Other vaccines made from inactivated viruses include typhoid, paratyphoid, whooping cough (pertussis), cholera, plague, and influenza.

Toxoids

There are other vaccines known as toxoids. These are effective against diphtheria and tetanus toxins. Toxoids are prepared from the poisons or toxins given off by certain microorganisms.

Combined Vaccines

Various vaccines have been combined to ensure immunization against several diseases at the same time. One such combination is the DPT vaccine, a combination of diphtheria, pertussis, and tetanus toxoids.

Autogenous Vaccines

Autogenous vaccines are made from cultures of bacteria isolated from an infected person. Such vaccines can be prepared, for example, from the pathogens in a staphylococcal boil. These bacteria are killed and then injected back into the same patient. This process ensures greater antibody formation, especially in the treatment of antibiotic-resistant staphylococcal infections.

IMMUNE SERUMS

Immune serums, such as gamma globulin, are used to produce passive immunity. The blood serum from an immune animal or human is injected into the body. This serum contains the antibodies produced by the subject. Antibodies work immediately to destroy the toxins produced by the bacteria. This type of immunity usually lasts only for several weeks. Such animal serums have on occasion been known to result in lethal complications due to a severe allergic response to the animal serum in the recipient.

Some examples of immune serum globulin given to minimize or prevent viral infections include those for viral hepatitis, both hepatitis A (HAV) and hepatitis B (HBV), measles, and rubella. Vaccinia immune globulin, zoster immune globulin, and mumps immune globulin may be given to children who are particularly immunologically deficient because of treatment with immunosuppressive drugs. Human rabies immune globulin is started at the same time that active rabies immunization is begun.

Antitoxins

To produce an antitoxin, horses, cattle, sheep, goats, and rabbits are inoculated or vaccinated with the toxin in question to produce an immune serum. Antitoxins are used for treatment of diphtheria and tetanus.

The diphtheria antitoxin is prepared in the following way. Toxins produced by diphtheria germs grown in laboratory cultures are injected into a healthy horse. These toxins cause the cells of the horse to produce antitoxins. The process is continued until the blood of the horse contains a large amount of antitoxin. Some of the blood is taken from the immune horse, and the serum (or watery part) is separated from the cells and used to develop the antitoxin. After refining and testing, the serum becomes an immune serum or diphtheria antitoxin, and is ready to be injected into the bodies of human beings.

Antitoxins for other diseases are prepared in similar ways. Some people react violently to injections of certain immune serums, which is known as serum sickness; it is caused by the horse serum, which acts as a foreign antigen, rather than by the specific antibodies contained in the horse serum. Symptoms include hives, swelling and pain in the joints and glands, and high fever.

PROPER HEALTH CARE

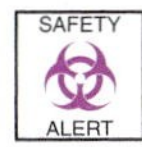

Health care professionals who are responsible for preparing and injecting vaccines and serums must follow manufacturers' instructions scrupulously for the injection, storage, and dating of these materials. Some viruses, such as the Sabin vaccine, are live, and they may be rendered ineffective or, worse, overly effective—actually producing disease—if they are not properly used and stored. The rabies immune globulin serum must be injected partly intramuscular and partly at the site of the bite to achieve its maximum effectiveness.

A serum is more correctly known as **antiserum,** or immune serum. It is in fact blood serum, containing preformed antibodies from an immune animal or person. A vaccine, on the other hand, contains the pathogen, pathogen extract, or toxin needed for antibody production. This is how vaccines provide active and lasting immunization against certain diseases. Antiserums are required for the treatment of disease. Though they take effect almost immediately, their immunity lasts only from 3 to 5 weeks because the injected serum, with its antibodies, is later eliminated from the body.

Some bacterial antigens used for vaccine production are shown in Table 17–1.

Immunity may last for a few months or many years. The duration of immunity acquired by vaccination varies with the antigen, the dose of vaccine, and the age and health of the individual. Immunity to hepatitis B was once thought to be lifelong, but it may last only 6 to 10 years.

Vaccines should be stored in a refrigerator and should not be removed more than 1 hour before use.

Boosters

Some immunizations will produce enough immunity to last a good many years or even a lifetime. Such is the case with the measles-mumps-rubella (MMR) and polio series of immunizations given during infancy and early childhood. Others, such as tetanus, require a periodic **booster** to bring the antibody levels back up to higher protective levels to continue preventing disease, should the individual come in contact with the causative organism *Clostridium tetani.*

Table 17–1 Vaccines and Immune Sera

Vaccine	Pathogen	Antigen	Inoculation
Cholera	*Vibrio cholerae*	Nonviable bacteria	Two doses at 7- to 10-day intervals, followed by one stimulating dose every 4 to 6 months by subcutaneous injection.
Diphtheria	*Corynebacterium diphtheriae*	Toxoid (modified form)	Two or three doses at 4-week intervals at age 9 months, followed by a stimulating dose at 6 years if necessary.
Bubonic plague	*Yersinia pestis*	Nonviable bacteria	Two doses at 7- to 10-day intervals, followed by a stimulating dose every 4 to 6 months.
Whooping cough (pertussis)	*Bordetella pertussis*	Nonviable bacteria	Three doses at 3-week intervals at age 1 month or more.
Smallpox	Variola virus	Attenuated virus	Introduction to skin cells by multiple puncture.
Tetanus	*Clostridium tetani*	Toxoid	Two doses at 4-week intervals. A stimulating dose at time of injury.
Typhoid	*Salmonella typhi*	Nonviable bacteria	Three doses by subcutaneous injection at 7- to 10-day intervals. A stimulating dose every 6 to 12 months.
Typhus	*Rickettsia prowazekii* *Rickettsia typhi*	Rickettsia	Three doses at 7- to 10-day intervals by a subcutaneous injection, followed by one stimulating dose every 4 to 6 months.
Yellow fever	*Arbovirus*	Attenuated virus	A subcutaneous injection good for 10 years.
Red Measles Mumps German Measles	Rubeola Paromyxovirus Rubella	Nonviable viruses	Two doses, one at 15 months, one at age 4 to 6 years.
Polio	Polio virus	Attenuated virus	Four doses, one at 2 months, 4 months, 18 months, and 4 to 6 years.

CHILDHOOD IMMUNIZATIONS

Vaccines to prevent some of the most devastating and communicable diseases are available and should be given to children starting in infancy. Thanks to worldwide intervention and a strong vaccination policy, smallpox disease has been eradicated, and physicians are no longer routinely vaccinating children for this insidious disease. In fact, a parent would be hard-pressed to find a physician willing to vaccinate against smallpox anymore. Children are immunized against diphtheria (D), pertussis (P) or whooping cough, tetanus (T), polio—oral and live (OPV), measles (M), mumps (M), Rubella (R) or German measles, Haemophilus Influenza type B (Hib), hepatitis B (HBV), and a tuberculosis skin test (TB). These immunizations are administered before the start of school, and usually annually or biannually thereafter. The series of these immunizations are given as shown in Table 17–2.

Table 17–2 Schedule of and Recommendations for Receiving Immunizations

	HBV	DTP	DTaP	MMR	OPV	HIB	VAR	TD
Birth	X							
1 month								
2 months	X	X			X	X		
4 months		X			X	X		
6 months	X	X			X	X		
12 months		X		X		X	X	
15–18 months		X	X					
4–6 years		X	X	X	X			X and every 2 years thereafter
11 years				X				X and every 2 years thereafter
15 years		X (DT) Only & T. every 10 years						X and every 2 years thereafter

HBV	DTP	MMR	DTaP	OPV IPV	HIB	VAR	TD
Hepatitis B virus	Diphtheria-tetanus-pertussis	Measles-mumps-rubella	Diphtheria tetanus acellular pertussis	Live oral poliovirus vaccine, Inactivated poliovirus vaccine	Haemophilus Influenza type B, conjugate	Varicella (chicken pox)	TB skin test (Tine or Mantoux)

The new polio vaccine inactivated polio virus (IPV) is a potentially less risky option than receiving a live virus preparation in the OPV. Additionally, an acellular pertussis vaccine has been developed for use only with the fourth and fifth booster doses of diphtheria and tetanus. This combination vaccine is known as the DTaP vaccine. Acellular pertussis, unlike its predecessor, is more purified and is unlikely to cause some of the adverse reactions (fever, tenderness, swelling, soreness, drowsiness, fretfulness, and anorexia) of the whole-cell pertussis vaccines.

It is vitally important that parents complete the immunization series for their children prior to the children starting school. Table 17–2 illustrates the Centers for Disease Control and the American Academy of Pediatric Physicians recommended ages and vaccination requirements.

SUMMARY

In this chapter we see the importance of immunity and how immunizations can provide the necessary protection from numerous diseases. Beginning with Dr. Edward Jenner and his discovery of the cowpox virus, to protection from the dreaded smallpox, to the eradication of this disease through continued immunizations worldwide, we have seen the great importance of immunizations. There are several types of immune serums: Some are made from live organisms and some are made from attenuated (weakened) or dead organisms. Because of the inherent risk with injecting a live microorganism, great efforts are underway to develop more vaccines from dead antigens. We have seen the success of this effort with the development of the new acellular pertussis vaccine. Even though it is not to be given in place of the first three doses, it has been proven effective for the fourth and fifth doses. Today immunization for hepatitis B and haemophilus B are commonplace. A promising chicken pox vaccine is now on the market.

STUDY AND DISCUSSION

- Explain why a health care professional must be thoroughly familiar with the principles of immunization.
- Identify the sterile precautions used by doctors and health care experts in the mass inoculation programs against poliomyelitis and influenza.
- What is a booster shot?
- Upon what factors does the duration of immunity depend? Give details.
- Prepare library reports on the discovery of the methods of vaccination for the following diseases. Name the scientist who is responsible for the discovery in each case:

  a. smallpox c. poliomyelitis e. typhoid fever
  b. rabies d. influenza f. anthrax
- Prepare a report describing how immunity is produced in one of the following diseases. State whether it is passive or active immunity. Name the specific animals and cultures used in the laboratory for the immunization.

a. diphtheria
b. lockjaw
c. scarlet fever
d. smallpox
e. rabies
f. influenza (epidemic of 1957–1958)
g. poliomyelitis (Salk vaccine or Sabin vaccine)
h. cholera
i. bubonic plague
j. whooping cough
k. typhoid fever
l. paratyphoid fever
m. typhus fever
n. yellow fever

REVIEW QUESTIONS

A. General Questions: Provide complete answers to each of the following.

1. List six ways by which the body protects itself against infection.

2. Name six diseases that may be controlled by vaccination.

3. Identify three diseases for which antitoxins are used in emergency cases.

4. What is an attenuated organism?

5. Name two ways of attenuating pathogens.

6. What types of vaccines are made from attenuated live pathogens?

7. What is DPT vaccine?

8. What is an autogenous vaccine?

9. What is an immune serum?

10. State differences and similarities between an immune serum and a vaccine.

B. Multiple-Choice Questions: Select the letter of the choice that best answers the question.

1. Vaccines are _____ .
   a. prepared from live or attenuated organisms
   b. weakened microorganisms
   c. gamma globulin inoculations
   d. prepared from horse serums
2. Combination vaccines include _____ and _____ .
   a. BCG
   b. DPT
   c. MMR
   d. SS
   e. HSI
3. _____ is no longer a threat to the world's health problems.
   a. Tuberculosis
   b. Polio
   c. Pertussis
   d. Smallpox
4. Examples of attenuated live pathogens include _____ .
   a. rabies, polio, cholera, and mumps
   b. mumps, cholera, plague, and typhus
   c. typhus, rabies, measles, and mumps
   d. typhoid, cholera, plague, and pertussis
5. Examples of killed pathogens include _____ .
   a. rabies, polio, cholera, and mumps
   b. mumps, cholera, plague, and typhus
   c. typhus, rabies, measles, and mumps
   d. typhoid, cholera, plague, and pertussis

C. Completion Questions: From the following list of terms fill in the blanks with the correct choice.

virulent	attenuated	toxoids	antibodies
antitoxins	Salk	Sabin	rabies
smallpox	cholera	tetanus	typhus

1. Organisms that are weakened or thinned are referred to as ____________ organisms.

2. ____________ are vaccines prepared from weakened poisons given off by some bacteria, such as diphtheria.

3. The ____________ polio vaccine was made from a live virus.

4. The ____________ vaccine is harvested from embryonated duck eggs.

5. The ____________ vaccine is prepared from a nonviable bacteria.

D. Matching Questions: Match the terms in Column I with their corresponding terms in Column II.

Column I		Column II
_______	1. variola	a. German measles
_______	2. pertussis	b. lockjaw
_______	3. varicella	c. polio
_______	4. rubella	d. cowpox
_______	5. rubeolla	e. red measles
_______	6. tetanus	f. chicken pox
_______	7. infantile paralysis	g. smallpox
_______	8. vaccinia	h. whooping cough

SECTION THREE

ACHIEVEMENT REVIEW

A. Select the word or expression that best completes each statement.

1. A disease transmitted by mosquitoes is _____ .
   a. rheumatic fever　c. typhus fever
   b. typhoid fever　d. yellow fever
2. The virus disease that continues to cause the greatest number of absences from school each year is _____ .
   a. measles　c. poliomyelitis
   b. mumps　d. colds
3. Vaccination is used to control _____ .
   a. anemia　c. poliomyelitis
   b. hemophilia　d. diabetes
4. A toxin is a substance that _____ .
   a. improves health　c. kills bacteria
   b. is harmless　d. is produced by bacteria
5. Jenner developed a way of making people immune to _____ .
   a. cancer　c. smallpox
   b. malaria　d. tuberculosis
6. Oysters sometimes transmit _____ .
   a. malaria　c. typhoid fever
   b. rabies　d. yellow fever
7. Weakened, live virus is used to prevent _____ .
   a. arthritis　c. smallpox
   b. athlete's foot　d. diphtheria
8. When a person has appendicitis, the blood shows an increase in the number of _____ .
   a. antitoxins　c. red blood cells
   b. platelets　d. white blood cells
9. Disease organisms are engulfed and destroyed in the blood or lymph by _____ .
   a. fibrin　c. red blood cells
   b. platelets　d. white blood cells
10. A contagious disease is _____ .
    a. anemia　c. cancer
    b. diabetes　d. the common cold
11. A disease spread by the bite of a flea is _____ .
    a. malaria　c. poliomyelitis
    b. bubonic plague　d. typhoid fever
12. Of the following diseases, the one that is communicable is _____ .
    a. cancer　c. rickets
    b. diabetes　d. tuberculosis

13. Poisons produced in the body by invading bacteria are called _____ .
    a. antitoxins
    b. germicides
    c. toxins
    d. vaccines
14. Poisons from disease-producing bacteria are counteracted by _____ .
    a. antitoxins
    b. fibrinogen
    c. germicides
    d. red blood cells
15. A disease often contracted by drinking polluted water is _____ .
    a. measles
    b. the common cold
    c. typhoid fever
    d. yellow fever

B. Match each word or term in Column I with the statement in Column II which is best associated with it.

Column I	Column II
_______ 1. influenza	a. ragweed pollen
_______ 2. deep wound	b. rabies
_______ 3. typhus fever	c. white corpuscles
_______ 4. cowpox	d. disease carrier
_______ 5. allergy	e. malaria
_______ 6. bite of mad dog	f. immunity
_______ 7. ameboid movement	g. diphtheria
_______ 8. Typhoid Mary	h. smallpox
_______ 9. anopheles mosquito	i. lockjaw
_______ 10. toxoid	j. droplet infection
	k. bite of a flea

C. Insert the term or expression that best completes each statement.

1. A person who is not susceptible to a disease is said to be _______________ .

2. A toxin that has been weakened by chemicals but can still make the body produce antitoxins is known as a _______________ .

3. Yellow fever can be transmitted by the_______________ .

4. Chemical substances in the blood that cause bacteria to clump are called _______________ .

5. Diseases that result from oversensitivity to foreign proteins are called _______________ .

6. The body's first line of defense against disease organisms is the _______________ .

7. The general name for the chemical substances in the blood produced by the cells of the body that fight bacteria and their products is _______________ .

8. An individual's inborn resistance to a disease is known as _______________ .

9. The two types of acquired immunity are ________________ and ________________.

10. Vaccination was first used by ________________.

11. The hairs in the nose and windpipe form a first line of defense by ________________.

12. A person may develop his or her own immunity either by ________________ or by ________________.

13. The animal used in the laboratory for the production of diphtheria antitoxin is the ________________.

14. Antibodies that cause bacteria to dissolve are known as ________________.

15. Antibodies that act on bacteria and make them ready to be ingested by white blood cells are called ________________.

16. List five routes through which bacteria may enter the body.

17. Name three routes through which bacteria may leave the body.

18. Mobile phagocytes are wandering cells in the blood called ________________.

19. When the body is injured, the mobile phagocytes ________________ in number.

20. The ________________ has a special ability to form antibodies and antitoxins.

21. The lymph nodes remove bacteria from the ________________ and ________________.

22. An invasion of the body by pathogenic bacteria may result in ________________.

23. A ________________ infection is one that is restricted to one area.

24. A ________________ infection is one that has spread to many parts of the body.

25. A________________ period is the interval between the time bacteria enter the body and the first signs of disease.

26. A creamy white mixture of cell fluid containing dead leukocytes and bacteria is called ________________ .

27. The ability of a person to resist disease is known as ________________ .

28. ________________ immunity occurs when the body itself is active in producing antibodies that protect it from disease.

29. Recovering from a disease usually results in ________________ immunity.

30. Passive immunity occurs when ________________ are injected into the body.

31. Immunity produced in this way is of very ________________ duration.

32. ________________ are substances that stimulate the body to form protective substances or antibodies.

33. Two common responses to invasion are ________________ and ________________ .

34. John Enders successfully produced a new vaccine for protection against ________________ .

35. Another vaccine for poliomyelitis besides the Salk vaccine is the _____ . This new vaccine is different from the Salk vaccine because it is given _____ and it contains _____ .

SECTION 4

Methods of Destruction of Microbiological Material

CHAPTER 18

Physical and Chemical Agents of Destruction

OBJECTIVES

After completing this chapter, you will be able to:

- discuss the various physical means of destroying bacteria.
- describe how bacteria are destroyed by chemical means.
- list some common antiseptic and disinfectant preparations used by health care professionals.
- describe the similarities between universal precautions and standard precautions.

KEY WORDS

autoclave
bactericides
bactericidal
bacteriostatic
disinfectants
disinfection
filterable virus
filtrate
germicidal
germicides
HEPA
in vitro
in vivo
laminar airflow
lyophilization
phenol coefficient
pipette
sodium hypochlorite
steam sterilizer
sterilization
thermal death point
thermal death time
thermolabile

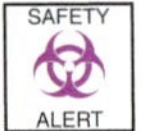

There are many bacteria that cause disease and food spoilage. Every health care professional should be knowledgeable about the different methods of destroying bacteria as well as any other microorganisms that may be harmful. We have examined methods of growing or demonstrating the presence of organisms, but one must be able to prevent their growth and multiplication in the health care environment. Just as certain antibiotics can either kill bacteria or merely inhibit their growth, removing certain criteria of an organism's growth conditions can also inhibit their growth. But when the objective is to kill or destroy the microorganism, inhibition of their growth is not sufficient. Procedures that kill microorganisms are **bactericidal** and those that merely inhibit their growth are **bacteriostatic.**

Sterilization is the only **in vitro** method of ensuring complete destruction of bacteria so that they may not multiply later when favorable growth conditions return. Sterilization methods may be by physical or chemical means. Physical methods employ instrumentation to accomplish the end point, whereas chemical methods utilize the liquid chemicals to destroy microorganisms. The destruction or inhibition of bacteria by chemicals is generally called **disinfection.** Many chemical agents in the form of antiseptic or disinfectant solutions can be used to check the growth of microorganisms and to destroy them.

STERILIZATION

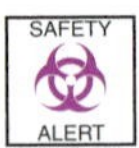

Sterilization is the total destruction of all forms of microorganisms. This is an *absolute* term; there is no "range" or "degree" of sterility. The following discussion details the different types of physical agents of destruction. These include cold temperature, drying, radiation, heat, moist heat, incineration, filtration, and ultrasonic waves (Table 18–1).

Cold Temperature

Neither cold nor freezing is a reliable method of killing bacteria. Low temperatures do slow bacterial growth, temporarily preventing the ability to multiply rapidly and produce toxins. Freezing produces a bacteriostatic effect, keeping bacteria in a state of suspended animation. When the temperatures rise above the freezing point, however, the bacteria will start to grow again and reproduce.

Cold cannot be used to cure disease, but it can help reduce the possibility of a disease advancing to a critical stage. An example is the "freezing" of the appendix with ice packs. This is a temporary means of arresting appendicitis until the appendix can be safely removed.

Freezing is also a good method of preserving certain foods. Putting bacteria in suspended animation keeps them from acting to decompose and spoil the food.

Many bacterial cultures and biological specimens are preserved by rapid freezing to very low temperatures. Most, like the typhoid bacillus, will resume growth and reproduction upon thawing. Some pathogens, however, can be killed by freezing. These include the ones that cause gonorrhea, meningitis, and syphilis.

TABLE 18–1 Summary of Physical Agents for Destruction of Microorganisms

Method	Application	Limitations
Dry heat		
Hot-air oven	Sterilizing materials damaged by or impermeable to moisture, such as glass, metal, oils, sharp instruments	Destroys materials that cannot tolerate high temperatures for prolonged periods of time
Incineration	Destruction and disposal of contaminated objects that cannot be reused	Size of incinerator must be adequate to incinerate the largest load quickly and completely. There is air pollution.
Filtration		
Fiberglass (HEPA) filters	Disinfection of air within an enclosure, such as in a cubicle or room	Expensive
Membrane filters	Sterilization of heat-sensitive biological fluids	Biological fluids must be relatively free of suspended particles.
Moist heat		
Autoclave	Sterilization of instruments, linens, liquids and other mediums, treatment trays and utensils, culture mediums, microorganisms	Ineffective against heat-sensitive materials and against microorganisms in materials impervious to steam
Boiling water or free-flowing steam	Sanitizes bedding, clothing and dishes, and destroys non-spore-forming pathogens	Cannot ensure complete sterilization after one exposure
Physical cleaning		
Ultrasonic waves	Effective in decontaminating delicate cleaning instruments	Procedure not effective alone, but is an adjunct to enhance the effectiveness of other methods.
Washing	Hands, skin, objects	Reduces but does not kill all microorganisms
Radiation		
Ionizing radiations	Sterilization of heat-sensitive medical equipment and other surgical materials	Expensive and requires special facilities for use
Ultraviolet light	Disinfect surfaces and to control airborne infection	Must penetrate to be effective (does not pass through transparent glass or opaque objects; irritate eyes and skin; low penetration)

Drying

We learned in Chapter 4 that moisture is needed for bacterial growth. Drying can be useful in preventing the growth of some bacteria. By removing all moisture, one of the essential ingredients needed for bacterial growth is removed. Thus, growth is inhibited.

The effectiveness of drying in killing organisms depends on many factors, or variables. We must consider the kind of organisms, the number of cells to be killed, the thickness of the article to be sterilized, the temperature used, and the presence or absence of oxygen. Some bacteria, like those that produce meningitis and gonorrhea, are killed by drying within a few hours. Tuberculosis bacilli can withstand drying for several days or longer.

Spore-forming bacteria can withstand drying almost indefinitely. One investigator reported that anthrax bacteria were alive after 40 years of drying in a glass bottle. Therefore, drying is not a very effective method for sterilization. On the other hand, it does serve its purpose by killing most of the active forms of bacteria. It is especially useful for preserving milk, fruits, and cereals. Biological preparations, including antibiotics, serums, toxins, and pure cultures of microorganisms, as well as certain foods, are often preserved by being frozen and then dried in a vacuum. This process is known as **lyophilization.**

The health care professional should be aware of the presence of dried viable bacteria in dried blood, excrement, and pus. These bacteria can be found just about anywhere: in dust and on bedding, clothing, surgical dressings, and windows. Precautionary measures include damp-dusting furniture, wet-mopping floors, and proper disposal of dressings. Otherwise, the dried microbes can easily be spread throughout the environment.

Radiation

Sunlight.

Direct sunlight has a powerful **germicidal,** or destructive, effect on microorganisms living on the surface of the skin and clothing. Sunlight is composed of three rays: long infrared (heat) rays, visible light rays, and the short ultraviolet (UV) rays.

Ultraviolet light.

The long infrared rays have a minimal effect on bacteria, and the visible light rays only inhibit bacterial growth. It is the ultraviolet rays that have a germicidal effect on microorganisms. Because these UV rays do not penetrate matter, they are effective only against airborne and surface microbes.

UV lamps are now found in hospital rooms where patients have contagious diseases. They are also used in newborn nurseries, operating rooms, cafeterias, and classrooms. In addition, such biological preparations as antitoxins, toxins, serums, and vaccines are sterilized with UV rays.

It is important to use caution with UV lamps. Exposure of the eyes or skin to UV rays can result in serious burns. Repeated overexposure to UV rays is a potential cause of skin cancer.

Beta, gamma, and X rays.

Beta rays, gamma rays, and X rays (roentgen rays) are lethal to all forms of life, including microorganisms. These rays have considerable energy and penetration power, which makes them useful in the sterilization of food packages and heat-sensitive surgical equipment. They are also effective in the treatment of diseases such as cancer.

Obviously, great care must be observed when using such powerful rays on patients. The rays must be precisely focused on the specific area to be treated, or normal neighboring cells may be damaged or killed.

Heat

Heat is by far the most effective of the physical agents of sterilization. High temperatures are more destructive than low temperatures. The length of time an article is subjected to the temperature is important; the longer the time, the more effective it will be in killing bacteria. The time is not counted from the moment the flame is lighted but from the time the particular desired temperature or pressure has been reached. The higher the temperature used, the shorter the time required (and vice versa).

The time and temperature combination required to kill a particular organism under laboratory conditions is called the **thermal death point** or **thermal death time.** This will vary with each organism, with the number of organisms present, and with the surroundings of the bacteria, such as the medium and amount of moisture.

Heat may be used to sterilize objects in the form of dry or moist heat.

Dry Heat Methods

Open flame. The open flame of a Bunsen burner or stove may be used to sterilize objects that have come in contact with microbes. We are all familiar with the common procedure of sterilizing a needle with a flame when it is to be used to remove a splinter. We learned earlier to sterilize the inoculating needle in this way.

Incineration. Disposable articles that have come in contact with pathogens can be incinerated after use. The incineration temperature must be kept high enough to guarantee the immediate ashing of materials as they are fed into the flames. A dry heat incinerator should never be overloaded with moist or protein-laden materials such as feces, pus, or vomitus. Overloading causes the "lumping" of incompletely burned material and the entrapment of moisture and contaminating pathogens within the moist surfaces. Thus, incinerating chambers must be large enough to accommodate the maximum load introduced and still be able to maintain high temperatures to ensure complete and immediate incineration and sterilization of the largest loads. Incineration is generally used to destroy bandages, carcasses, infected laboratory animals, and other refuse from infected patients.

Hot-air oven. Dry heat from an oven is commonly used for sterilizing laboratory glassware, petri dishes, sheets, towels, gauze, powders, fats, oils and waxes, needles, and sharp instruments. Dry heat is less effective than moist heat, so a higher temperature must be used. It would take 320°F (160°C) for at least 1 hour to kill all bacteria. Dry heat is used for articles that would be injured by moist heat, such as gauze. Oils and powders used in medical treatment must be sterilized with hot air because steam cannot penetrate them.

Moist Heat Methods

Boiling water. Boiling water (212°F; 100°C) is another means of destroying organisms. An article boiled in water for 20 minutes may be free from active bacteria, but not from spores. To ensure that spores have also been killed, articles should be boiled three more times, for 30 minutes each, at 24-hour intervals. This lengthy process will permit the spores to emerge and be destroyed. Articles must be completely covered by the boiling water.

The boiling water method can be used for instruments, foot tubs, treatment trays, bedpans, urinals, and douche and enema apparatus. It is also effective in disinfecting linens and dishes of patients and for drinking water.

Steam under pressure (pressure cooker and autoclave). The best method for sterilizing equipment and supplies by physical means is by moist steam under pressure. An ordinary pressure cooker operates on this principle and may be used to sterilize objects at home. The hospital counterpart of a pressure cooker is the **autoclave,** or **steam sterilizer.** It is a large, airtight chamber in which steam is generated from water by applying heat.

This is the only sterilization method that ensures the killing of both spores and active cells. The autoclave operates at 15 pounds of steam pressure for 15 to 20 minutes. (Longer periods may be used if desired.) As the pressure is increased, the temperature is also increased; it can rise to 250.8°F (121.6°C) under 15 pounds of pressure, as compared with the 212°F (100°C) for ordinary boiling water. The autoclave is the only acceptable method of destroying bacteriological and other microbiological waste generated in a microbiology laboratory.

Moist, pressurized steam may be used to sterilize any highly contaminated trays, articles, bacteriological cultures, aprons, rubber gloves, rubber tubing, surgical instruments, and contaminated glassware. It also can be used for sterilizing home-canned foods. Gas sterilizers are also effective in killing microorganisms. *Note:* Heat may discolor metals or dull sharp instruments.

Filtration

Filters are used in laboratories to remove bacteria and other large microorganisms from animal serum, solutions of antibiotics, enzymes, sugar, and vitamins. These fluids are both **thermolabile** (destroyed by heat) and susceptible to radiation, so the common methods of sterilization cannot be used.

Filters of various pore sizes can separate a variety of microorganisms from the liquids or gases in which they are suspended. These include bacteria, cells, large viruses, and products of bacterial growth (enzymes and exotoxins). The material that passes through the filter is the **filtrate.** The small viruses that pass through into the filtrate are known as **filterable viruses.**

There is a large assortment of filters from which a health care professional may choose. Kinds of filters include an asbestos pad in the Seitz filter, diatomaceous earth in the Berkefield filter, porcelain in the Chamberland-Pasteur filter, sintered glass (made from fused uniform glass particles), thin plastic films, and the newer cellulose membrane or molecular filters.

A new type of filter, the membrane or molecular filter, has been developed. The pores of a membrane filter are of a uniform, specific, and predetermined size. These filters are made from biologically inert cellulose material. They are circular membranes of about 150 μm thickness and contain millions of microscopic pores of a very uniform diameter. Thus, membrane filters can be made with pore sizes ranging from about 0.01 to 10 μm. These filters are widely used in industry and in laboratories to sterilize fluid materials. They have also been used in the microbiology laboratory to identify microbes from water samples and other materials.

The development of the high-efficiency particulate air (**HEPA**) filters has made it possible to deliver clean air into an enclosure such as a cubicle or a room. HEPA filters are made up of cellulose acetate (the filter medium) pleated around aluminum foil. These filters remove particles as small as 0.3 μm. The HEPA filters coupled with a system of **laminar airflow*** are widely used to deliver bacteria-free and dust-free air into a room.

Although replaced mostly by metal or plastic caps, cotton plugs are often still used to close flasks, test tubes, and pipettes. Air and other gases pass through the cotton, but most microorganisms are entrapped in the cotton fibers (unless the cotton is wet).

Ultrasonic Waves

Ultrasonic waves are used for cleaning delicate equipment and glassware. An ultrasonic cleaner is a vessel filled with fluid, usually water, through which short sound waves pass. These waves will mechanically dislodge any particles or solvent from instruments and glassware. To be completely effective, however, ultrasonic cleaning must be followed by another form of sterilization.

ANTISEPTICS AND DISINFECTANTS

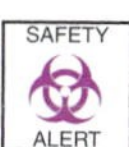

The various chemicals used as antiseptics or disinfectants can be classified into three groups: (1) **disinfectants**—compounds (such as cresol) used liberally on environmental surfaces to kill bacteria found within bodily excretions and in the environment; (2) **germicides**—compounds (such as iodine) applied directly to the skin or tissues either for disease prevention or treatment; and (3) **bactericides**—preparations taken internally for the treatment of infections (e.g., penicillin and sulfonamides) (Table 18–2).

Chemical

Several chemicals are used in a variety of situations to achieve a sterile field or to sterilize a contaminated area. Under OSHA's rule on Occupational Exposure to Potential Blood-borne Pathogens it is recommended that a 0.5% **sodium hypochlorite** solution (a 10%

*Laminar airflow is a unidirectional airflow system in which a stream of air is passed through a bank of HEPA filters. The air is subsequently delivered into an enclosure so that the entire body of air moves with uniform speed along parallel flow lines. The laminar-airflow system is widely used in the aerospace and electronics industries. This gives a high degree of cleanliness, which is necessary for product reliability.

TABLE 18–2 Some Chemical Disinfectants, Their Uses, and Recommended Strengths

Chemical	Uses	Common Recommended Strength
Phenol (carbolic acid)	Disinfects instruments, utensils, clothing, linen, sinks, toilets, excreta, floors; protective handwash for health care personnel	5% standard disinfectant
Lysol	Disinfects excreta, sinks, toilets, utensils; effective as a general disinfectant	2%–5%
Bichloride of mercury	Disinfects instruments, glassware, rubber articles; used in antiseptic ointments	0.1% (1 to 1000)
Formaldehyde (Formalin)	Disinfects excreta, linen, dishes, instruments, rubber gloves; tissue preservation and fumigation	1.5%–10%
Chlorine	Disinfects water supply, sewage, pools, bedpans, toilets, floors	Varies with amount of organic matter present
Ethyl or isopropyl alcohol	Preparation of skin prior to an injection or operation (scrubbing up); disinfects thermometers	70%
Hydrogen peroxide	Cleanses skin wounds, irrigates wounds; mouthwash, gargle	3%–20%
Iodine	Treats parasitic skin diseases, disinfects water, air (iodine vapors), food, utensils	2%
Mercurochrome	Wounds, abrasions, cuts	1%–2.5%
Metaphen	Skin	2%–5%
Argyrol (silver compound)	Infection of mucous membranes of eye, nose, throat, bladder (mild antiseptic)	10%–25%
Hexylresorcinol	Wounds, mouthwash, gargle	33⅓%
Acidine dyes: acriflavine and proflavine	Burns, wounds, ophthalmic applications, bladder irrigation	2%–3%
Sodium hypochloride	Spills, equipment, work areas	0.5%
Household bleach	Spills, equipment work areas	10%
New Products for hands.		
Alcare®	hand cleansing	lotion c̄ alcohol & aloe
	hand cleansing	gel c̄ alcohol & aloe
Ultra safe®	hand cleansing	waterproof skin protectant
Antec®	Spills, counters, work area, equipment	1/50–1/200
	Bactericidal	

dilution of common household bleach in water) be used to wipe up spills of blood. This chemical will kill human immunodeficiency virus, hepatitis B viruses, and even tuberculosis germs. The longer the wet solution remains on the contaminated spill the better the germicidal effects of the solution. Iodine, povidone, and betadine are routinely used to sterilize tissue surfaces before drawing blood cultures and before surgical procedures. Some chemicals have only a bacteriostatic effect, such as isopropyl alcohol. Others, including phenolic agents, 70% ethanol, and Alcide (a commercial product moderately effective on spores) have varying degrees of effectiveness and are frequently used to wipe down outer surfaces of equipment and work areas in the laboratory. Today's safety standards recommend the use of bleach in a spray bottle to clean work areas, equipment, and spills. It is advisable to spray this disinfectant on a regular basis inside centrifuges and other containers used to store, hold, or carry blood samples.

Antiseptic solutions are used to check the growth of bacteria. They may be used safely on the skin or inside the body. For example, boric acid solution is a mild antiseptic. A disinfectant, however, has the strength to kill bacteria. It is used to disinfect instruments, equipment, floors, and bathrooms. It is not to be used on the skin or inside the body.

Effectiveness

Some antiseptics and disinfectants are better than others in destroying bacteria. This can be shown by a simple experiment, as described later in this chapter. The effect of an antimicrobial chemical depends upon three factors: the type of material to be treated, the types of microorganisms, and environmental factors.

Type of material to be treated. A potent disinfectant is generally used on contaminated objects and utensils. However, this same disinfectant would prove too strong and poisonous for direct application to human skin and tissue. In other words, the chemical used should be compatible with the material to be treated. The antimicrobial agent should be nonpoisonous to animal and human tissue, and noncorrosive and nonstaining to objects being treated.

Types of microorganisms. The ideal, universal antimicrobial agent effective against all microbes does not exist. Some, however, are more effective than others in their ability to kill microbes. Spore-forming microbes, for instance, and others like the hepatitis virus and the tubercle and leprosy bacilli, are strongly resistant to most common disinfectants. By contrast, vegetative (growing) microbes are much less resistant. So the health professional must consider the specific microbe(s) to be killed when selecting a chemical disinfectant. The amount of time and proper concentrations needed to kill certain microbes should also be taken into account.

Environmental factors. Temperature, time, concentration, and pH all tend to influence the effectiveness of a chemical agent. Disinfectants and antiseptics work against pathogens by breaking up the cell membrane of the pathogen, neutralizing bacterial toxins and enzymes, and damaging the DNA material.

The standard disinfectant used by bacteriologists for determining the killing strength of another disinfectant is phenol (carbolic acid). The **phenol coefficient** is the killing power of a germicide toward a test organism as compared with that of phenol under identical conditions. For example, if a certain disinfectant is said to have a phenol coefficient of 50%, it has half the germicidal effect of carbolic acid. All health care personnel should be familiar with this standard.

Soap and water are most widely used for the mechanical removal of debris that protect and help organisms to grow. Health care providers should always wash their hands thoroughly before and after coming into contact with patients or when handling contaminated objects.

SAFETY PRECAUTIONS

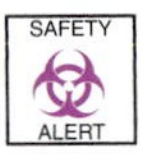

It is vital that health professionals understand the nature and the solution strengths of chemicals being used to destroy microbes. Since almost all these agents are poisonous, they would obviously be very harmful if used either in a stronger solution or for the wrong purpose. When mixed, solutions must be labeled with the name, the strength, and the date the solution was made. All chemicals should be kept under lock and key or otherwise inaccessible to children and untrained adults.

Microbiology laboratories are unique environments that can pose serious biological harm if safety precautions are not strictly adhered to. Since the nature of clinical specimens received from patients may pose a health hazard to personnel, microbiologists must be meticulously cautious in handling specimens. Once, thirty-one persons contracted typhoid fever all traceable to the strain received in a bacteriology laboratory for proficiency testing. In another instance, the last few cases of smallpox in the world were acquired by workers in another part of the building that housed the smallpox research. The principal investigator was so distraught at the thought that possible safety violations in his laboratory were the cause of these cases that he committed suicide. Today, with concern for the spread of the human immunodeficiency virus and hepatitis B, hepatitis C, and other highly infective diseases, all health care providers are cautioned to follow the U.S. Centers for Disease Control (CDC) safety precautions concerning the handling of all patient and contaminated materials. Infection control measures or medical asepsis include procedures and practices that all health care professionals use to prevent the spread of disease. These procedures are known as universal precautions and were enacted as law in June 1992 under the Occupational Safety and Health Administration (OSHA) Final Rule, titled "Occupational Exposure To Bloodborne Pathogens."

The universal precautions format has been updated and fine-tuned by the CDC to include practices intended for compliance by all health care professionals who come in contact with patients of any type. These new standard precautions combine many of the basic principles of universal precautions with techniques known as body substance isolation (BSI), a set of guidelines maintaining that personal protective equipment/clothing will be worn for contact with all body fluids regardless if blood is visible. The result has been the formation of standard precautions. These precautions are designed to reduce the risk of transmission of microorganisms from both recognized and unrecognized sources of infection. These sources include blood, all body fluids, secretions, excretions, nonintact skin, and mucous membranes.

The success of these prevention measures will be only as good as the health care practitioners' conscientious effort to practice them. A complete review of standard precautions, universal precautions, OSHA's Bloodborne Pathogen rule, and the Clinical Laboratory Act of 1988 (CLIA 88) regulations can be found in Appendix C.

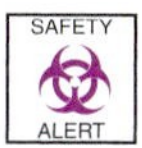

Essentials of Universal & Standard Precautions

1. Use appropriate barrier precautions to avoid skin and mucous membrane exposure. This includes wearing gloves at all times and masks, gowns or aprons, and goggles if there is a risk of splashes or droplet formation.
2. Change gloves with each and every patient contact. Wash hands immediately after glove removal and after any contamination.
3. Take special care when handling needles, scalpels, or other sharp objects. Needles should not be cut or broken. Resheathing of needles is permissible only when a one-handed technique is available. Dispose of sharp objects in hard-walled containers.
4. Use disposable mouthpieces or other ventilation devices with one-way valves when performing resuscitation measures.
5. Do not mouth **pipette.**
6. Refrain from handling patients or patient care equipment if you have open sores or weeping dermatitis.
7. Transport specimens in leakproof containers.
8. Decontaminate all spills immediately with 10% bleach solution.
9. Use properly marked biohazard infectious waste containers (red or orange) to dispose of biohazardous waste. Protect custodial and housekeeping staff by autoclaving before disposing.

SUMMARY

This chapter describes methods of destroying microorganisms. Physical means include sterilization by autoclave, boiling, incineration, filtration, and ultraviolet light. Each of these methodologies has varying degrees of effect on microorganisms. It is certain that autoclaving and incineration will kill everything, provided proper procedures are followed. Chemical methods include the use of antiseptics and disinfectants. Their effectiveness is variable. Most disinfectants are applied topically, such as iodine for cuts and bleach for laboratory benchtops and equipment. These are called germicides. Bactericides, on the other hand, include antibiotic therapy. Some antibiotics will kill the bacteria (bactericidal) and some only stop further growth of the bacteria (bacteriostatic). It is essential that all health care practitioners wash their hands after each and every patient contact and when handling microbiological specimens. The Centers for Disease Control (CDC), the Occupational Safety and Health Administration (OSHA), and the Clinical Laboratory Improvement Act of 1988 (CLIA 88) have published numerous guidelines, policies, and rules for the prevention of the transmission of potentially infective materials. Universal and standard precautions, if practiced consistently by all health care workers, would eliminate all worker contaminations.

STUDY AND DISCUSSION

- Explain how you would disinfect each item shown:

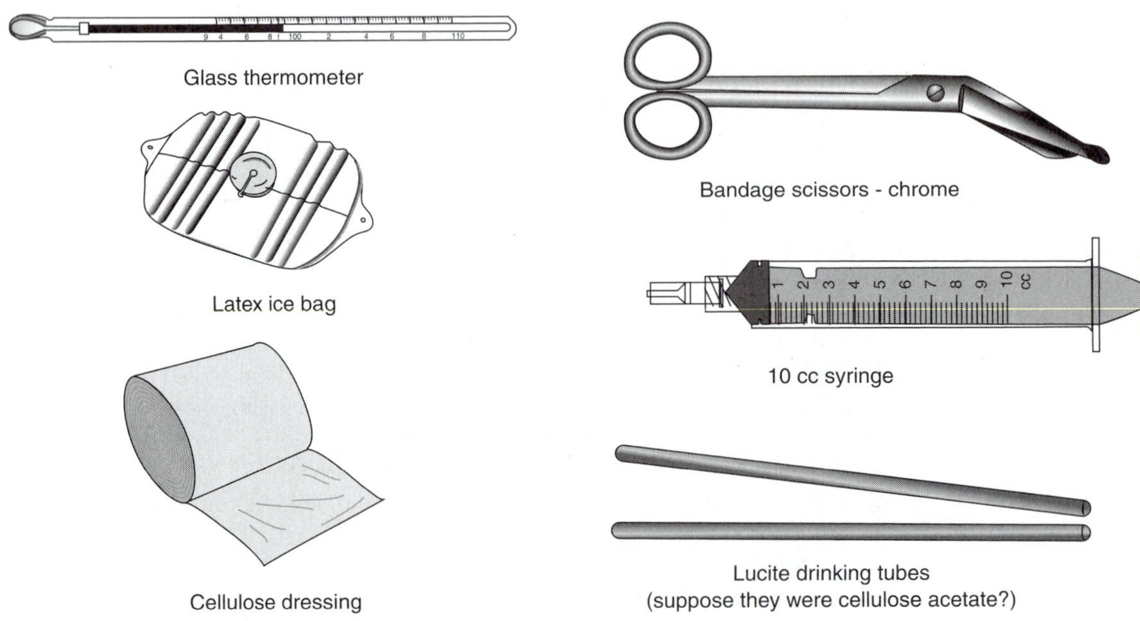

- Give three examples of situations in which you would use a method of physical sterilization in the home. Describe each method.
- Sterilize a roll of gauze in a home pressure cooker. Explain the process step by step.
- Explain what happens if you fail to refrigerate the unused part of a frozen-food dinner and it begins to decay.
- Explain why time is an important factor in the sterilization process.
- In the operating room, doctors and other health care professionals wear gowns and caps that have been sterilized. They also wear sterile gauze masks over their mouths and noses and sterile gloves on their hands. Explain the reasons for these precautions.
- Prepare a report of any one of the germ-free life research centers in the United States, France, Japan, or Sweden. See *The World of Microbes Encyclopedia of the Life Sciences*, vol. 4.
- Discuss how the length of time in which an article remains in a disinfectant affects the bacteria.
- What chemicals are used for disinfectants or antiseptics for the following?
  a. Hands of doctors and nurses before an operation
  b. Skin of a patient before operation
  c. Thermometers
  d. Scalpels
  e. Irrigating infected wounds
  f. Eyewashes
  g. Mouthwashes
  h. Vaginal douches

i. Bladder irrigations
j. Enemas

- Explain the steps you would take to sterilize a thermometer after removing it from the mouth of a patient.
- Discuss the dangers involved in using chemical solutions that are stronger than recommended. Specifically, discuss iodine, phenol, and bichloride of mercury.

Procedure 18–1 Experiment with Chemical Agents

Equipment and Materials Needed

Sterile agar
3 disinfectants:
  Carbolic acid, 5% solution
  Lysol, 2%–5% solution
  Bichloride of mercury, 0.1%

7 petri dishes

Autoclave
3 antiseptics:
  Tincture of iodine, 2%
  Boric acid, 2%–5%
  Alcohol, 70% solution

Method

1. Expose each of seven petri dishes of sterilized agar to dusty air in the same room for 5 minutes.
2. Cover one of the exposed dishes without pouring any chemical into it.
3. Into each of the other six (exposed) dishes, pour a different antiseptic or disinfectant. Cover and label correctly. Incubate all dishes for 24 hours.

Observations and Conclusions

1. Which chemical seemed to check the growth of bacteria least of all?
2. Which chemical seemed to check the growth of bacteria most of all?
3. Complete the following table to show the varying effectiveness of the antiseptics and disinfectants used.

Petri Dish with	No. of Colonies After 24 Hours' Incubation	No. of Colonies After 48 Hours' Incubation	No. of Colonies After 72 Hours' Incubation
No chemical			
Iodine			
Alcohol			
Lysol			
Carbolic acid			
Bichloride of mercury			

4. Compare the growth and number of colonies in each petri dish with your control on three successive days.
5. Which of the six chemicals used was the most effective in controlling the growth of bacteria?

REVIEW QUESTIONS

A. General Questions: Provide complete answers to each of the following.

1. You are boiling some instruments to disinfect them. You intended to let them boil for 20 minutes. They have been boiling for 10 minutes when somebody drops several used instruments in with yours. How does this affect your disinfection time?
2. Name four agents of physical destruction of bacteria.
3. Of the four agents you have named, which is the most effective?
4. Which type of heat would you use to ensure that you killed all spores as well as bacteria?
5. Which type of heat would you use to sterilize medicated oils and powders?
6. How long should ordinary articles be boiled in the home to kill bacteria?

7. Why would you use an autoclave to sterilize dishes?

8. Name one method that might be used to kill bacteria in the air of an operating room.

9. Does the process of sterilization kill all bacteria?

10. What is meant by a *bacteriostatic effect* on bacteria?

11. Explain the process of lyophilization.

12. Why should a health care worker wet-dust and wet-mop in the room of a patient?

13. What type of sun rays have a germicidal effect on microorganisms?

14. Where can UV lamps be found, and why?

15. Explain why health professionals who operate UV lamps must be cautious.

16. What are beta, gamma, and X rays used for?

17. What can filters separate out from liquids or gases?

18. Name four different types of filters.

19. Why is ultrasonic cleaning ineffective by itself?

20. Why should a dry heat incinerator never be overloaded?

21. What are HEPA filters, and what does the acronym HEPA signify?

22. What is meant by laminar airflow?

23. A health care worker is preparing a medicine that must be administered hypodermically to a patient. No disposable syringes are available; however, the patient has a needle and glass syringe. First the needle and the syringe are boiled. Before injecting the medication, the skin of the patient's arm is cleansed with 70% alcohol. Explain the bacteriological principles involved.

24. Name five antiseptic solutions that may be used on the skin.

25. Explain what is meant by a 10% solution.

26. Explain how the strength or concentration of a solution affects its antimicrobial power.

27. Give an example of a frequently used chemical that may be both a disinfectant and an antiseptic. Explain how this is possible.

28. Explain why there is no ideal, universal antimicrobial agent.

29. How are antimicrobial agents effective in their destruction of microbes?

B. Multiple-Choice Questions: Select the letter of the choice that best answers the question.

1. Freezing produces a _____ effect on bacteria.
   a. bactericidal
   b. bacteriostatic
   c. lyophilized
   d. germicidal
2. Sterilization _____.
   a. inhibits the growth of all microorganisms
   b. kills bacteria but not viruses
   c. kills all microorganisms
   d. destroys pathogenic microorganisms
3. Included as germicides are _____.
   a. heat, infrared rays, and beta rays
   b. heat, ultraviolet rays, and X rays
   c. infrared rays, ultraviolet rays, and X rays
   d. visible light rays, heat, infrared rays
4. Lyophilization removes _____.
   a. dried blood
   b. water
   c. food
   d. pus
5. Antibiotics are classified as _____.
   a. disinfectants
   b. germicides
   c. bactericides
6. The recommended germicide for blood spills is _____.
   a. iodine
   b. betadine
   c. isopropyl alcohol
   d. household bleach
7. Disinfectants suitable for cleansing wounds include _____.
   a. phenol, lysol, hydrogen peroxide, and iodine
   b. mercurochrome, hydrogen peroxide, and proflavine
   c. chlorine, sodium hypochlorite, and phenol
   d. metaphen, alcohol, lysol, argyrol
8. Disinfectants suitable for cleaning work areas and spills include _____.
   a. phenol, lysol, hydrogen peroxide, and iodine
   b. mercurochrome, hydrogen peroxide, and proflavine
   c. chlorine, sodium hypochlorite, and phenol
   d. metaphen, alcohol, lysol, argyrol
9. According to universal precautions protocol it is permissible to _____.
   a. wear personal protective clothing when leaving the lab
   b. pipette by mouth provided the pipette tip is stuffed with nonabsorbent cotton
   c. carry urine samples for culture to the lab in a leakproof container
   d. resheath a needle as long as you are very careful
10. Personal protective clothing means _____.
    a. wearing a lab coat over street clothes while working in the lab
    b. wearing an impermeable lab coat at all times while working with hazardous materials
    c. wearing a uniform and a lab coat at all times while working in the lab
    d. wearing an impermeable lab coat as well as gloves and eye protection if indicated while working in the lab

C. Completion Questions: From the following list of terms fill in the blanks with the correct choice.

bactericidal	bacteriostatic	disinfection
in vivo	in vitro	autoclave
HEPA	germicide	disinfectant
thermolabile	thermostable	heat resistant

1. Procedures that inhibit the growth of bacteria are referred to as being ______________.

2. Procedures that are performed in test tubes or petri dishes are ______________ while those experiments occurring in living organisms are ______________.

3. To sterilize by steam under pressure is to ______________ the substance.

4. A chemical substance that destroys or inhibits bacterial growth is called a ______________.

5. Filters may be used to remove bacteria from solutions that may be ______________.

D. True/False

_____ 1. Needles may be resheathed if one hand is used.

_____ 2. Spills must be decontaminated with 30% bleach solution.

_____ 3. All employees are required to receive hepatitis B vaccines when first hired.

_____ 4. Latex gloves may be washed as you wash your hands in order to save time.

_____ 5. The employer may choose to supply all protective clothing, gloves, gowns, and shields.

_____ 6. Biohazard signs are red or orange.

_____ 7. Facilities that generate more than 50 pounds of biohazardous waste per year must engage a biohazard waste management company to properly dispose of that waste.

_____ 8. In cases of possible exposure to HBV or HIV it is recommended that blood samples be drawn from both the health care worker and the patient, if known to determine baselines.

_____ 9. Lab coats worn at the work bench may be worn to the lunch area provided the coat has not been designated as an impermeable personal protective covering.

_____ 10. Health care employees must wash their hands before leaving the laboratory for the day.

E. Matching Questions: Match the terms in Column I with their corresponding terms in Column II.

Column I	Column II
_______ 1. hot air oven	a. destruction of disposable things
_______ 2. membrane filters	b. disinfect air in a room
_______ 3. autoclave	c. sanitize dishes
_______ 4. ultrasonic waves	d. controls airborne infection
_______ 5. incineration	e. sterilize linens
_______ 6. HEPA filters	f. sterilize medical equipment
_______ 7. soap and water	g. sterilize glass
_______ 8. boiling water	h. sterilize heat-sensitive biologicals
_______ 9. ionizing radiation	i. cleaning delicate instruments
_______ 10. ultraviolet light	j. hands, skin

CHAPTER

19 Chemotherapeutic Agents

OBJECTIVES

After completing this chapter, you will be able to:

- identify the general characteristics and action of antibiotics and other chemotherapeutic agents.
- identify the action of antibiotics and other chemotherapeutic agents on microorganisms.
- state the general characteristics of antibiotics.
- match a disease with the most common antibiotic treatment.
- describe the mode of action of some common antibiotics.

KEY WORDS

antibiotics	*Candida albicans*	in vivo
antibiotic sensitivity test	competitive inhibition	narrow-spectrum antibiotics
broad-spectrum antibiotics	in vitro	

Our reliance on drugs and chemicals to treat disease dates back nearly five centuries. In 1495, mercury was first used to treat syphilis. Unfortunately, this and similar experiments that followed proved harmful to the patient. But the search continued for chemotherapeutic agents that were effective as well as safe.

The work of Paul Ehrlich marked the beginning of modern chemotherapy in 1910. The famous "606" compound he synthesized was both effective against syphilis and safe for the patient. Compound "606" is an arsenical compound. Its trade name is Salvarsan, and its chemical name is arsphenamine. This drug was commonly used to treat syphilis until 1935, when penicillin was refined.

Since then literally thousands of chemotherapeutic agents have been developed or synthesized for the treatment of disease. These are drugs or chemicals that fight infectious diseases by arresting or destroying pathogens **in vivo** (within a living organism).

Antibiotics are chemotherapeutic agents that are the product of living microorganisms. Tiny amounts of antibiotics are effective in killing pathogens. Research on and development of new antibiotics is an important part of a microbiologist's work (Figure 19–1). Today many antibiotics are synthetically manufactured. Most natural antibiotics

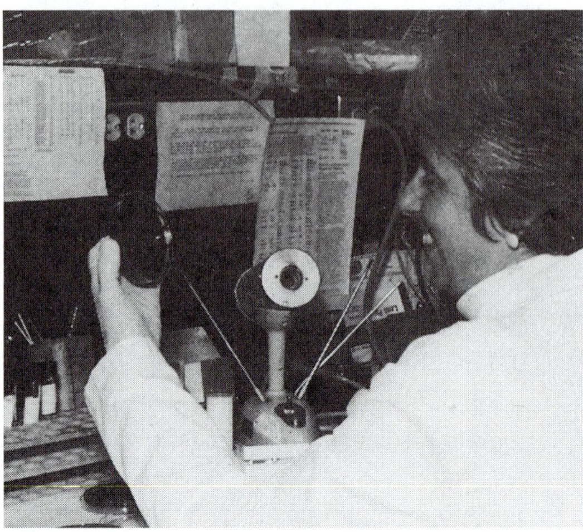

Figure 19–1 Microbiologist examines morphology of culture plates

are derived from chemical substances produced by a variety of fungi. Antibiotics may be bacteriostatic or bactericidal and are usually only effective against bacterial invaders. Antiviral and antifungal agents are most often synthetically produced.

Chemicals used **in vitro** (outside an organism's body) are not chemotherapeutic. These include the antiseptics, disinfectants, and germicides discussed in Chapter 18.

CHEMOTHERAPEUTIC AGENTS

- Synthetic compounds (the sulfa and nitrofuran drugs)
  1. Sulfa drugs
     a. sulfanilamide
     b. sulfadiazine
     c. sulfisoxasole, Gantrisin, etc.
  2. Nitrofuran drugs
     a. furoxone
     b. furalin
     c. furadantin
- Naturally occurring (antibiotics)
  1. penicillin
  2. streptomycin
  3. chloramphenicol
  4. tetracycline
  5. erythromycin
  6. novobiocin
  7. neomycin
  8. polymyxin
  9. bacitracin
  10. nystatin

Mode of Action

There are three ways in which chemotherapeutic agents inhibit or kill bacteria without harm to the host (Table 19–1). **Competitive inhibition** occurs when the metabolism of a

Table 19–1 Some Disease-Causing Microorganisms, Their Related Drug or Antibiotic Treatments, and Their Modes of Action

Disease	Bacteria	Drug or Antibiotic Treatment	Mode of Action
Anthrax	*Bacillus anthracis*	Erythromycin	Interferes with protein synthesis
		Penicillin	Inhibits cell-wall synthesis
		Tetracycline	Interferes with protein synthesis
Boils, carbuncles, pneumonia, septicemia	*Staphylococcus aureus*	Lincomycin	Inhibits protein synthesis
		Penicillin	Inhibits cell-wall synthesis
		Vancomycin	Inhibits cell-wall synthesis
Botulism	*Clostridium botulinum*	Kanamycin	Induces abnormal protein synthesis
		Penicillin	Inhibits cell-wall synthesis
Cholera	*Vibrio cholerae*	Chloramphenicol	Interferes with protein synthesis
		Streptomycin	Produces abnormal protein synthesis
Diphtheria	*Corynebacterium diphtheriae*	Lincomycin	Inhibits protein synthesis
		Penicillin	Inhibits cell-wall synthesis
Gangrene, wound infections, gastroenteritis	*Clostridium perfringens* and any *Salmonella* species	Kanamycin	Induces abnormal protein synthesis
		Penicillin	Inhibits cell-wall synthesis
		Ampicillin	Inhibits cell-wall synthesis
		Chloramphenicol	Interferes with protein synthesis
		Tetracycline	Interferes with protein
		Clindamycin	Interferes with protein synthesis
Gonorrhea	*Neisseria gonorrhoeae*	Penicillin	Inhibits cell-wall synthesis
		Tetracycline	Interferes with protein synthesis
		Sulfisoxazole	
Leprosy	*Mycobacterium leprae*	Kanamycin	Induces abnormal protein synthesis
		Novobiocin	Affects DNA formation
Meningitis	*Neisseria meningitidis*	Penicillin	Inhibits cell-wall synthesis
	Haemophilis influenzae		
	Cryptococcus neoformans	Amphotericin B	Damages cell wall

Table 19–1 Continued

Disease	Bacteria	Drug or Antibiotic Treatment	Mode of Action
Pertussis (whooping cough)	*Bordetella pertussis*	Ampicillin Penicillin Tetracycline	Inhibits cell-wall synthesis Inhibits cell-wall synthesis Interferes with protein synthesis
Plague	*Yersinia pestis*	Streptomycin Tetracycline	Produces abnormal protein synthesis Interferes with protein synthesis
Pneumonia	*Klebsiella pneumoniae* *Streptococcus pneumoniae*	Colistin Kanamycin Neomycin Penicillin	Causes cell membrane deterioration Induces abnormal protein synthesis Induces abnormal protein synthesis Inhibits cell-wall synthesis
Rocky Mountain spotted fever	*Rickettsia rickettsii*	Chloramphenicol Tetracycline	Interferes with protein synthesis Interferes with protein synthesis
Strep throat, scarlet fever, rheumatic fever	*Streptococcus pyogenes*	Erythromycin Lincomycin Penicillin	Interferes with protein synthesis Inhibits protein synthesis Inhibits cell-wall synthesis
Syphilis	*Treponema pallidum*	Erythromycin Penicillin Tetracycline	Interferes with protein synthesis Inhibits cell-wall synthesis Interferes with protein synthesis
Tetanus (lockjaw)	*Clostridium tetani*	Kanamycin Penicillin	Induces abnormal protein synthesis Inhibits cell-wall synthesis
Thrush	*Candida albicans*	Amphotericin B	Damages cell wall
Tuberculosis	*Mycobacterium tuberculosis*	Isoniazid Streptomycin	Competitive inhibition Produces abnormal protein synthesis

Table 19–1 Continued

Disease	Bacteria	Drug or Antibiotic Treatment	Mode of Action
Typhoid fever	*Salmonella typhi*	Ampicillin	Inhibits cell-wall synthesis
		Chloramphenicol	Interferes with protein synthesis
		Tetracycline	Interferes with protein synthesis
Urinary infections	*Escherichia coli*	Ampicillin	Inhibits cell-wall synthesis
		Kanamycin	Induces abnormal protein synthesis
		Sulfonamides	Competitive inhibition

bacterium is blocked by an agent that mimics a nutrient needed by the bacteria. Thus, the bacteria are tricked into accepting the chemotherapeutic agent instead. As a result, microbial growth is interrupted and the bacterium later dies.

The sulfonamide drugs work in this manner. They inhibit folic acid synthesis in microbes needing para-aminobenzoic acid (PABA) to make folic acid. The lack of folic acid, in turn, arrests cellular growth. Human cells, however, are not affected by this process.

Damage to the cell wall of a bacterium can be induced with penicillin. Penicillin is especially effective in killing gram-positive bacteria such as staphylococci and streptococci and also in killing some gram-negative bacteria such as gonococci. It works by interfering with bacterial cell wall synthesis. This weakens the cell wall, causing the bacteria to lyse and die. Penicillin is safe for humans, because human cells do not have cell walls.

Inhibition of protein synthesis is yet another mechanism of certain chemotherapeutic agents. For example, the tetracyclines, chloramphenicol, erythromycin, and lincomycin interfere with the process of protein synthesis. Here again, bacteria are destroyed with no harm to the human host.

Antibiotics can be subdivided, depending on whether they act against a single group of bacteria or more than one. The **narrow-spectrum antibiotics** act against only one group. **Broad-spectrum antibiotics** are effective against many gram-negative and gram-positive bacteria. Broad-spectrum antibiotics include tetracycline, kanamycin, neomycin, streptomycin, ampicillin, and chloramphenicol.

Naming of Chemotherapeutic Agents

It should be pointed out that many of the same antibiotics are processed by different drug companies. As a result, similar chemotherapeutic agents have been given different trade names. In fact, certain trade names are so commonly used that the original terms have been disregarded. Today, prescriptions are often made out using these trade names. Table 19–2

Table 19–2 Generic and Trade Names of Drugs

Generic Names	Trade Names
Chloramphenicol	Chloromycetin
Tetracycline	Achromycin Panmycin Steclin Sumycin Tetracyn
Erythromycin	Erythrocin Ilotycin
Novobiocin	Albamycin Cathomycin
Neomycin	Kantex

gives examples of common trade names that are used more often than the generic names. Trade name drugs are often more expensive than the generic counterpart.

Other Considerations

Antibiotics are made in many different forms, including pills, capsules, throat lozenges, liquids, and ointments. They are administered in several ways: by mouth, by injection, and by local application.

Most antibiotics should be kept refrigerated; however, there are exceptions to this rule. Each antibiotic product has instructions as to its proper storage and expiration date. The health care professional must follow these instructions for the safety of the patient.

Although this practice is rapidly disappearing, antibiotics are sometimes given in combinations of two or more at a time. The penicillin-streptomycin combination is an example of two drugs that may be combined.

Harmful Aspects of Antibiotics

Antibiotics, if not properly controlled, can become more harmful than beneficial. Great care must be taken to observe and report signs due to the following possible effects:

- Accumulation of different strains of bacteria, which become increasingly resistant to the action of antibiotics. The best example of this is the so-called hospital staph. These strains have developed due to the indiscriminate use of antibiotics and as a result nosocomial infections such as *Staphylococcus aureus* frequently recur in hospitals, especially in nurseries, where the patients are most vulnerable. Another disease, gonorrhea, has also experienced the wide use of penicillin and as a result the bacteria has mutated, producing strains that are resistant to penicillin. These penicillinase-producing *Neisseria gonorrhoeae* (PPNG) are best treated with sulfisoxazole. Today, antibiotic-resistant strains of tuberculosis are leading to new epidemic levels of this disease. Resistant strains have always been prevalent when only one antibiotic is taken. Coupled with the long-term therapy required and the vast numbers of medications that need be taken, some with unpleasant side effects, it is often difficult to convince patients that without all three medications they will not get well, especially when they feel better when not taking nausea-producing drugs.

- Elimination of normal bacteria from a certain area of the body. This allows disease-producing microorganisms in the same area to gain a foothold. An example is the killing of intestinal bacteria by overuse of antibiotics, with the resulting overgrowth of a pathogenic fungi (***Candida albicans***).
- Toxicity. Some antibiotics are very toxic and therefore their dosages are carefully monitored.
- Other adverse effects, depending upon the antibiotic used. Included are such effects as allergic reactions (skin eruptions, asthma), digestive reactions (nausea, vomiting, loss of appetite, diarrhea), nerve damage, and kidney damage.

ANTIBIOTIC SENSITIVITY TESTING

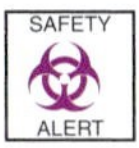

Laboratory tests have been devised to assist the physician in choosing an antibiotic. Laboratories will usually run two or more procedures to determine the bacteria's susceptibility to various antibiotics. The oldest and most common procedure is known as the Kirby-Bauer **antibiotic sensitivity test** (see color plate #29). Once the organism has been at least tentatively identified, a few colonies are taken from a pure isolate and inoculated into a broth media and allowed to grow for several hours to the turbidity of a McFarland standard. Once the desired turbidity of broth has been reached (i.e., when the bacteria are in their stationary or lag phase, 1×10^9/milliliter), a swab is used to inoculate the broth culture onto Mueller-Hinton agar (a special media ideal for the growth of most bacteria and optimal diffusion of the antibiotic-soaked filter disks). The entire plate is streaked with the swab so as to yield a blanket of growth completely covering the plate. Once the plate has been inoculated, filter disks soaked in different antibiotics are dropped onto the plate, usually from a dispenser, although they may be hand dropped using sterile forceps. It is advisable to tap each disk to secure them to the media so that when the plate is covered and turned upside down for overnight incubation at 37°C (98.6°F) the disks will not fall off. It is customary for a laboratory to keep separate dispensers for gram-positive and gram-negative organisms, because antibiotic choice is first determined by the organism's Gram-staining characteristics before source of infection.

The next day, the antibiotic sensitivity is determined by the ring of inhibition of no growth around the antibiotic disk. The antibiotic is able to diffuse into the media before the bacteria have a chance to grow. Therefore, if the bacteria are "sensitive" to the drug, there will be no growth for a zone of approximately 8 to 25 millimeters around the disk. If the organism is "resistant" to the drug, the organism will grow right up to the edge of the filter disk. Other more accurate and precise methods of antibiotic sensitivity may be performed in hospital and reference laboratories. The minimum inhibitory concentration (MIC) and the minimum bactericidal concentration (MBC) tests involve the addition of a standardized growth of the organism to be tested to varying dilutions of the antibiotics in question. After an overnight incubation, visual turbidity is noted. The first tube containing no visible growth is said to be the MIC. All tubes showing no visible growth are then subcultured onto plated culture media and incubated again overnight. The first dilution showing no growth on the plate is then the MBC. These techniques can be purchased commercially using microtiter dilution trays. They are fast and accurate but can be expensive. The plates come premade with varying dilutions of different antibiotic panels on them. Using specially made inoculating needles, all ninety-six wells of a microtiter plate can be simultaneously inoculated, saving much time. Special care must be taken in the storage and incubation of the plates to prevent drying of the same amounts of antibiotic in the tiny wells.

It should be noted that test results conducted in vitro do not always parallel in vivo actions. For example, a drug found to be resistant during laboratory testing may well be sensitive to the bacteria in the body because that bacteria is causing a urinary tract infection and antibiotics are much more concentrated in urine. On the other hand, they are much lower in spinal fluid than in serum.

Some antibiotics are particularly toxic; therefore, their levels in serum must be monitored. Some of these drugs include gentamicin, tobramycin, and vancomycin. They are frequently used to treat very resistant infections, particularly among dialysis and immunosuppressed patients. Predose and postdose levels are determined by drawing blood samples at approximately 30 minutes before a dose of antibiotic is infused and then again at a specified time when the drug has reached its peak level in the body. In this way, the physician can determine if the patient is absorbing all of the dosage given. If a patient is not absorbing all of the drug given and levels are not being monitored, dose after dose would be given, escalating the amount of antibiotic beyond the toxic limits. In summary, the physician has the last word on antibiotics of choice, but the microbiologist can provide valuable assistance so that the wisest choice can be made.

SUMMARY

This chapter describes some of the more common antibiotics and matches them with certain diseases they are used to treat. It also describes the basic actions of antibiotics. Most antibiotics either inhibit cell-wall synthesis or inhibit protein synthesis as their method of destroying bacteria. It should be noted that not all antibiotics are meant to kill bacteria. Some simply inhibit the growth of the microorganism to further prevent its multiplication. Antibiotics are either broad spectrum or narrow spectrum in association with the numbers and kinds of groups of bacteria. For example, penicillin is a narrow-spectrum antibiotic because it is used most effectively against gram-positive organisms, whereas ampicillin is a broad-spectrum antibiotic and is effective against both gram-positive and gram-negative organisms.

STUDY AND DISCUSSION

- Do some additional reading about specific antibiotic effects.
- Read the biography of Dr. S. Waksman or another discoverer of antibiotics. Prepare a short report for the class.

- Investigate newspaper and magazine articles on *Staphylococcus aureus*, the golden killer.
- Perform the antibiotic sensitivity test outlined in the experiment instructions.

Procedure 19–1 Experiment Using Antibiotic Sensitivity Disk

Equipment and Materials Needed

Sterile petri dishes
Sterile swabs
Sterile tubes containing 15 milliliters of nutrient agar
Red glass-marking pencils (one for four persons)
Small forceps

Sensitivity disks containing the following antibiotic agents available in vials of 50 each; the high concentrations are best for this experiment:

penicillin	tetramycin	neomycin
streptomycin	erythromycin	bacitracin
chloramphenicol (Chloromycetin)		

Cultures of the following nonpathogenic bacteria (one for four persons):

Staphylococcus albus
Sarcina lutea

Method

1. Pour a nutrient agar plate using sterile technique. (These may be prepared beforehand.)
2. Let it cool until firm and then invert. Allow it to stand until quite hard (20 to 30 minutes) or put it in refrigerator for about 10 minutes.
3. Using one of the above cultures and a sterile swab, cover the surface of one of the prepared plates so that there is a thin layer of the bacteria over the whole area of the plate. (Instructor may demonstrate this first.)
4. Using the red marking pencil, divide the bottom of the petri dish into four or six sections, and identify each section.
5. Using forceps that are flamed each time in a Bunsen burner, put one of each of the sensitivity disks in the center of each of the sections, leaving one section without a disk. This is the control section. Press the disks gently into the agar. Incubate overnight at 98.6°F (37°C).
6. Note the growth of the organisms at the region of the antibiotic disks.

Observations and Conclusions

1. Use the following designations to compile your results:
   a. If there is a ring of inhibition around the antibiotic sensitivity disk, the organism is sensitive to that antibiotic.
   b. If there is no ring of inhibition around the antibiotic sensitivity disk, the organism is resistant to that antibiotic.

2. Compare your results with those of other students and the instructor.
3. What does the experiment demonstrate?
4. How do the results correlate with use of the same antibiotic in a patient's body?

REVIEW QUESTIONS

A. General Questions: Provide complete answers to each of the following.

1. Penicillin is a broad-spectrum antibiotic. Explain in your own words what this means.

2. What precautions must be observed in the storage of antibiotics?

3. The doctor has prescribed sulfadiazine for a patient who is under your care. What adverse effects might you observe?

4. What is the difference between in vitro and in vivo?

5. Name four synthetic chemotherapeutic agents and four naturally occurring chemotherapeutic agents.

6. How do chemotherapeutic agents work against pathogens?

7. Explain the difference between a broad-spectrum antibiotic and a narrow-spectrum antibiotic. Give examples of each.

8. Name five antibiotics that will interfere with protein synthesis in a bacterium.

B. Multiple-Choice Questions: Select the letter of the choice that best answers the question.

1. Most natural antibiotics are derived from _____ .
   a. fungi
   b. flowers
   c. herbs and spices
   d. all of the above
2. Narrow-spectrum antibiotics include _____ .
   a. penicillin
   b. ampicillin
   c. neomycin
   d. kanamycin
3. Culture media most suited for Kirby-Bauer sensitivity testing is _____ .
   a. nutrient agar
   b. 5% sheep blood agar
   c. Mueller-Hinton agar
   d. chocolate agar
4. The McFarland standard represents a growth of approximately _____ of bacteria per milliliter of broth.
   a. 1×10^6
   b. 1×10^8
   c. 1×10^3
   d. 1×10^9
5. Several methods of determining antibiotic susceptibility levels are used. Methods inoculating numerous small wells simultaneously are called _____ .
   a. Kirby-Bauer
   b. minimal inhibitory concentration (MIC)
   c. minimal bactericidal concentration (MBC)
   d. microtiter dilution

C. Completion Questions: From the following list of terms fill in the blanks with the correct choice.

penicillin	salvarsan	sulfisoxasole
rifampin	amphotericin B	minimal inhibitory
gentamycin	tetracycline	minimal bactericidal
ampicillin	tobramycin	peak
trough		

1. The first antibiotic used to treat syphilis was ____________ .

2. To successfully treat tuberculosis, long courses of streptomycin, isoniazid, and ____________ are given to patients for 2 years or more.

3. The first tube in a series of tubes incubated with a given antibiotic to show no visible growth of bacteria is called the ____________ concentration level.

4. Two of the most toxic antibiotics include ____________ and ____________.

5. Because of the toxicity of some antibiotics it is important to monitor their levels so that the patient will not become overmedicated with these poisons. Blood samples are drawn before the dose is given to determine the ____________ level and blood samples are drawn again 30 minutes after the antibiotic has been given to determine the ____________ level.

D. Matching Questions: Match the diseases in Column I with their antibiotic of choice in Column II. Although some antibiotics may be used in treating more than one disease listed, each antibiotic listed should be used only once.

Column I		Column II
_______	1. leprosy	a. ampicillin
_______	2. plague	b. sulfisoxazole
_______	3. strep throat	c. streptomycin
_______	4. pertussis	d. chloramphenicol
_______	5. pneumonia (*Klebsiella*)	e. vancomycin
_______	6. gonorrhea (PPNG)	f. penicillin
_______	7. botulism	g. clindamycin
_______	8. anthrax	h. kanamycin
_______	9. diphtheria	i. erythromycin
_______	10. Rocky Mountain spotted fever	j. lincomycin
_______	11. cholera	k. isoniazid
_______	12. carbuncles, boils	l. sulfonamides
_______	13. gangrene	m. colistin
_______	14. urinary infections	n. novobiocin
_______	15. tuberculosis	o. tetracycline

SECTION 4

ACHIEVEMENT REVIEW

A. Answer the following questions, giving the bacteriological explanation for your answer.

1. How would you sterilize oils and ointments?

2. Explain briefly how a patient is protected from infection by contact with doctors and other health care personnel in an operating room.

3. Describe the method for sterilizing rubber gloves such as those you wear in the operating room.

4. Explain why shaving the operation site is necessary.

B. Match each word or term in Column I with the statement in Column II that is best associated with it. (Some letters are used more than once.)

Column I

_______ 1. physical agents of sterilization
_______ 2. toxic conditions produced by bacteria
_______ 3. sterilization of ointments
_______ 4. carbolic acid
_______ 5. boric acid
_______ 6. freedom from bacteria
_______ 7. disinfection of mattresses, pillows
_______ 8. moist steam under pressure
_______ 9. heating milk to 145°F (63°C)
_______ 10. sterilization in an open flame

Column II

a. inoculating needle
b. pasteurization
c. autoclave
d. ultraviolet rays
e. asepsis
f. antiseptic
g. phenol coefficient
h. hot air
i. sepsis

C. Insert the word or expression that best completes each statement.

1. A five percent (5%) formalin solution contains ______________ part(s) formalin and ______________ part(s) water.
2. A dilute solution of ______________ may be used for wet dressings.
3. The most widely used cleansing agent is ______________ .
4. The only certain way of destroying the spores of disease germs is by ______________ .
5. The invasion of any item by disease bacteria is known as ______________ .
6. The time and temperature combination required to kill a particular organism under laboratory conditions is called the ______________ .
7. Generally speaking, an article boiled in water for ______________ minutes should be free from active bacteria, but not from spores.
8. The kitchen appliance that uses steam pressure is the ______________ .
9. The use of an ______________ in a room may help control bacteria in the air.
10. A sterile bandage is one that is ______________ .
11. A chemical used to kill germs is called a ______________ .
12. A ______________ is a chemical that kills germs but may not be used on the skin.
13. A disinfectant may also be called a______________ .
14. A vapor used to kill bacteria is called a ______________ .
15. The name of a chemical used to disinfect sinks is _____ .

D. Indicate which of the following statements are true (T) and which are false (F).

1. Exbiota are microorganisms that live in space. _____
2. Asepsis refers to the presence of germ life. _____
3. A sterile bandage is one that is free from pathogenic organisms. _____
4. An antiseptic is a chemical agent that prevents the growth of germs. _____
5. An antiseptic is a germicide. _____
6. A deodorant is used for cuts and wounds. _____
7. Infection is the invasion of the body tissues by pathogenic bacteria. _____
8. Sepsis is a toxic state produced by bacteria. _____
9. Infection is the destroying of harmful germs in the body. _____
10. To be sterile, water must be heated to 150°F (66°C). _____

11. Boric acid solution is used as a germicide. ______
12. Phenol is also known as carbolic acid. ______
13. Metal instruments, glass, towels, and linens may be sterilized by boiling for 5 minutes. ______
14. Adding a small quantity of baking soda to water in which instruments are boiled will keep them bright. ______
15. Disinfectants may be used on the human body. ______
16. Sterilization is essential to destroy microorganisms and prevent infection. ______
17. Physical agents that destroy bacteria are heat, light, and disinfectants. ______
18. Freezing is a reliable method of sterilization. ______
19. Time is of no consequence in the sterilization process. ______
20. Time is counted from the moment the flame is lighted. ______
21. Needles may be sterilized by being placed in a direct flame for an instant. ______
22. All bed linens, towels, and clothing used on patients having contagious diseases must be burned. ______
23. To sterilize by baking, articles must remain in the oven at a temperature of 320°F (160°C) for at least an hour. ______
24. The boiling point of water is 212°F (100°C). ______
25. Pasteurization of milk does not kill all the bacteria present. ______
26. The most effective method of sterilization is exposure to direct steam. ______
27. Pressure sterilizers are not essential equipment in a modern hospital. ______
28. Spore-forming bacteria can be destroyed by exposure to steam at 5 pounds of pressure for 20 minutes. ______
29. The opposite of sepsis is toxin. ______
30. Drying is a good method of preserving foods. ______
31. Direct sunlight has a destructive effect on some microorganisms. ______
32. Disinfectants do not kill bacteria. ______
33. Ultraviolet rays are the longest rays of sunshine and are thus able to penetrate deeply into materials. ______
34. Exposure to direct sunlight for several hours is a successful means of disinfecting items such as mattresses, pillows, and blankets. ______
35. Streptomycin is used in the treatment of tubercular patients. ______

36. A disinfectant solution may be changed to an antiseptic by dilution in some cases. _____
37. Antiseptic solutions are excellent chemical agents used to kill bacteria. _____
38. Antiseptics are also known as germicides and bactericides. _____
39. Disinfectants are used for sterilizing instruments. _____
40. A solution containing sodium chloride is an antiseptic. _____
41. A 10% solution of formalin is used to wash the hands. _____
42. Mercuric chloride is extremely dangerous to use because it is very poisonous. _____
43. Argyrol is an antiseptic used to prevent the growth of bacteria in the mucous membranes of the eyes, nose, and throat. _____
44. Lysol may be used either as an antiseptic or a disinfectant, depending on the strength of its solution. _____
45. Chlorine is a good disinfectant for cleaning wounds. _____
46. Mercurochrome, merthiolate, and mercuric chloride are safe antiseptics to be used on unbroken skin. _____
47. It is not important for the health care professional to remember percentages of solutions. _____
48. Solutions made up should always be labeled. _____
49. It is rarely necessary to keep chemicals under lock and key, as they are harmless. _____
50. Thermometers may be disinfected by soaking in alcohol for an hour. _____
51. A 10% formalin solution is made by using one part formalin to nine parts water. _____

SECTION 5 PUBLIC HEALTH MICROBIOLOGY

CHAPTER 20 Air, Food, Milk, Water, Soil, and Sewage Control

OBJECTIVES

After completing this chapter, you will be able to:

- List the most effective methods for preventing the spread of airborne diseases.
- Name the most common sources of contaminated milk.
- Identify the several means of avoiding milk contamination.
- List some diseases typically transmitted from cows and through human or other contamination.
- Describe the two methods of pasteurization.
- List the most common types and causes of food poisoning.
- Explain in detail how food poisoning can be prevented.
- Explain how water can be made safe so that it will not be a source of infection.
- Describe the ways in which disease can be prevented through proper control of the soil and sewage disposal.

KEY WORDS

Clostridium botulinum	high-temperature short-time (HTST) method	low-temperature holding (LTH) method
droplet nuclei		
flash method		

KEY WORDS (cont.)

petri dish counter
plate count
potable
ptomaine

AIR

Air is a poor medium for microbial growth, because it does not contain enough of the food and water microorganisms need. However, air is an excellent carrier of airborne microbes. Microbes can be carried on dust, air currents, large droplets, particulate matter, and droplet nuclei from a source of infection. **Droplet nuclei** occur when tiny liquid droplets evaporate. In addition, coughing and sneezing can spread microbes through the air, permitting droplet infection.

When a great number of people are crowded into small quarters, viruses and respiratory parasites may be readily transferred by the air. A healthy person may sit by someone who is infected. The infected person gives off microorganisms by exhaling, coughing, and sneezing. These microorganisms can gain entrance into the body through the respiratory tract. When the resistance of individuals is low, infection soon occurs and the person contracts the disease. The common cold is an example of a disease spread in this manner.

Crowded schoolrooms, movie theaters, or any room where many people are gathered have more microorganisms per square inch than open or well-ventilated places. A constant supply of fresh air can clean and rid enclosed areas of the impurities from respiration and perspiration, which helps to decrease the chance of infection.

Methods of Control

There are various methods used to control the level of organisms in the air. The best choice depends on the number of people and the type of activity in the room.

- Ultraviolet rays from UV lamps work well against airborne microbes. Their effectiveness, however, is limited to direct contact with the particle carrying the microbes. Also, precautions must be taken to protect the eyes and skin of both patients and health care professionals from direct contact with UV rays.
- Chemical agents can reduce airborne microbes. These chemical agents are sprayed in an aerosol; the vapors kill airborne microbes on contact. An effective aerosol should be highly germicidal, effective at normal temperature and humidity, nontoxic to living organisms, and nonstaining and noncorrosive to objects.
- Filtration is yet another method of removing airborne microbes. Filters are generally made from cotton, glass, or other fibrous substances. They are in common use in air-circulation systems. Some filters can also be used to sterilize culture media or to remove particles as small as viruses. By varying the pore size, these "millipore" filters are very useful when other methods of removing microbes may be detrimental to the media.

The health care professional should be familiar with the following fundamental principles of disinfection to prevent airborne diseases from spreading.

- Cover the mouth when coughing or sneezing.
- Use disposable tissues when coughing or sneezing.
- Wash and sterilize objects (for example, dishes and utensils) used by a patient with a respiratory disease.
- Always wash hands after treating any patient.
- Use a mask that acts as a barrier to, or a filter of, bacteria, when appropriate.
- Use a damp or oiled mop and dustcloth when dusting to prevent dust from flying about. Then use a vacuum cleaner.
- Expose pillows and mattresses to sunlight and air. Ventilate the room.

MILK

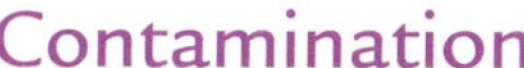

Contamination

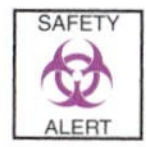

Milk, unlike air, is an excellent medium for bacterial growth. It contains carbohydrates, fats, proteins, minerals, vitamins, and water. Under the proper conditions, milk can serve as a bacterial carrier.

Even when drawn from the udder of a healthy cow, milk contains many microbes. Before milk reaches the consumer, it is further contaminated by a number of other sources. Unless the milk is promptly cooled to 50°F (10°C), the bacteria it contains will multiply rapidly and make it turn sour. Milk is most commonly contaminated by:

- *Diseased cows.* Milk drawn from an infected udder will contain pathogenic microbes.
- *Unclean milking areas.* The sanitary conditions of the milking area influence the microbial flora of the air. If the area is dusty or dirty, there is a strong possibility that the milk will become contaminated.
- *Improper or poor storage of milk in storage tanks or milk cans.*
- *Dairy workers with infected or unwashed hands.*
- *Unsanitary milking equipment.* Milk cans, milking machines, storage tanks, and other equipment will contaminate milk if not properly cleaned and sanitized.

Disease

Three cattle diseases can be transmitted to people through contaminated milk: brucellosis, Q fever, and bovine tuberculosis. Subsequent contamination may occur during the milking or storage process. Milk can then also be a carrier of such disease as botulism, diphtheria, bacillary dysentery, septic sore throat, scarlet fever, typhoid fever, and undulant fever.

In the United States today there is little danger of epidemics of such diseases. Strict local and state controls over the production and pasteurization of milk have been set up by boards of health. A number of rigid standards must now be met by the milk producer to protect the consumer. These standards include:

- examination of cows by inspectors at periodic intervals
- regular inspection of barns and equipment

- health examinations of workers
- pasteurization
- proper cooling of milk before and after pasteurization
- maximum bacterial counts permitted in milk that is to be sold

Dating of milk containers also helps protect the consumer.

Pasteurization

Pasteurization was named after Louis Pasteur, the founder of modern bacteriology. It is a process that destroys pathogenic or harmful bacteria. Milk boiled for 20 minutes effectively kills all bacteria. However, this affects the vitamin and fat content of the milk, not to mention its taste. Pasteurization kills about 90% of the bacteria found in milk, while getting rid of all the pathogenic bacteria. Thus, pasteurization has been judged more desirable than boiling.

We have all heard of pasteurization, but how does it actually work? There are in fact two methods of pasteurizing milk. One method is to draw milk from the cow and immediately chill it to a temperature below 50°F (10°C). Later, when the milk reaches the pasteurization plant, it is heated to 145°F (63°C) for 30 minutes. Finally, it is rapidly cooled back down to 50°F (10°C). This process is known as the **low-temperature holding (LTH) method.** The second method is called the **high-temperature short-time (HTST) method,** or **flash method.** Milk is made to flow in a thin film over electrically heated metal plates. It is heated to 160°F (71°C) for 20 to 30 seconds, then rapidly cooled.

Bacterial Counts

To further protect the consumer, public health laboratories will conduct bacterial counts on milk. Bacterial counts are made by taking a sample of milk and diluting it with sterile water. Next, a pour plate is made using a suitable medium and agar. The plate is incubated overnight while the bacteria multiply. From each bacterium present in the original milk sample, a colony will develop. The colonies are counted, and an estimate is made of the number of bacteria. To make the counting easier, the petri dish may be divided into squares, or a magnifying device called a **petri dish counter** is used. Counting the colonies on the plate is known as the **plate count** (Figure 20–1).

State sanitary codes have established specific minimum requirements for different grades of milk. Their criteria are based on conditions at the various dairy farms and plants and on the results of chemical and bacteriological tests on the milk.

Grade A pasteurized milk is drawn from disease-free cows. It has a maximum bacterial count of 200,000 per milliliter after milking and handling. Following pasteurization and at time of delivery the bacterial count must not exceed 30,000 per milliliter.

Certified milk is produced according to the strictest standards of the American Association of Medical Milk Commissions. These standards are so exacting that even raw milk can be delivered directly to the consumer. The bacterial count of this milk is no more than 10,000 per milliliter; it is the purest milk available.

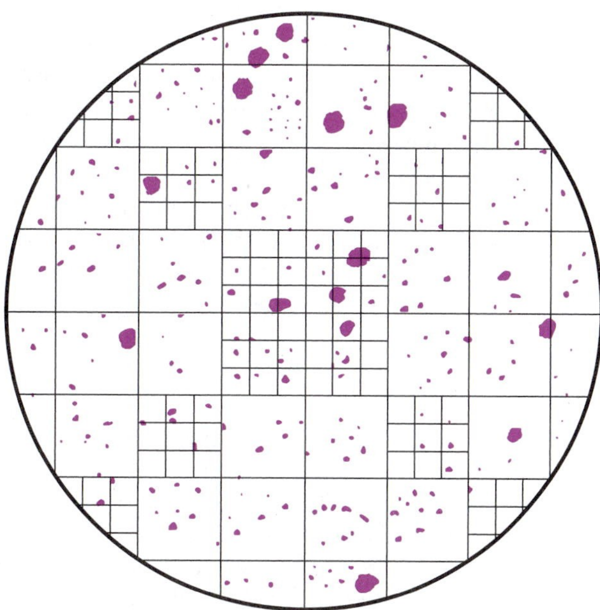

Figure 20–1 Bacterial plate count

FOOD

Food poisoning is a condition caused by eating foods that contain toxins or poisons or disease-producing bacteria. Toxins or poisons are produced by certain organisms, or they may be independent of any bacteria. Raw shellfish, meats, cream-filled pastries, raw milk, and canned products eaten without being cooked are the most common sources of food poisoning.

Bacteria that Cause Food Poisoning

Staphylococcus is a bacterium found in foods such as cream puffs, custards, milk, fish cakes, and chicken salad. This bacterium may be transmitted by a cook or server who has a pimple, boil, or lacerated finger. Therefore, people with these kinds of infections should avoid direct handling of food. People suffering from septic sore throat can infect foods with *Streptococcus* by coughing or sneezing.

Clostridium botulinum is the source of botulism, a highly fatal disease. This bacterium, which is anaerobic and lives in soil, is usually harmless if swallowed. But its toxins, produced in foods that have been improperly preserved, may cause death. Botulism can be prevented by processing food in such a manner that all spores are killed (for example, in a pressure cooker), and by heating home-preserved foods before tasting them.

Boiling for 15 minutes usually destroys toxins. The best method of preventing botulism is to discard—without tasting—all foods that show any change in appearance or odor.

An antitoxin exists for the *Clostridium* toxin; to be effective, it must be given immediately after having swallowed the contaminated food.

Salmonella causes food infections, gastroenteritis, typhoid fever, and paratyphoid fever, an acute illness of short duration. These bacteria may be transmitted by such foods as contaminated poultry, insufficiently cooked meats, raw eggs, raw salads, greens, cold cuts, fish, and potato salad.

Other bacteria, such as those that cause bacillary dysentery and cholera, can be transmitted by contaminated foods and human carriers. Amoebic dysentery is caused by parasites, not by bacteria. Nevertheless, this disease can be contracted by eating such contaminated foods as raw lettuce or celery grown in contaminated soil.

Food Spoilage

All raw foods carry microorganisms. Fortunately, most of these organisms are nonpathogenic. Microorganisms will cause decay and spoilage when left at room temperature. Therefore, raw foods should be thoroughly cleaned, washed, and refrigerated. Cooking kills bacteria; the use of a pressure cooker kills spores as well as bacteria.

We have discussed in earlier chapters that foods may be preserved by canning, freezing, pickling, salting, drying, and preserving in heavy syrup. Once preserved food is opened or defrosted, unused portions must be refrigerated just like fresh food.

Commercial food preservation is usually safe, because it is done under fully controlled conditions. Home preservation of foods, however, poses certain risks. One such example is canning. Canned foods can retain bacteria and spores if not properly preserved. This may result in food poisoning.

Ptomaine poisoning is a popular but incorrect term for bacterial food poisoning. **Ptomaines** are actually products of decomposition of materials that are so far spoiled that no human could eat them.

A major cause of food spoilage is the contamination of food by fungi and molds.

Prevention of Food Poisoning

As we have seen, pathogenic bacteria may come from diseased food handlers, contaminated soil and water in which food was grown, unclean containers, markets, stores, kitchens, unclean hands and clothing, and insects. The health care professional needs to be familiar with local sanitary codes. Strict adherence to all regulations, both in and out of the hospital, should always be insisted upon. In addition, certain basic safety measures can be explained to nonprofessionals who prepare or serve food.

SAFETY ALERT

The spread of foodborne diseases can be prevented by taking these precautions:

- Exclude carriers and persons with infections from kitchens.
- Prepare and store food in clean kitchens that are free from insects, rodents, or other animals.
- Use clean utensils, dishes, and containers.
- Allow the preparation of food only by persons who have clean hands and clothing.
- Adequately refrigerate food before and after preparation.
- Promptly serve cooked or much-handled food.

- Promptly and properly dispose of uneaten foods.
- Use only fresh, first-quality foods.
- Routinely examine anyone who comes in contact with foods at any time, especially those working in fast-food chains—the inexperienced youth who may not yet have the concern that "cleanliness is next to godliness."
- Use proper food-preservation methods.
- Serve fresh foods when possible.
- Thoroughly clean hands and fingernails after use of sanitary facilities.
- Wash the hands before and after handling or eating food.
- Use sanitary methods of disposing of human wastes.
- Use sanitary methods of disposing of oral and nasal discharge in tissues.
- Wash and rinse dishes in water heated to at least 176°F (80°C).

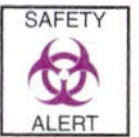

When a patient with a communicable disease is discharged from a hospital or clinic, the room must be thoroughly disinfected. This is the responsibility of the health care professional, who should always take the following steps:

- Give the patient a thorough soap and water bath in the room, including washing the hair and cleaning the nails.
- Incinerate all papers, magazines, and trash.
- Thoroughly scrub the floors and furniture with disinfectant.
- Wash all bed linens, blankets, and dishes, using methods of thorough sterilization (boiling, autoclaving).
- Expose each side of the mattress to direct sunlight for at least 6 hours, or use ethylene oxide gas.
- Use plastic covers on mattresses and pillows.
- Open the windows to let the room air out for a few days, if possible. Use an ultraviolet lamp, if available.
- Boil or disinfect all enamelware, glassware, instruments, and rubber articles.

MEAT AND EGGS

In the last few years much attention has been drawn to meat-packing and slaughter houses because of the high rate of meat and poultry contaminations with strains of *E. coli, Salmonella,* and *Campylobacter.* Legislation passed in 1967 and 1968 merely required inspections to be based on sight, smell, and touch. Microbiological testing for unseen contaminants was not required. In July 1996 the USDA Food Safety Inspection Service (FSIS) began implementing the newly approved Pathogen Reduction and Hazard Analysis and Critical Control Point (HACCP) system, to focus on prevention of food safety problems instead of providing symptomatic treatment after the problems occur. Large plants were required to implement an HACCP system by 1 January 1998. Smaller plants have until the summer of 1999 to comply. Because *E coli* is the most common fecal contaminant and the one receiving the most publicity, testing began January 1997 for all personnel. Plants are required to identify critical control points during processing where contamination is likely to occur. These points can then be targeted to eliminate or reduce safety hazards. Plant-specific standard operating procedures (SOPs) for sanitation were to have been established to keep facilities and equipment clean.

In other studies it has been discovered that there is a particular salmonella that is found in eggs before they hatch. *Salmonella enteritidis* ingested by the hen finds its way to the unborn egg, where it seems to cause no harm. It does not affect the egg at all. It is when the eggs are eaten, or left on serving trays (for numbers to multiply) to be later served, that the disease process begins with the person eating the contaminated eggs. As a precaution all eggs should be stored at 45°F and never left out.

WATER

The control of water, soil, and sewage is regulated by municipal authorities in most cities and villages. These agencies employ bacteriologists and other technologists for this purpose. People living in outlying areas, however, such as farmers, often must provide for their own water supply and sewage disposal.

Water is a major resource in the maintenance of human life. We need it for bathing, cleaning, cooking, drinking, growing crops, and the disposal of wastes. However, water can be one of the greatest carriers of disease. Cholera, dysentery, typhoid, and infectious hepatitis, for instance, can all be spread by water.

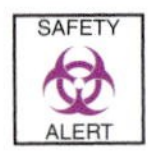

The source of contamination from biological pollution is human wastes. This can result directly from improper sewage disposal, or even from flies that come in contact with sewage or human excreta. A knowledge of water purification is needed prior to setting up methods of sewage disposal.

The water supply of a community may come from any of the following sources:

- *Surface water from lakes, rivers, and streams.* These water sources can also be contaminated by chemical pollution from industrial sites. We have all heard or read about serious cases of illegal pollutant dumping, inadequate—if any—treatment of industrial wastes, and the indiscriminate use of pesticides. In addition, surface waters can be contaminated biologically through soil microbes and raw fecal wastes.
- *Groundwater from shallow wells.* Pollution may occur from surface drainage during floods, or from cesspools, outhouses, and septic tanks.
- *Deep wells.* Properly sealed deep wells are usually safe because the surface water is filtered when it enters.

Water that is free from algae and suspended matter may still not be **potable** (safe to drink). It may contain protozoa and bacteria that can cause dysentery or typhoid fever. Such bacteria and protozoa are carried by the water, but originally they must have come from a person infected with the disease, or from a carrier.

Drinking water must be treated to be free of pathogenic bacteria. Water may contain other impurities besides bacteria. For each type of impurity, a specific treatment is given (Table 20–1).

The American Public Health Association has established standards for making tests at all stages of purification in municipal treatment plants. Tests are performed by bacteriologists, who determine the kinds and numbers of bacteria present. The number is determined by a plate count somewhat similar to that used for milk.

TABLE 20–1 Methods of Removing Impurities from Water

Common Impurities	Method of Removal
Solids, floating bodies, fish, leaves, twigs	Screening
Organic matter in solution and suspension (clay, mud, soil)	Sedimentation (settling), filtration, coagulation with alum
Gases (odors) in solution	Aeration (forcing a fine spray into air), absorption with activated carbon
Inorganic salts	Chemical softening
Algae and protozoa (fishy odors)	Copper sulfate
Pathogenic bacteria	Chlorination

If something unforeseen, like a flood, should cause good water to become polluted, emergency treatment of the water can be done in the home. One method is to boil the water for at least 20 minutes. Also, water may be disinfected by adding small quantities of sodium hypochlorite, calcium hypochlorite, or tincture of iodine (four drops of iodine in one gallon of water). Local health authorities publish directions and quantities of disinfectant solutions during an emergency.

SOIL AND SEWAGE

Soil is filled with microscopic organisms, most of which are useful. Some, however, are pathogens, such as those that cause lockjaw, food poisoning, and gas gangrene. The intestinal organisms that cause typhoid fever and dysentery can be introduced into the soil by polluted water and human excreta. Hookworm eggs, common in soil, have been found in areas near outdoor toilets.

Sewage disposal is thus an important health consideration. Homes in rural areas often have cesspools and septic tanks. These are designed to allow the solid matter to settle. In large cities, sewage is generally held for 12 to 30 hours. This permits anaerobic bacteria to decompose the organic matter and make it harmless. Many kinds of protozoa and bacteria play a useful part in this decomposition of organic matter.

Large cities treat their sewage in various ways to make it harmless. These methods include screening, separation, filtration, aeration, chlorination, and biological treatment by introducing bacteria that actually feed upon and decompose the organic matter.

SUMMARY

The method of choice for preventing the spread of airborne disease varies with the size of the area to be protected, the hazards of the preventive measure, and the toxicity of the preventive agent. Ultraviolet light is ideal for small areas, but one must be careful to protect the skin and eyes from overexposure. Chemicals in the form of aerosols are also very good especially if they are germicidal and nontoxic. Filtration can be a good way to remove particles from the air. This method is especially useful for sterilizing culture media that cannot be autoclaved. Milk is an excellent growth medium for bacteria. It is easily contaminated by improper pasteurization, diseased cows, poor storage procedures, unsanitary milking habits, and failure of dairy workers to work with no infections or clean hands. To protect us from these potential infective sources it is important that cows and barns be inspected regularly, that workers obtain regular health exams, that milk is properly pasteurized and cooled, and that bacterial counts on milk be taken regularly to ensure the noncontamination of milk.

Milk can be pasteurized by one of two methods, the low-temperature holding (LTH) method or the high-temperature short-time (HTST) method.

Food poisoning is readily caused by a number of organisms, including *Staphylococcus, Clostridium, E. coli,* and *Salmonella.* Food should be thoroughly cooked and not left out at room temperature for a long time. Always wash hands before preparing foods and do so in a clean environment. Periodically check food handlers for carrier states and be sure they adhere to all sanitary rules. Never serve foods from a can that is bulging or expels gas when opened. These are but a few of the precautions that can be taken to prevent food poisoning.

Maintaining clean water is a requirement of municipal agencies. Water is tested regularly for impurities. In rural areas farmers should be sure that contaminated streams do not get into their well water supply, and they should have their water tested regularly. Because human and animal waste is the major source of water contamination, it is imperative that the sewage system not pollute the drinking water supply. In rural areas, septic tanks and cesspools should be well away from the home and checked routinely for leaks. City water treatment and sewage facilities use a variety of procedures including screening, separation, filtration, aeration, chlorination, and introducing certain bacteria that actually feed upon and decompose the organic matter.

STUDY AND DISCUSSION: AIR

- Explain how the wearing of a mask helps to control bacteria in the surgical or operation room and in the sick room.
- Explain why a mother who has a cold should wear a mask when nursing her baby.
- Perform the following experiment.

Procedure 20-1 Bacteria in the Air

Equipment and Materials Needed

Microscope	Agar	7 Petri dishes

Method

1. Prepare and sterilize agar and petri dishes as learned earlier.
2. Keep one petri dish unopened as a control.

3. Open each of the other petri dishes in the following places. Keep each dish exposed for 5 minutes.
   a. In a crowded classroom, with windows and doors closed and the ventilating system turned off.
   b. In a well-ventilated room containing three people.
   c. In the center of a room where a dry duster is being used.
   d. In the center of a room being dusted with a damp duster.
   e. In a room that is being swept.
   f. In a room where a vacuum cleaner with a filter is being used.
4. Close, label, and incubate all dishes for 24 hours.

Observations and Conclusions

1. In the following chart record the number of colonies found in each plate.

DISH	A	B	C	D	E	F
No. of colonies						

2. Examine the colonies under the microscope and note varieties.

3. What conclusions would you note relative to decreasing the transfer of infection by control of the air? Compare dish A with B, C with D, and E with F.

STUDY AND DISCUSSION: FOOD

- The following case of food poisoning is taken from real life. Explain how it most likely occurred, and how you would have prevented it.

  A number of guests had refreshments at the home of Mr. and Mrs. Soapless. These facts were later discovered:

  1. Some guests became ill from food poisoning.
  2. Chicken salad was eaten by everyone who became ill.
  3. The chicken for the salad had been cooked the previous day, sliced, and placed in an earthen jar while the chicken was still warm.
  4. The jar of chicken was allowed to stand in the kitchen overnight, unrefrigerated.
  5. The person who prepared the salad had an infected finger.
  6. Cultures of *Staphylococcus* were obtained from the infected finger and the chicken salad.
  7. Toxins were obtained from broth cultures of the newly isolated *Staphylococcus*. They produced illness when injected into a lab animal.

- You are dealing with a patient who has typhoid fever. Explain how you would sterilize the following:
  a. dishes
  b. thermometer, tongue depressor
  c. bedpan, urine, feces
  d. linens, gowns
  e. unfinished food
  f. magazines, newspapers
- You have canned some string beans at home. When you open them, you are not quite sure that they are safe. What would you do to be absolutely sure there was no botulism present?
- Typhoid Mary was a cook who left a trail of typhoid fever outbreaks wherever she was employed. Explain how this occurred.
- Open a can of vegetable soup. Listen to the noise of the inrushing air. Why are canned foods usually packed under vacuum?
- Arrange a field trip to your local department of health. Report on your local sanitary code for prevention of food contamination.
- Perform the experiment on transmission of bacteria by the hands.

Procedure 20–2 Transmission of Bacteria by the Hands

Equipment and Materials Needed

Agar	Incubator	Basin
4 petri dishes	Bacteria	Water
Autoclave	Culture	

Method

1. Prepare and sterilize agar in petri dishes.
2. Four students immerse the fingers of their right hands in the basin of water, to which has been added a culture of bacteria selected by the instructor for this experiment. The students allow their fingers to dry without touching any other object. Now, these procedures are performed:
   a. One student draws the fingertips of the right hand lightly across the surface of the agar.
   b. Another student washes his or her hands just as before a meal, dries the hands with a sterile towel, and then draws the fingertips across the agar of a second dish.
   c. A third student scrubs his or her hands with soap, water, and a brush. The student should be sure to clean beneath the nails, as is done before assisting in an operation. This procedure is continued for 5 minutes; the student then dries hands with a sterile towel. Now the student draws the fingertips lightly across the surface of the agar of a third dish.
   d. A fourth student proceeds as in (c); after 5 minutes, the student immerses the right hand in a hand disinfectant solution such as is used in a hospital. Both hands are then dried with a sterile towel, and the fingertips are drawn lightly across the surface of the agar of a fourth dish.
3. All plates are labeled, incubated, and examined after 24 hours.

Observations and Conclusions

1. Observe each of the four petri dishes for types and number of colonies. List your results in this chart.

DISH	A	B	C	D	E	F
No. of colonies						
Types of bacteria						

2. Explain the value of scrubbing hands and immersing them in a disinfectant.

3. Under what circumstances would you:
   a. Wash your hands with soap and water?

   b. Scrub your hands for 5 minutes with soap, water, and a brush?

   c. Use a disinfectant after scrubbing your hands?

4. Capture an ordinary housefly, and let it walk across a sterile agar plate. Keep another sterile agar plate unopened as a control. Put the plates away in a warm place for a day. Observe and report the results.

STUDY AND DISCUSSION: MILK

- Visit a nearby pasteurization plant and report on it as a class project.
- Investigate local board of health regulations concerning the protection of milk.
- Explain how typhoid fever could be spread through contaminated milk.
- Perform the following experiment.

Procedure 20–3 Bacteria in Milk

Equipment and Materials Needed

Petri dish and cover
Melted agar
Magnifying glass
Pipette
Milk

Method

1. Keep the milk in the refrigerator until ready to use. If not homogenized, mix thoroughly.
2. Sterilize the petri dish, cover, and pipette. Sterilize the agar.
3. Pour the melted agar into the sterile petri dish.
4. Using the sterile pipette, place one milliliter (1 ml) of milk in the dish of melted agar.
5. Place the cover on the dish and carefully shake the contents.
6. With a pencil, divide the cover of the petri dish in halves, quarters, and eighths as shown.

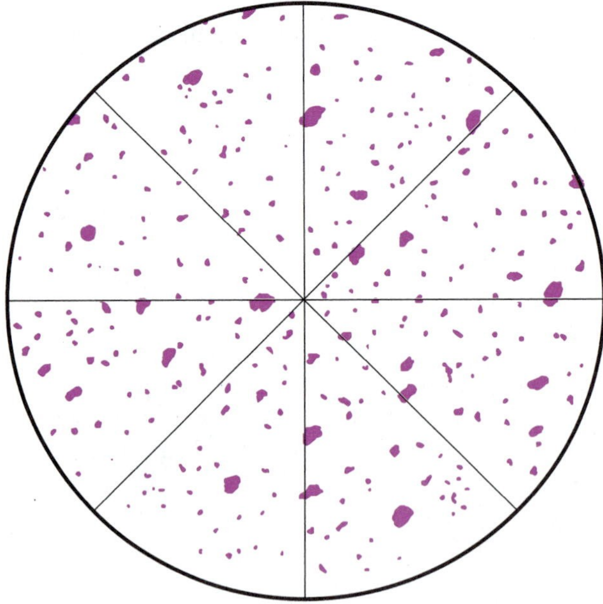

7. Incubate for 4 or 5 days at room temperature, or overnight in a 37°C incubator.
8. Using a magnifying glass, count the number of bacterial colonies in one section (one-eighth) of the dish. Multiply the number by eight to get the number of bacteria per milliliter of milk.

Observations and Conclusions

1. How many bacteria did you find in 1 ml of milk?

2. Explain why the above number is only an estimate.

3. Is your count within the number allowed in your state for that particular grade of milk?

4. Why are there so many bacteria in the milk even though it is certified or pasteurized?

5. Why is the plate count too slow a method to prevent a quantity of contaminated milk from getting on the market?

6. How is the bacterial count useful in checking disease spread by pathogenic bacteria in milk?

STUDY AND DISCUSSION: WATER, SOIL, AND SEWAGE

- Organize a field trip to a modern sewage disposal plant. Report on safety measures used to safeguard the health of local residents.
- Plan a field trip to a modern water purification plant. Report on all the treatment measures used.
- Explain how ice may spread intestinal diseases.
- Explain why a traveler to a foreign country may be required to be inoculated against typhoid fever.
- Exhibit a glass of water that has been allowed to stand overnight.
  a. Taste the water, and describe the taste to the class.
  b. Pour the water back and forth from one glass to another about ten times, to aerate it.
  c. Taste the water again, describing any difference in its taste. Is it improved?
- Demonstrate sedimentation, filtration, and coagulation, referring to the experiments described below.

- Referring to the experiments described below, demonstrate how microorganisms can be killed by:
  a. use of copper sulfate
  b. use of chlorine
  c. use of boiling water
- Suggested experiments demonstrating environmental control
  1. Sedimentation, filtration, and coagulation
     a. Pour some muddy water into each of the three beakers, A, B, and C.
     b. Permit beaker A to stand for 30 minutes to illustrate sedimentation.
     c. Pour the water from beaker B through a glass funnel filled with clean sand. Define filtration and filtrate.
     d. To beaker C, add a teaspoon of alum, then stir. Show how the alum coagulates and, in so doing, drags down or settles the mud.
  2. Use of copper sulfate to kill microorganisms
     a. Exhibit some spirogyra in a glass of water. Explain that such algae impart a fishy taste to water.
     b. Have the students observe a filament of spirogyra under the microscope. Have them note that it is alive.
     c. Add a small crystal of copper sulfate to the glass of water containing the spirogyra. Allow it to stand for a day.
     d. The following day have the students again observe some of this algae under the microscope. Have them note its condition, dead or alive.
     e. Explain that the fishy odor and taste of water may sometimes be removed by passing the water over activated carbon and then aerating it.
  3. Use of chlorine to kill microorganisms
     a. Place a drop of water containing some paramecia on a microscope and have the students observe the movements of these microorganisms.
     b. Lift the cover slip on the slide carefully and inject into the water a very small drop of water to which you had previously added some chlorine.
     c. Have the students observe how quickly the chlorine kills the protozoa.
  4. Use of boiling water to kill microorganisms
     a. Boil a test tube containing some of the paramecia.
     b. Place a drop of the boiled water under the microscope and have the students observe that the protozoa have been killed.

Procedure 20–4 Experiment: Bacteria in Water

Equipment and Materials Needed

Petri dish and cover
Melted agar
Pipette
Sample of tap water
Magnifying glass

Method

1. Sterilize the petri dish, cover, and pipette.
2. Heat the agar.
3. Pour the melted agar into the sterile petri dish.

4. Using the sterile pipette, place 1 ml of tap water in the dish of melted agar.
5. Cover the dish immediately.
6. Carefully rotate the petri dish on a flat surface to mix the contents.
7. With a pencil, divide the cover of the petri dish in halves, quarters, and eighths.
8. Incubate for 2 or 3 days at room temperature.
9. Using a magnifying glass, count the number of bacterial colonies in one section (one eighth) of the dish.
10. Multiply the number by eight to get total number of bacteria per milliliter of water.

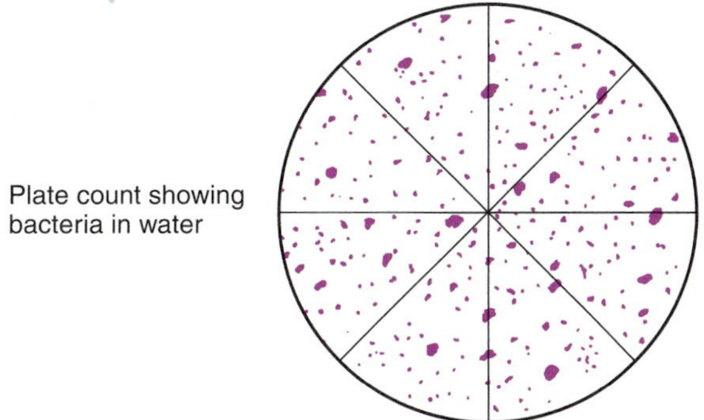
Plate count showing bacteria in water

Observations and Conclusions

1. What was the estimated number of bacteria per milliliter of water?

2. What kind of bacteria are present in tap water?

3. How is this test useful in checking the spread of disease through water?

4. When was this test conducted and by whom?

REVIEW QUESTIONS

A. General Questions: Provide complete answers to each of the following.

1. Name five diseases that can be transmitted by the air.

2. What are some methods of disinfecting the air?

3. What makes air an excellent carrier of microbes?

4. Why should we wash our hands with soap and water before preparing food?

5. Why should home-canned foods be boiled for 20 minutes before using?

6. Name six foods that are often responsible for food poisoning.

7. Name two bacteria that may cause food poisoning.

8. Name three different ways in which food can become contaminated.

9. Why must all workers who handle food have periodic health examinations?

10. Why is refrigeration of food necessary both before and after foods have been cooked?

11. The illustration shows the path made by a fly on a petri dish. Explain how the fly contaminated the petri dish.

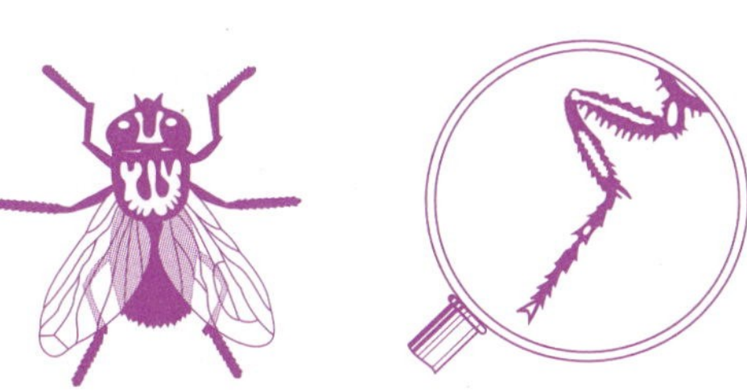

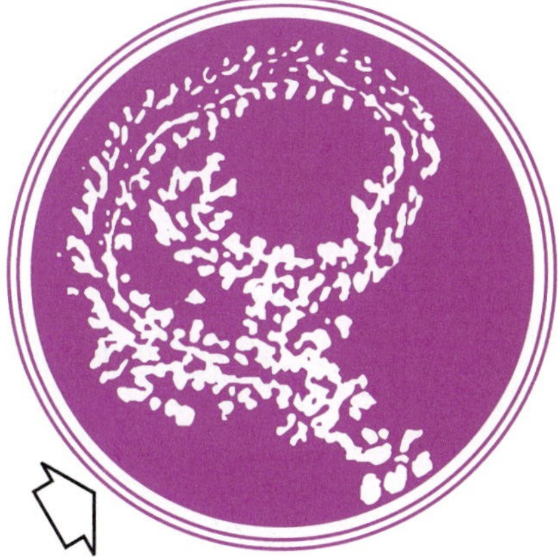

A fly walked around on this petri dish. Can you see how its legs can carry enough bacteria to make a trail like this?

12. What is meant by a bacterial count?

13. List four ways in which bacteria may contaminate milk.

14. Name six diseases that may be transmitted by contaminated milk.

15. Explain why milk should be refrigerated when not in use.

16. What measures are taken to prevent disease being spread by bacteria in milk?

17. Describe the two pasteurization methods.

18. Does pasteurization kill all of the bacteria in milk?

19. Why is it necessary to take frequent bacterial counts of milk samples?

20. Name and describe the differences between Grade A milk and certified milk.

21. What is potable water?

22. Name two diseases commonly spread by water.

23. Explain how a flood might contaminate normally pure water.

24. Name three substances that might be used to treat water for home consumption during an emergency.

25. What is the safest method of treating water from an unknown source?

26. Explain how some bacteria and protozoa can be useful in sewage disposal.

27. Name two anaerobic bacteria found in soil that may affect puncture wounds.

28. When would anaerobic bacteria from the soil be likely to cause infection?

29. What is the greatest danger of poorly disposed sewage?

B. Multiple-Choice Questions: Select the letter of the choice that best answers the question.

1. Prevention of the spread of airborne droplets is easily effected by _____ .
   a. covering the mouth when coughing or sneezing
   b. coughing into a filter to contain the microorganisms
   c. spraying a chemical aerosol when one coughs or sneezes
   d. setting up ultraviolet lamps around the work area
2. Milk contamination occurs when _____ .
   a. cows are diseased
   b. the milking areas are not clean
   c. the grocer fails to refrigerate the milk upon arrival
   d. the milk is not properly pasteurized
   e. all of the above

3. Pasteurization kills _____ .
   a. all bacteria
   b. most bacteria
   c. all pathogens
   d. most pathogens
4. Milk ready for the consumer can have no more than _____ .
   a. 1,000 bacteria per milliliter
   b. 10,000 bacteria per milliliter
   c. 30,000 bacteria per milliliter
   d. 200,000 bacteria per milliliter
5. The purest milk contains _____ .
   a. 1,000 bacteria per milliliter
   b. 10,000 bacteria per milliliter
   c. 30,000 bacteria per milliliter
   d. 0 bacteria per milliliter

C. Completion Questions: From the following list of terms fill in the blanks with the correct choice.

droplet nuclei	botulism	cooking	drying
toxins	salmonella	pickling	canning
food poisoning	dysentery	salting	

1. Food poisoning is usually caused by _____ produced by the culprit bacteria.
2. _____ is frequently a cause of food poisoning found in canned food.
3. Evaporated liquid drops containing microorganisms are called _____ .
4. Parasites such as the amoeba can cause _____ .

D. Matching Questions: Match the foods and conditions in Column I with their corresponding methods of preserving without spoiling in Column II.

Column I		**Column II**
_______	1. kills spores	a. salting
_______	2. kills bacteria	b. pickling
_______	3. raisins	c. drying
_______	4. salt pork	d. canning
_______	5. meat	e. pressure cooker
_______	6. fruits	f. freezing
_______	7. cucumbers	g. preserving in heavy syrup
_______	8. tomatos	h. boiling
_______	9. beef jerky	i. dehydration

CHAPTER 21

Health and Safety Measures Practiced in Health Care Facilities

OBJECTIVES

After completing this chapter, you will be able to:

- explain the importance of practicing sanitary measures in a health care facility.
- identify the sources of infections that can occur in health care facilities.
- describe methods of controlling infection within a health care facility.
- describe the key features of the standard precautions guidelines.
- explain how the standard precautions guidelines differ from universal precautions.
- describe the purpose of standard precautions and state five examples of how health care practitioners should practice standard precautions.
- differentiate between the six levels of personal protective equipment requirements.

KEY WORDS

asepsis
bacteremia
endoscope
epidemic
endoscopy
epidemiologist
fomites
infection-control practitioner (ICP)
mutate
nosocomial infection
opportunistic pathogen

In the microbiology laboratory, biosafety level protocols have been established by CDC and the National Institutes of Health (NIH) to guide personnel in the handling of infectious material. These guidelines set rules for the safe handling of microorganisms. Table 21–1 describes the biosafety levels with examples. At each level specific precautions are recommended, each being more complex than the previous level. Since the advent of the human immunodeficiency virus, and the emergence of hepatitis as a blood-to-blood contagion, particular care has been given to the protection of health care professionals to protect themselves from autoinoculation (self-infection). For example, most facilities do not even work with level 4 pathogens. These most dangerous organisms are restricted to sites at the CDC or other NIH facilities.

Table 21–1 Summary of Recommended Biosafety Levels for Infectious Agents

	Level 1	Level 2	Level 3	Level 4
Agents present that can cause:	No known disease in healthy adults	Associated with human disease by autoinoculation, ingestion, or mucous membrane exposure	Disease with serious or lethal consequences; aerosol transmission of exotic agents	High risk; life-threatening disease; agents are dangerous; toxins transmitted by aerosol or unknown route
Laboratory practices	Standard lab procedures	Limited area access, biohazard warning signs, sharps precautions, and written decontamination procedures	Controlled access to the area; baseline serum testing of workers; decontamination of all waste and lab clothing before laundering	Clothing exchange before entering area; shower upon exit; all materials to be decontaminated after exit
Primary barriers & safety equipment used	None required	Personal protective equipment (PPE): lab coat, gloves, face protection if needed, splash or aerosol guards	Respiratory protective measures	Full body air supplied, positive pressure personal suit
Secondary barriers & facilities needed	Open bench top, sink required	An autoclave to the environment	Physical separation from access, self-closing, double doors, air exhaust is not recirculated	Separate isolated zone of building a dedicated vacuum and decontamination system
Examples of some organisms encountered	Bacteria: fungi viruses and parasites that are very unlikely to cause disease: saphropytes and micrococcus	Bacteria: bacillus, *E. coli*, pseudomonas, salmonella, chlamydia staphylococcus, streptococci Viruses: HIV, hepatitis yellow fever Fungus: *Candida albicans*, cryptococcus Parasites: *Guiardia Cryptosporidium*, ascaris, tapeworms	Bacteria: anthrax, tuberculosis, brucella, rickettsia Fungus: histoplasma Viruses: HIV, hantaan, yellow fever (wild type), equinine encephalitis, HIV isolates	Bacteria: none Fungi: none Parasites: none Viruses: ebola, lassa, smallpox (variola), Crimean-Congo hemorrhagic fever

The need for strict sanitary measures in any type of health care facility is therefore readily seen. People who are host to all kinds of pathogenic microorganisms are gathered under one roof—the possibility of transfer of bacteria is great. We have learned how fast bacteria can be transmitted and how fast they multiply. Thus, no carelessness can be allowed in the environmental control of microorganisms. Carelessness on the part of one hospital worker—nurse, doctor, cook, attendant, or cleaning person—could result in serious illness or even the death of many people.

For example, at a Maryland medical center in the late 1970s, six cancer patients had blood poisoning. This occurred because they had received transfusions of blood platelets from a donor who had an undetected bone marrow infection. In Oklahoma, patients receiving respiratory therapy contracted a serious bronchial and lung infection, and eleven died because their inhalation devices were contaminated. In yet another case, seven patients in a Pennsylvania hospital came down with severe gastrointestinal infections after they were examined with improperly sterilized **endoscopes.**

These three "mini**epidemics**" are examples of how hospital infections are spread through carelessness or the use of improper aseptic techniques.

Miniepidemics are examples of a hazard occurring in the central supply areas, delivery rooms, intensive-care units, nurseries, operating rooms, and wards of even the best health care facilities. These types of infections, acquired during a patient's care and treatment in a medical facility, are called **nosocomial infections.*** Nosocomial infections hit 1.5 million Americans hospitalized each year, causing the deaths of about 15,000 patients.

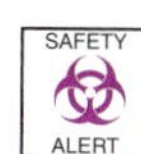

Nosocomial infections can occur despite the use of new antibiotics and disinfectants. There are several reasons for this problem.

1. The overuse of broad-range antibiotics, even for the smallest of infections. This allows **opportunistic pathogens**† to **mutate** or change and develop a resistance to the antibiotics.
2. With an increased reliance on antibiotics, sometimes there is a corresponding decrease in the proper use of aseptic procedures.
3. Increased use of antiinflammatory drugs and immunosuppressant agents, anticancer chemotherapy, antilymphocytic serum, ionizing radiation, and steroids.
4. Overcrowding of health care facilities and understaffed and overworked personnel often lead to lax procedures.
5. Improper cleaning of dialysis and respiratory equipment.
6. Carrier states of health care workers, particularly for *Staphylococcus aureus.*
7. Use of more complex and lengthy surgical procedures.
8. Increase in the number and type of health care providers, some of whom are unaware of the importance and value of aseptic and sterile procedures.

Even if only one of these factors occurs, it is enough for opportunistic pathogens to take hold and cause diseases, infections, and other health problems. Obviously, sick and debilitated persons in a health care facility are more vulnerable to the effects of opportunistic pathogens. Measures must be taken to protect them and the health care personnel who attend to them from contracting any infections from opportunists. These opportunistic pathogens are *Escherichia coli, Proteus* and *Pseudomonas* species, *Staphylococcus aureus,* and *Streptococcus pneumoniae.* They cause such nosocomial infections as burn, respiratory, surgical, and wound infections. Nosocomial infections add, on the average, 7 days to a patient's stay in a health care facility. This problem plays a role in the high cost of health

**Nosocomial* comes from the Greek word for *hospital.*

†Opportunistic pathogens are microorganisms that have the ability or potential to produce a disease in a host organism who is sick, debilitated, or weak.

and hospital care. The seriousness of the threat of nosocomial infections has led to the development of a new health care specialty: the **infection-control practitioner (ICP).** Teams of ICPs—which include doctors, specially trained nurses, **epidemiologists,*** and technicians—work in many health care facilities. They help to track lurking bacteria, fungi, and viruses; monitor sterilization techniques; and prevent nosocomial outbreaks. With the hospitalization of increasing numbers of patients who are immunocompromised, the threat of nosocomial infections is even a larger threat. These patients are in a state of lowered resistance, whether due to the effects of immunosuppressant drugs, anticancer chemotherapy, radiation therapy, or AIDS and therefore are more vulnerable to all sorts of secondary nosocomial and opportunistic infections.

The threat of catching a nosocomial infection is greatest in the major research and teaching facilities. Generally, the patients are more sick and debilitated and more surgical procedures are performed.

Persons who are most vulnerable are (1) patients with such chronic, debilitating diseases as cancer, diabetes, and kidney disorders, (2) premature and newborn infants, (3) women in labor and during childbirth, (4) the elderly, (5) burn and surgical patients, (6) paralyzed patients, (7) patients with a weakened immune system, as in AIDS, (8) patients receiving treatment with anticancer chemotherapy drugs, antilymphocyte serum, radiation therapy, and steroids, and (9) patients receiving antirejection drugs following organ transplantation.

Two separate studies have shown that nosocomial infections developed in 36% of all patients spending time in intensive-care units. Intensive-care patients who remained for more than a week contracted nosocomial infections 90% of the time.

The most frequently encountered nosocomial and opportunistic infection sites tend to be the upper and lower respiratory tracts, the urogenital tract, and blood. Suctioning of tracheotomy patients, insertion of urinary catheters, and cleansing of surgical wounds require the most detailed care to prevent the introduction of *Staphylococcus, Clostridium, Proteus,* and *Pseudomonas* infections. Urinary-tract infections generally account for 30% to 40% of the nosocomial infections. Infected surgical wounds are next, followed by respiratory infections, including pneumonia and **bacteremia** (infection of the bloodstream). Bacteremia is the most serious of the nosocomial infections, with a death rate of 20% to 25%.

PREVENTING THE SPREAD OF DISEASE

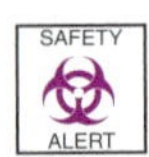

The best way to prevent the spread of disease by all members of the health care team is to practice good handwashing techniques, follow the universal precautions, and practice good safety techniques in the laboratory and throughout the health care facility. The records of modern health care facilities show that the danger of infection can be lessened by conscious effort on the part of medical and health care personnel. In this chapter, the various ways in which health care personnel can help to prevent the spread of disease are given. These measures have already been described in earlier chapters.

Body secretions from an infected person contain large numbers of pathogenic bacteria. A health care professional, for example, may be directly responsible for the transfer of

*An epidemiologist is an individual trained in the systemic study of epidemics.

organisms because of daily contact with the body secretions of patients. It is the duty of all health care personnel to practice sanitary precautions in their work to prevent the spread of infection to patients, other health care workers, visitors, and themselves. It is even possible to reinfect a patient by careless practices.

Microorganisms can be transmitted within a hospital by direct contact with a patient, direct contact with a carrier, or indirect contact with a patient through air, **fomites,** food, or hands.

Let us start with a review of some of the universal precautions.

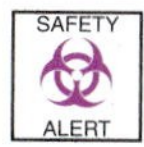

Standard and Universal Precautions

Universal precautions. In an effort to curb the transmission of AIDS, hepatitis B, and other infectious diseases, in 1985 the CDC issued guidelines known as Universal Blood and Body Fluid Precautions or simply universal precautions. It is now known that consistent use and adherence to these guidelines greatly minimizes the risk of infectious disease transmission. At the recommendation of the CDC, health care providers were to consider every patient potentially infectious for AIDS, hepatitis B, and other bloodborne pathogens and to routinely and consistently use the techniques of universal precautions as a means of infection control.

While most of the basic tenets of universal precautions have now been incorporated into the new standard precautions, it is nonetheless important to know and understand the primary preventive measures of these 1985 recommendations.

Following is a summary of the CDC's universal precautions and guidelines for control of AIDS, hepatitis B, and other infectious diseases:

1. Consider all (patients') blood and body fluids to be contaminated.
2. Always wash hands before and after (patient) contact.
3. Always wash hands if contaminated with blood or body fluids.
4. Wear gloves when handling or touching blood, body fluids, body tissue, mucous membranes, nonintact skin, or contaminated equipment and supplies.
5. Wear gloves when performing venipuncture and other blood access treatments or procedures.
6. Change gloves after each patient contact.
7. Wash hands after glove removal. Gloves do not replace handwash technique.
8. Wear gloves, gown, mask, and goggles/face shield if splashing of blood or body fluids can occur or if exposure to droplets of blood or body fluids is a possibility. Examples of this are wound care and **endoscopy.**
9. Use extreme caution when handling needles, scalpels, and other sharp instruments (sharps) during procedures and when handling them after procedures are completed. Dispose of sharps in an approved puncture-proof container that should be located as close as practical to the work area.
10. Use a mouthpiece if performing cardiopulmonary resuscitation even though saliva has not been implicated in transmission of human immunodeficiency virus (HIV), the virus that causes AIDS.
11. Clean blood and body fluid spills with agency disinfectant or a 10% solution of sodium hypochlorite (household bleach).

12. Report needlesticks, splashes, and contamination by wounds or body fluids. Follow up with employee health services, physician, and other appropriate personnel.
13. Health care workers with open lesions (injury or wound) or dermatitis (skin rash) should avoid direct contact with patients and their supplies and equipment until healed.
14. Laboratory specimens and their containers are modes of disease transmission and gloves should be worn during handling.
15. Pregnant health care providers should be especially careful to adhere to the guidelines so as to protect themselves and the unborn child.

Standard precautions. The CDC spent several years researching, improving, and developing recommendations to protect health care providers, patients, and their visitors from infectious diseases. This intensive period of research resulted in standard precautions, a set of infection control guidelines that should now be utilized by all health care professionals for all patients.

Standard precautions combine many of the basic principles of universal precautions with techniques known as body substance isolation (BSI), a system that maintains that personal protective equipment should be worn for contact with all body fluids regardless if blood is visible. Although BSI was developed not by a federal or state agency but by a private hospital, its techniques nonetheless have been adopted by many health care facilities.

The rationale behind developing the new standard precautions was that while universal precautions and body substance isolation provide a good degree of protection, the CDC recognized that both could be improved upon. Advantages of the new standard precautions are that they include all of the major recommendations of universal precautions and body substance isolation, while incorporating new information; they simplify medical terminology to be as user friendly as possible; they use new terms to avoid confusion with existing infection control and isolation systems; and they are intended to protect all patients, all health care providers, and all visitors.

According to the CDC, standard precautions are "designed to reduce the risk of transmission of microorganisms from both recognized and unrecognized sources of infection in hospitals" (CDC, 1994). They apply to:

1. blood
2. all body fluids, secretions, and excretions regardless if they contain visible blood
3. nonintact skin
4. mucous membranes

To be effective, standard precautions must be practiced conscientiously at all times. Although standard precautions were intended primarily for use in acute care facilities such as hospitals, they can and should be applied in other types of facilities including the ambulatory care settings (Lindh et al., 1998).

Transmission-Based Precautions

When the CDC was in the process of developing a new guideline for isolation precautions in hospitals, the agency arrived at what it terms two tiers of precautions. The first tier is called the standard precautions, discussed earlier, designed for all patients regardless of their diagnosis or presumed infection status. The second tier of precautions is intended for patients diagnosed with or suspected of specific highly transmissible diseases. These are known as transmission-based precautions.

Transmission-based precautions condense the seven existing categories of isolation precautions developed by the CDC in 1970 into three sets of precautions based on routes of infection. Released in 1996 to complement standard precautions, transmission-based precautions reduce the risk of airborne, droplet, and contact transmission of pathogens and are always to be used *in addition to* standard precautions.

These airborne, contact, and droplet precautions also list specific syndromes that can appear in adult and pediatric patients who are highly suspicious for infection. They identify the appropriate transmission-based precautions to be used until a diagnosis can be made. Remember that these precautions are for specific categories of patients and are to be used in addition to standard precautions, which are used for all patients.

Transmission of HIV and HBV. HIV and HBV are transmitted essentially through the same means. Contracting either disease requires direct contact with the virus living in infected blood and body fluids. The viruses are transmitted primarily through the following means:

- Sexual contact with an infected person (heterosexual, homosexual, or bisexual). The virus enters through the vagina, rectum, penis, or mouth.
- Sharing needles for intravenous (I.V.) drug use with an infected person.
- Receiving blood or blood products from an infected person (all blood collected for transfusions is routinely checked for HIV and HBV; therefore, risk from this source is now rare).
- Intrauterine infection of the fetus by a pregnant infected woman.
- Percutaneous (needle-stick) injuries to healthcare personnel causing exposure to infected blood or body fluid.

Despite the similarities between HIV and HBV, the risk of contracting HBV is greater than contracting HIV. For example, HIV infection following an accidental needlestick is approximately 1%, while HBV infection following an accidental needlestick can be as high as 30% (Lane, 1993).

Blood and Body Fluids

In all infection control efforts, it is important to understand what is meant by blood and body fluids. Specifically, they are described as the blood, secretions, and excretions of a patient. Examples of blood and body fluids and some of the areas in which medical assistants may become exposed to them are:

Blood

- specimens drawn during venipuncture
- open wounds of any kind
- epistaxis, or nosebleeds
- vaginal bleeding, including menses (menstruation), lochia (discharge following childbirth), and hemorrhage
- feces and vomit or other body fluids with or without blood

Vaginal secretions
- physiological leukorrhea (normal vaginal discharge)
- vaginitis

Cerebral spinal fluid
- fluid aspirated, or withdrawn, during a lumbar puncture
- leakage of fluid due to trauma to the brain and/or spinal cord

Synovial fluid
- fluid aspirated during arthroscopic procedures

Pleural fluid
- fluid aspirated during thoracentesis, a surgical puncture of the thoracic cavity
- fluid leakage due to chest trauma

Pericardial fluid
- fluid around the heart exposed during cardiac surgery or due to cardiac trauma

Peritoneal fluid
- fluid exposed during abdominal surgery (least likely fluid that medical assistant will come into contact with)

Semen
- seminal fluid as a laboratory specimen for sperm count in examination for fertility level

Amniotic fluid
- fluid aspirated during amniocentesis, a surgical puncture of the amniotic sac
- vaginal leakage during pregnancy, labor, and delivery

Sputum
- material coughed up and expectorated from the respiratory tract

Saliva
- oral mucous gland fluid in mouth during oral/dental procedures
- any other body fluid visibly contaminated with blood

Thus far, only blood and blood products, semen, vaginal secretions, and possibly breast milk have been directly linked to transmission of HIV, and the virus is not spread casually nor through close family contacts. There is no vaccine to protect individuals from HIV.

HBV has been found in blood and blood products, vaginal secretions, semen, and saliva. Infection can spread through close family contacts, kissing, sexual contacts, intrauterinely, and during delivery. An infant may become a chronic carrier, one who has no symptoms but can transmit disease. If there has been an exposure to the virus, a prompt injection of immunoglobulin, an antibody, will help provide protection from the virus. Hepatitis B vaccine is available and the series of three injections usually immunizes an individual from an attack of hepatitis B.

Other Safety Precautions

In addition, in the microbiology laboratory the following safety precautions are standard procedure.

1. Keep work areas clean by spraying with 10% bleach at the end of each shift.
2. Always set culture plates face down to avoid moisture from the lid falling on the media.

3. When opening a plate to examine it, pick it up from the upside-down position on the work bench and leave the lid remaining on the counter.
4. Do not pass an open plate to a colleague to look at. Let him or her pick it up from the closed position on the bench.
5. Sterilize inoculating loops immediately after use. Use care to avoid spattering in the flame. It is best to use an incinerator system that has a protective shield to prevent spatters.
6. To transfer inoculum from a broth tube to a plate or another broth tube, one hand (left if you are right-handed) should hold the broth tube while the other holds the inoculating loop between the thumb and index finger as the ring and pinkie fingers hold the cap (right hand if you are right-handed). The broth tube is flamed immediately after removing the cap and again after the inoculum has been obtained. The broth is immediately recapped by moving the tube to the pinkie and screwing the tube into the cap. The broth tube is then set into a rack and the plate to be inoculated is picked up in the hand that held the broth tube. This technique avoids contamination of the work area, broth tube, and cap as well as avoiding undue motion of the hand holding the inoculating loop.
7. When a sterile container is opened, care should be taken to minimize the time the open container is exposed to the air.
8. To remove swabs, gauze, etc. from a sterile container, use sterile forceps and quickly replace cover. Never lay the sterile cap or cover down on the counter.
9. No food, drink, or gum chewing should be permitted in lab or work areas.
10. Incinerate all waste before disposing of it.
11. Maintain separate enclosed areas for tuberculous, fungus, and virus work.
12. Do not pipette any reagent, broth culture, etc. by mouth.

ASEPSIS

All health care personnel, including administrative supervisors, custodial and maintenance personnel, medical, nursing, and technicians, have the common goal of disease cure, control, and prevention. To this end, the basic goal that must be achieved by all is cleanliness. In a clean environment, **asepsis** can be established and maintained where necessary. There are two types of asepsis practiced in a health care or hospital facility—medical asepsis and surgical asepsis.

Medical Asepsis

Medical asepsis is a condition in which pathogenic organisms, but not necessarily all others, are excluded from the immediate area. The scope of medical asepsis is illustrated in Table 21–2.

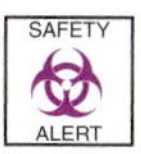

Surgical Asepsis

Surgical asepsis involves the exclusion of all microorganisms from the immediate area around a patient's open wound and all objects coming into contact with the wound. This is needed to prevent the contamination of deep tissues with microorganisms.

Table 21–2 Scope of Medical Asepsis

Examples of Control Measures That Destroy or Limit the Spread of Pathogens		
Practiced by the Individual	**Enforced by the Community**	**Additional Measures Against a Known Communicable Agent**
Covering mouth when coughing	Disposal of garbage and sewage	Separating an infected person from others—isolation technique
Sneezing and coughing into disposable tissues Washing hands before handling food	Controlling pests, such as mosquitoes and rodents Licensing food handlers	Using precautions and controls, such as gowns and masks Sterilizing or disinfecting items used by the infected person
Washing dishes and glassware thoroughly Using individual items of personal care, such as towels, toothbrush, comb, etc.	Regulating drinking-water plants Regulating interstate food transportation	Reporting the illness to the proper community agency
Wiping eyes or removing foreign particles with clean tissues or handkerchiefs Expectorating into disposable wipes Washing hands after elimination	Establishing immunization regulations for foreign travel Recommending and enforcing health programs in public schools Inspecting health-related facilities: food-serving establishments; canning and food-packaging plants; recreation areas	Using special precautions, depending upon the mode of transmission of the organism (i.e., if through respiratory secretions, intestinal excretions, blood, or drainage from a wound). Such precautions might include the burning of secretions, the disinfection of excreta, and the sterilization of dishes.

Surgical asepsis includes the following:

- The area of the patient's skin to be operated on is shaved if necessary and thoroughly cleansed and scrubbed with soap and antiseptic.
- The surrounding surgical area is covered with sterile linen drapes, creating a sterile surgical field, if the surgery is extensive.
- The surgeon and all assisting personnel must scrub their hands and forearms for 10 minutes with a germicidal soap.
- All surgical personnel must wear sterile caps, masks, gowns, gloves, and shoe covers to prevent microorganisms from any part of their body from shedding into the operating room.

- All surgical instruments, dressing, and sutures must be sterilized.
- Any surgical item that cannot be autoclaved is penetrated with a disinfectant.
- The operating room's floors, walls, and equipment are thoroughly cleaned, disinfected, or sterilized.
- A proper stream of fresh, filtered air must be constantly delivered, circulated, and drawn out to ensure proper ventilation.
- Used and contaminated surgical instruments and supplies, damaged gloves, and moist, saturated masks are all replaced with sterile ones.

The idea of surgical asepsis is applicable not only in an operating room but in many other situations as well. These include postoperative surgical wounds for several days after surgery, or until the tissues surrounding the wound have healed well enough to maintain natural barriers against infection. Delivery rooms practice surgical asepsis to prevent infection of injured mucous membranes. It is also practiced in nurseries to protect vulnerable newborn infants from infections. Each health care facility must follow specific, strict guidelines with respect to infection control. These guidelines are from the Centers for Disease Control and Prevention (CDC) of the U.S. Public Health Service. The guidelines form a national policy, which is described in a manual called *Guideline for Isolation Precautions in Hospitals.*

General Principles of Infection Control

One of the many basic concepts of infection control is through the technique of isolation. Isolation of the patient is essential for one of two reasons: (1) to prevent the communicability or spread of pathogenic microorganisms to susceptible individuals, or (2) to protect an already sick or susceptible patient from exposure to pathogens.

Isolation Techniques

Depending upon the state of health and vulnerability of a patient, there are several types of isolation techniques. One set of isolation techniques is used for the severely compromised (vulnerable) patient, another for the surgical patient, and yet others for patients with respiratory problems, burns, as well as those with wounds and infections.

Isolation procedures for the severely compromised patient. The advances of modern medicine and technology have produced dramatic cures or treatments for diseases that were once fatal. However, some of these treatments, which may involve chemotherapeutic drugs or mechanical instruments invading the body, are used over a long time. This increases the patient's vulnerability to infection(s). Patients included in this category are cancer patients, those with severe burns, leukemia patients, premature infants, and patients receiving a transplant or radiation, steroid, or antimetabolite therapy. Techniques involved in protecting compromised patients from nosocomial infections include the following:

- The room is cleaned, scrubbed, and disinfected before the patient is admitted.
- When possible, a compromised patient is kept in a private room.

- Compromised patients should be especially separated from patients with infections or communicable diseases.
- *All* personnel entering the patient's room should wear sterile caps, gowns, and masks to avoid transmission of microorganisms into the room from their clothing and from their respiratory tract or hair.
- All health care personnel must properly wash their hands before, during, and after patient care.

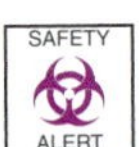

Precautions to be taken with the surgical patient. Generally the surgical patient who shows no signs of overt infection before or after surgery does not need isolation. However, the surgical wound itself is isolated with a good, sterile dressing. Postoperative patients with infective diseases must be isolated so they do not pose a threat to compromised patients or patients with unhealed wounds. Also, these patients should be isolated in a private room with a private bath. This helps to contain the pathogens within a definite area and thus lessens contagion to other patients.

Two other vital sterile techniques involve the proper use of paper gowns and masks.

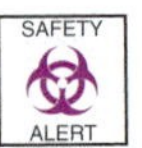

Gowns. A clean, dry, fresh gown is worn not only in the operating room but also in the isolation room. Any individual entering an isolation room must wear a clean, fresh gown, which is discarded after each use. For a gown to be a completely protective garment, it must be ample in size and easily fastenable. This ensures that the wearer's arms and clothing are protected from contamination by pathogens. A clean, fresh gown should be worn by each person who enters either an isolation room or an operating room on each occasion, and thrown away after each use. Under no circumstances should a moist and soiled gown be worn. A moist area is a favorable growth environment for pathogens, which can then contaminate the clothing under the gown. Today, gowns worn as outer protective covering are fluid impermeable per OSHA's final bloodborne pathogen rule.

Masks. Masks must be worn in the operating room and in an isolation room of a respiratory infection patient. Respiratory infection patients must be masked if they are taken to another area of the health care facility for treatment. Health care personnel who care for a respiratory infection patient must be masked for self-protection. The effectiveness and protection of a mask is short-lived, because the warm exhaled air from the mouth and nose cause the mask to get moist. A used mask should be discarded immediately, or laundered and autoclaved. Today, most health care facilities find it faster to use paper masks. They are discarded after use, thus saving on the cost, labor, and time of laundering and sterilization. When a used mask is handled, the hands should be washed immediately.

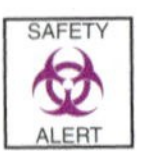

Handwashing. Our hands touch so many things that they also transfer disease-producing organisms. When someone touches the patient or anything in the patient's environment, some of the bacteria will be transferred to that person's hands. Even when gloves are worn, hands must be washed after contact with an infected patient and after touching excretions and secretions. Hands should be washed and gloved before doing invasive techniques and before dressing or touching wounds and patients who are especially sensitive to infection. Hands are also washed between patient contacts in newborn nurseries and in intensive-care units. Thus, the number of bacteria on the hands is decreased through washing and the use of antiseptics. It is impossible to kill all the bacteria on the hands, as disinfectants would destroy the skin cells.

The following are measures to be used to lessen the transfer of organisms by the hands.

- The hands, the back, palms, fingers, and wrists are thoroughly washed with soap and water or antiseptics such as PhisoHex or Betadine.
- The hands are held down from the elbow so that dirty, contaminated water does not run up the arm while washing.
- The hands are thoroughly rinsed under running water.
- Hands are dried immediately with disposable paper towels. (They are preferable to cloth towels, which must be laundered and sterilized. Also a used, wet cloth towel can harbor pathogens.)
- The fingernails are kept short and clean. No bracelets, rings, or wristwatches should be worn by health care personnel caring for infectious patients.
- Gloves and forceps are used in handling contaminated objects.

Personal Hygiene

Because of their constant close contact with sick patients, health care personnel must pay careful attention to their personal hygiene. This not only protects their own health but lessens the spread of pathogens to patients and other health care personnel as well. Their clothes, hair, and skin should be kept clean and in good condition. When caring for patients, health care personnel should not wear street clothes, which harbor many microorganisms. The traditional white uniform and white duty shoes may be worn, because they are easily cleaned. However, colorful scrub pant and top outfits are increasingly popular. Once worn only in the operating room, scrubs allow for ease of movement, are simple to launder, and are generally less expensive to purchase than regular uniforms. Many health care facilities now provide them as well as launder them in response to OSHA's new rule on exposure to bloodborne pathogens. Uniforms and outer protective clothing should never be worn outside of the health care facility, and the health care provider should always have clean clothes when near the patient. Personal hygiene care includes:

- Daily showers with a mild deodorant soap
- Frequent shampooing of hair
- The use of a nongreasy lubricant or moisturizing cream or lotion to prevent excessive drying
- Fingernails kept short and clean
- Simple hairstyle, so frequent touching or fixing with the hands is avoided
- Long hair tied back and off the shoulders
- Proper and thorough handwashing always before and after patient contact
- Minimal wearing of jewelry

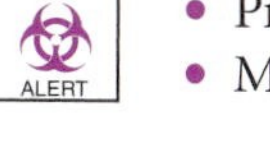

Occupational Safety and Health Administration's final rule, occupational exposure to blood borne pathogens. In addition to the above universal precautions, OSHA's Final Rule includes the following:

1. Facilities must establish an exposure control plan, which all workers will follow.
2. Employers must provide training for employees.

3. Universal precautions must be practiced by all.
4. Employers shall minimize the potential for exposure by employees by establishing engineering and work practice controls to minimize employee exposure. This includes accessible handwashing facilities, needle disposal sites, and antiseptic hand cleansers, gloves, and towels.
5. Food and drink are not permitted in lab areas and must not be stored with blood or other infectious materials.
6. Facilities that generate more than 50 pounds of hazardous waste per month must employ a biohazardous waste management source to dispose of the waste properly. It may not be sterilized only to be disposed in the regular trash disposal system. Facilities that generate less than 50 pounds per month may use normal trash disposal methods.
7. The employer will provide, at no cost to the employee, personal protective clothing, gloves, gowns, shields, goggles, masks, resuscitation bags, and hypoallergenic or powderless gloves as well as repair, replacement, and cleaning and/or disposal of the same.
8. Personal protective clothing may not be worn or taken out of the work area.
9. Gloves may not be washed or reused. No one must be discouraged from using them. Gloves are required when a worker has cuts or scratches on the hands, when performing a phlebotomy on a child or uncooperative patient, when performing a micropuncture, or when in training.
10. Caps, hoods, shoe covers, or boots are to be worn when gross contamination may be anticipated, as in surgery or the autopsy room.
11. In housekeeping, work areas will be kept clean and sanitary. Beds will be disinfected after hazardous contact. All bins, pails, etc. will be inspected and decontaminated as soon as possible. Broken glass will not be picked up by hand. Sharps will not be inserted into bed linens. Contaminated laundry will be bagged for transportation. Gloves will be provided to laundry workers.
12. Hepatitis B vaccination will be made readily available by the employer to all health care employees who may have potential exposure risk, at no cost to the employee.
13. In the case of possible HBV or HIV exposure (needle-stick injury, etc.) base-line blood samples may be drawn from the source as well as the employee so as not to harm patient privacy laws.
14. Universal biohazard signs will be used. Container colors may be red or orange.

OSHA has also published a companion piece to the Blood Borne Pathogens Standard—that of the Chemical Hygiene Plan.

The standard for occupational exposure to hazardous chemicals in the laboratory. The intention of this law is to heighten employee awareness of risks linked with chemical dangers. It serves to improve work practices through employee training and identification of hazardous chemicals that exist in the workplace. The use of protective equipment is utilized to protect employees from harmful chemicals.

Chemical Hygiene Plan. The Chemical Hygiene Plan (CHP) is the core of the OSHA safety standard. A written plan must specify the training and information requirements of the standard. Certain specific control measures such as fume hoods and glove boxes must be included in the plan. A designated employee is the chemical hygiene or safety officer. Provisions for housekeeping and maintenance of the facility are included. OSHA standards are not optional and penalties are imposed for noncompliance with the standard. Employers must take the time to meet the requirements not only to be in compliance with the law, but to protect employees as well.

All laboratories and ambulatory care settings, including physicians' offices, must comply with a chemical hygiene plan to meet the OSHA regulations. The only laboratories exempt from compliance are those that exclusively use methods that do not place employees at risk for exposure to chemicals that are hazardous. For example, there may be physicians' office laboratories (POLs) that perform only dipstick tests or use other commercially prepared kits in which reagents are not exposed and as a result they are exempt from compliance. The primary component of the OSHA standard is that a written chemical hygiene plan and program must be operational if chemicals are stored in a facility and handled by employees. Some examples of chemicals include, but are not limited to: stains, ethyl alcohol, sodium hypochlorite (household bleach), formaldehyde, fixatives, preservatives, injectables such as chemotherapeutic agents, acetone, and so on. Many laboratory accidents result in chemical-related illnesses ranging from eye irritation to pulmonary edema.

There are three primary goals that an employer must accomplish to be in compliance with the OSHA standard for chemical exposure:

1. There must be an inventory undertaken and a list compiled of all chemicals considered hazardous. The following information must be documented: the quantity of chemical stored per month or year; whether the substance is gas, liquid, or solid; the manufacturer's name and address; and the chemical hazard classification.
2. A material safety data sheet (MSDS) manual must be assembled. MSDS manuals are often supplied by the manufacturer when the chemicals are ordered and will give information regarding whether a chemical is hazardous. All other MSDS information must be requested from the manufacturer. The MSDS sheets must be alphabetized and indexed and be reviewed on a regular basis and modifications made. The manual must be available to all employees. The various chemicals are labeled using the National Fire Protection Association's color and number method. Their four colors are white, blue, red, and yellow.

   - White signifies the need for personal protective equipment (PPE).
   - Blue signifies a health hazard.
   - Red signifies a fire hazard.
   - Yellow signifies an instability hazard.

   Within each of the blue, red, and yellow categories are five levels of danger ranging from 0 (no unusual hazard) to 4 (a potentially fatal danger). White has its own levels of protective clothing requirements:
   a. gloves
   b. goggles, gloves
   c. goggles, gloves, apron
   d. face shields, gloves, mask

e. goggles, gloves, mask
f. goggles, gloves, apron, mask

3. The employer is required to provide a hazard communication educational program to the employee within 30 days of employment and before the employee handles any hazardous chemicals. The training program should consist of the location and identification of hazardous chemicals, how to read and understand the labels on the chemicals, where the MSDS manual is kept, when to use personal protective equipment, and procedures to follow for chemical spills. The training sessions must be documented, signed by the employer, and permanently retained in the employee record.

   Since January 1991 laboratories (including POLs) have a chemical hygiene plan (CHP) in place.

Air

In respiratory infections, it is not possible to destroy all the organisms while they are still in the nose and throat; these are bound to reach the air. As we have learned, covering the mouth and nose when coughing and sneezing can help prevent the spread of organisms. Other measures that decrease the number of microorganisms in the air include the following:

- Limit the number of persons in a room.
- Remove the bacteria from the floor and furniture by damp dusting. Floors can also be swept with oil-treated sawdust.
- Handle linens in a manner that will prevent raising dust.
- Introduce fresh air and sunlight when possible.
- Use individual cubicles or rooms with windows.
- Remove bacteria from the air by filtration, ultraviolet light, and germicidal vapors.

Masks that cover both the nose and mouth are of some value in preventing the transfer of bacteria. After use, masks should be disposed of promptly.

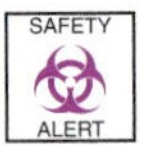

Fomites

Fomites (singular, fomes) are substances other than food that absorb and transmit infectious material. Examples of fomites are linens, clothing, dishes, bedpans, basins, thermometers, and other equipment and personal articles. The health care professional has the major responsibility for preventing infection by fomites. Prevention may be accomplished by properly disinfecting all fomites, by bagging and discarding disposable items, and by discarding any cracked dishes that could be traps for bacterial contamination. It is also important to use individual equipment for each patient; use disposable equipment when indicated. Place soiled linens and clothing in bags to be sent to the laundry.

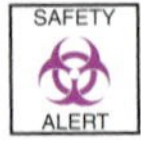

Food

Health care personnel must never bring food or drink into the work area. Food, drink, and snacks should be eaten in a designated break or lunch room, and food must not be stored in any refrigerator that may be used to store laboratory specimens.

Infection may be traced to food consumption. Methods of preventing the spread of infection through food are simple and effective. Preventive methods involve proper disposal of uneaten foods and the use of high-quality and unspoiled food. Proper cooking and storage of foods, sanitary methods of preparing foods, and frequent health examinations for food handlers are also important. The kitchen area and utensils must be kept clean.

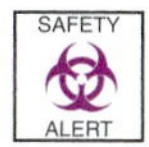

Human Carriers

Visitors, doctors, nurses, and other staff members continually come in contact with sick people and their environments. These health team members can become carriers because of this exposure. Carriers may not get the disease, but they can carry pathogenic organisms and transfer them to others who become ill because of low resistance. Infections of the throat are often transferred in this way. Especially susceptible to throat infections are premature infants, sick infants and children, and patients with open wounds. Women after childbirth, malnourished individuals of all ages, and persons weakened by illness are also susceptible to infection.

Smoking is no longer permitted in most health care facilities, but certainly smoking should not be permitted in any work areas. Equally important, but often not observed, is the refraining from applying makeup, cosmetics, and nail polish in the laboratory area. These activities foster unnecessary hand-to-face contact which can increase one's chances of transmission of microorganisms.

SUMMARY

Failure to adhere to the rules and guidelines of good sanitary measures introduces a very high risk of becoming contaminated with a potentially serious infection, which may even result in death. Many infections come right from the hospital. These nosocomial infections may be transmitted by a health care worker who is a carrier or by someone failing to adhere to the universal standards. To control the spread of infection, health care sanitation and protection of the health care professional guidelines are outlined in detail in the universal precautions and standard precautions guidelines. Although the two documents are similar, the standard precautions guideline is more user friendly with numerous universal drawings to accompany the text. Additionally, precautions for each type of potential contamination are divided into separate tables for quick reference. This document is also more self-explanatory than the universal precautions guideline.

The Occupational Safety and Health Administration (OSHA) regulations have been updated by adding a separate section on hazardous chemicals to the law. The Clinical Laboratory Improvement Act of 1988 (CLIA 88) has added additional tests to the waived tests category, including cholesterol testing using simple, user-friendly instrumentation, as well as pregnancy testing and group A streptococcus testing. A separate category on physician-performed microscopy (PPM) has been added to allow physicians to perform urine microscopic tests, Gram stains, and semen analysis tests. It is possible that yet another category will be added. CDC has recommended that this category fall between the waived test and moderately complex categories, further diluting the effectiveness of the regulation.

STUDY AND DISCUSSION

The following is an abstract of a report by the U.S. Public Health Service of an outbreak of dysentery involving 144 cases. This outbreak took place in a hospital in Miami, Florida, in 1943. Most of the cases occurred among nurses; a few occurred among waitresses and kitchen helpers.

The butcher admitted to being ill prior to the outbreak. General unsanitary conditions were found in the kitchen and in food handling, as was shown by these facts:

Butter was picked up by hand.
Waitresses used their fingers to wipe mayonnaise from dishes and replace it in the original container.
Cream was poured into a two-gallon tin that had no lid or handle.
Forty-six different people dipped their hands into the ice bin.
The paper towel container in the employee's washroom was empty.
Anyone who wanted to could use the refrigerators and food-storage areas at night.

1. Discuss how good hospital sanitation would have prevented this outbreak by analyzing each condition.
2. Discuss the procedures that a local health department would have to carry out if a typhoid carrier was discovered in the community.
3. What is a carrier? Describe the ways in which a person may become a carrier.
4. How would you prevent germs from spreading from a carrier to a well person?
5. Explain what aseptic procedures you would use after coming in contact with these diseases:

   a. tuberculosis
   b. septic sore throat
   c. diphtheria
   d. influenza
   e. pneumonia
   f. poliomyelitis
   g. typhoid fever
   h. food poisoning

REVIEW QUESTIONS

A. General Questions: Provide complete answers to each of the following.

1. Explain how you would destroy bacteria on dishes used by patients with communicable disease.

2. What are fomites?

3. List three examples of fomites.

4. Explain in what way a practical nurse or other health professional is responsible for preventing the transmission of disease in a hospital.

5. When opening a sterile jar, how is the lid placed on a table?

6. How is a sterile article removed from a jar?

7. How is the floor or furniture dusted in a patient's room?

8. Name three modern ways of removing dust from the air.

9. What is meant by a *nosocomial infection?*

10. Why do nosocomial infections occur in health care facilities?

11. What is an infection-control practitioner?

12. State the difference between medical asepsis and surgical asepsis. Give three examples of each.

13. What precautions are to be taken with a surgical patient?

14. Why are masks used? Why are health care facilities switching to paper masks?

15. What is the value of proper and thorough handwashing?

B. Multiple-Choice Questions: Select the letter of the choice that best answers the question.

1. Miniepidemics usually occur in _____ .
   a. private industry where there may be a limited number of tasks being performed by a few people
   b. in hospitals where several departments may exhibit a pattern of similar infections
   c. in hospitals where a single factor in one department may be traced to a pattern of similar infections
   d. in schools where a single factor such as head lice infects several of the classes in the building
2. Many nosocomial infections occur when _____ despite the utmost precautions to prevent them.
   a. antiinflammatory and immunosuppressant drugs must be used for long periods of time
   b. aseptic techniques become slack
   c. health care facilities become overcrowded
   d. reusable equipment is not properly cleaned

3. Expectorate means to _____ .
   a. cough
   b. sneeze
   c. spit phlegm
   d. blow your nose
4. In the operating room all personnel must wear _____ .
   a. gown, gloves, mask
   b. gown, gloves, mask, shoe covers
   c. gown, gloves, mask, shoe covers, head gear
   d. gown, gloves, mask, head gear
5. Mr. Jones has been diagnosed with tuberculosis and is on the appropriate treatment. He is ambulatory and needs to have another chest X ray. Should _____
   a. a portable X-ray machine be brought to his room?
   b. he go to the X-ray department in a wheelchair?
   c. he wear a mask and walk with an escort to the X-ray department?
   d. he and the escort wear a mask to the X-ray department?

C. True/False

_____ 1. When gloves are worn consistently, it is not necessary to wash your hands between each and every patient except when working in the nursery.

_____ 2. Jewelry should be kept to a minimum when caring for infectious patients.

_____ 3. Street clothes may be worn to and from work but not on duty.

_____ 4. Immunocompromised patients are best protected by being kept in a private room.

_____ 5. In the nursery it is necessary to wash your hands with a disinfectant such as Phisoderm as well as soap and water.

_____ 6. All postoperative surgical patients should be isolated for at least 24 hours.

_____ 7. When entering the room of a burn patient it is necessary to wear a gown, gloves, and mask to protect the patient from the health care worker's flora.

_____ 8. Long hair is permissible so long as it is combed and neatly groomed.

_____ 9. Rooms occupied by respiratory patients should be aerated with ultraviolet light and/or germicidal vapors in addition to routine cleaning.

_____ 10. Fomites include dry goods and food that may harbor and transmit infections from one patient to another if not properly handled.

_____ 11. Cracked dishes should be double sterilized before reusing.

_____ 12. Health care facilities must provide impermeable outer protective clothing as well as scrubs for their employees.

_____ 13. Proper handling and storage of food is as important as proper handwashing in preventing the spread of infection to patients.

_____ 14. Health care workers who may be designated as carriers of a potentially infectious organism such as *Staphylococcus aureus* must be treated and constantly monitored with nasopharangeal cultures.

_____ 15. It is acceptable practice to be permitted to apply nail polish while sitting at the nurses' station provided all duties have been completed.

_____ 16. Gloves may be reworn, provided they are washed with a disinfectant such as Phisoderm or Betadine.

_____ 17. To enter a room marked "Respiratory Isolation," only a mask need be worn.

_____ 18. It is illegal to transport some foods and plants from state to state.

_____ 19. Microbiology plates are stored right side up during incubation to allow for maximum growth potential.

_____ 20. Health care workers who smoke should do so outside so that the patients will not be able to smell the odor of smoke on their clothes or breath.

_____ 21. In the bacteriology laboratory the work benches must be sprayed with a disinfectant such as 10% bleach at least daily.

_____ 22. In transferring inoculum from a liquid broth culture to a sterile broth it is important to flame the sterile broth after adding the inoculum.

_____ 23. Epidemiologists and infection-control practitioners perform essentially the same job in a health care facility.

_____ 24. Today women in labor and childbirth have little need for concern for the possibility of acquiring a nosocomial infection.

_____ 25. Medical asepsis eliminates all microorganisms while surgical asepsis eliminates all pathogenic microorganisms.

SECTION FIVE

ACHIEVEMENT REVIEW

A. Underline the word or expression that best completes each statement.

1. People feel uncomfortable in an atmosphere where the humidity is 80% because _____ .
   a. they perspire
   b. they do not perspire
   c. evaporation of sweat is retarded
   d. evaporation of sweat is hastened
2. The best temperature for a room is _____ .
   a. 40°F (4°C)
   b. 82°F (28°C)
   c. 70°F (21°C)
   d. 55°F (13°C)
3. Of the four microbes given below, the one that is normally not a soil bacterium is _____ .
   a. gas gangrene bacillus
   b. the bacillus that causes botulism
   c. pneumonia bacillus
   d. tetanus bacillus
4. The microbe that can cause disease only if injected into the digestive tract is _____ .
   a. tetanus bacillus
   b. typhoid fever bacillus
   c. gas gangrene bacillus
   d. diphtheria bacillus
5. An example of the development of poisonous toxins in food as a result of bacterial activity is a _____ .
   a. staphylococcus
   b. diphtheria bacillus
   c. poliomyelitis virus
   d. spirillum
6. Custard-filled baked goods should be _____ .
   a. kept safely at room temperature
   b. warmed before serving
   c. individually wrapped
   d. kept under refrigeration after they have been baked
7. In recent years, the foods that cause outbreaks in botulism most often are _____ .
   a. milk
   b. home-canned foods
   c. commercially canned foods
8. The usual cause of an outbreak of salmonella food poisoning is _____ .
   a. salmon
   b. lack of salt
   c. contaminated foods
   d. overcooked foods
9. Amoebic dysentery is caused by _____ .
   a. a green plant
   b. bacteria
   c. a one-celled animal
   d. a spirillum
10. The responsibility of getting safe, clean food to the customer in a restaurant is that of _____ .
    a. the cook
    b. both the cook and the waitress

c. the manager
d. everyone who works in the restaurant

B. Match each word or term in Column I with the statement in Column II that is best associated with it.

Column I	Column II
_____ 1. contaminated articles	a. oiled or damp mop
_____ 2. used to kill germs in air	b. food poisoning
_____ 3. very susceptible to disease	c. medical asepsis
_____ 4. used to pick up sterile dressing	d. fomites
_____ 5. sanitation in patient's room	e. typhoid fever
_____ 6. freedom from disease bacteria	f. droplet infection
_____ 7. clean floors	g. ultraviolet lamp
_____ 8. sneezing and coughing	h. premature infants
_____ 9. infected excreta	i. sterile forceps
	j. nurses' responsibility

C. Insert the word or expression that best completes the following statements.

1. The spread of disease may be held to a minimum through environmental control of the following six items:

2. Bacteria will not grow in air because it does not contain enough _____ and _____ .

3. List four chief causes of contamination of milk.

4. Three diseases that can be transmitted through milk include _____ , _____ , and _____ .

5. Bacteria produce _____ or poisons in food that cause food spoilage.

6. List five common methods of preserving food so that bacteria will not multiply and decompose the food.

7. List two ways by which water may be purified in the home.

8. Name two methods of disinfecting the air in a room.

9. The substance commonly added to reservoirs to kill disease bacteria is _____ .

10. A health professional who is caring for a typhoid fever patient must _____ all articles in contact with the patient.

11. In the LTH method of pasteurization, milk is heated to _____ .

12. Undulant fever may be transmitted by contaminated _____ .

13. An incorrect term for bacterial food poisoning is _____ .

14. Name five precautions that should be taken to prevent disease caused by food poisoning.

D. Supply an answer for each of the following.

1. Describe the best way to sterilize infected dishes.

2. Explain why cracked dishes should be replaced.

3. Explain why paper cups are a safe way to serve drinks.

4. The single most effective means available to the health professional for interrupting the transmission of infections is _____ .

5. A person who has a communicable disease should be _____ from other people.

6. People who appear to be in good health, but carry the organism of a given disease in their bodies are called _____ .

7. A health care worker who is caring for a child with diphtheria should wear a _____ for protection.

8. List five communicable diseases.

9. List at least four ways in which the community can help to maintain sanitary conditions.

10. Name four ways in which an individual can help to prevent the spread of pathogenic organisms.

11. Name three special precautions that a health care professional can follow to prevent the spread of disease.

12. Name two measures used to decrease the transfer of infection by the hands.

APPENDIX A—SPECIMEN COLLECTION, TRANSPORT, AND STORAGE

ANATOMICAL AND SURGICAL PATHOLOGY SPECIMENS

1. Pathologist or physician will select suitable samples and put them directly into a sterile container for prompt delivery to the lab.
2. Tissue abscesses from brain, lung, pleural cavity, pelvis, liver, etc. must be cultured for anaerobic organisms.
3. Collect pus from the abscesses using a sterile needle and syringe, expelling all air from the syringe. Cork the needle to avoid oxygen contamination.
4. Inoculate on tryptic soy agar (TSA) with 10% sheep's blood aerobically. Anaerobically, use MacConkey and thioglycollate broth.
5. Prepare a sample for Gram stain evaluation.
6. Incubate overnight at 37°C.

BLOOD CULTURES

1. Select venipuncture site by palpation of the vein.
2. Using a circular motion, cleanse site with 70% isopropyl alcohol.
3. Let site air dry for 1 minute.
4. Using the same circular motion, cleanse the site with povidone iodine, iodophor, or iodine.
5. Let site air dry 1 minute.
6. Do not palpate the site again unless the gloved finger has been cleansed in the same manner as the venipuncture site.
7. Collect 10 to 20 ml of blood using a syringe and needle.
8. Immediately dispense the blood into the blood culture medium, whose rubber top has been cleansed and dried according to the manufacturer's directions.
9. Usually, blood culture bottles are inoculated in triplicate at timed intervals.
10. Incubate at 37°C. Examine daily for cloudy supernatant.
11. Subculture blood cultures onto chocolate agar and anaerobic blood agar at 24 hours, 48 hours, and then weekly for 21 days unless change is observed sooner.

PROCEDURES FOR USE OF SWABS IN OBTAINING ANY SPECIMEN

1. Select a product that comes with a saline or holding medium glass capsule in the tube.
2. Carefully remove cellophane outer cover.

3. With gloved hands, carefully remove the swab, handling only the holder and not the long cue stick.
4. Collect the sample by carefully touching the swab end to the area being tested. Rotate the swab around in ears and noses. For eyes, be careful not to injure the eye. For throat specimens, use a tongue depressor to hold the tongue down, and collect the specimen from the back of the throat in the tonsil areas.
5. In all cases, make sure the cotton tip of the swab is well saturated with material.
6. Immediately replace the swab in the holder without touching the cue stick.
7. Break the fluid capsule and let the material soak the end of the swab. This will keep the microorganisms viable until cultures can be set up.
8. Label the swabs with all pertinent information, such as patient name, identification number, date specimen taken, source of specimen, and physician name.
9. Deliver the specimens to the laboratory as soon as possible.

EAR CULTURES

1. The physician will collect samples from the inner ear using sterile equipment and culturettes.
2. Carefully cleanse the external ear with detergent to remove the normal bacterial flora before the sample is taken.
3. Inoculate on tryptic soy agar (TSA) with 10% sheep's blood, chocolate and MacConkey agar, and thioglycollate broth.
4. Prepare a sample for Gram stain evaluation.
5. Incubate overnight at 37°C.

EYE CULTURES

1. Collect cultures before application of any antibiotics or irrigation procedures.
2. Use a sterile culturette to collect purulent material from the lower cul-de-sac and the inner canthus of the eye.
3. Inoculate on tryptic soy agar (TSA) with 10% sheep's blood aerobically. Anaerobically, use MacConkey, chocolate, and thioglycollate broth.
4. Prepare a sample for Gram stain evaluation.
5. Incubate overnight at 37°C.

THROAT/NOSE CULTURES

1. Use a sterile culturette to collect tonsillar material by vigorously swabbing the areas of inflammation.
2. Using a tongue depressor will aid in the collection process.
3. Advise the patient to breathe regularly through the mouth to avoid gagging.
4. Inoculate on tryptic soy agar (TSA) with 10% sheep's blood aerobically.
5. Incubate overnight at 37°C.

SPUTUM SPECIMENS

1. A first-morning, deep-cough specimen is recommended.
2. Advise patient to raise sputum and expectorate into a sterile container.
3. Patients suspected of having a tubercular or fungal infection must use appropriate safety containers for collection to avoid aerosol spread of germs.
4. For mycobacteria, collect at least three daily specimens.
5. Deliver promptly to the lab to avoid overgrowth of normal respiratory flora.
6. Inoculate on tryptic soy agar (TSA) with 10% sheep's blood, and MacConkey and chocolate agar.
7. Prepare a sample for Gram stain evaluation.
8. Incubate overnight at 37°C.

BRONCHIAL WASHINGS

1. A physician will collect the washings using a bronchoscope.
2. Place the washings in a sterile container and deliver promptly to the lab.
3. Bacterial, fungal, mycobacterial, and parasitology studies are usually ordered on these samples.
4. Inoculate on tryptic soy agar (TSA) with 10% sheep's blood, MacConkey and chocolate agar, and thioglycollate broth.
5. Prepare a sample for Gram stain evaluation.
6. Incubate overnight at 37°C.

TRANSTRACHEAL ASPIRATIONS

1. Patients with a trachaeotomy or those on a respirator may require transtracheal aspirations.
2. The area around the trachaeotomy is well disinfected before a catheter is inserted, and sputum is suctioned from the trachea.
3. The sample is put immediately into a sterile container and transported to the lab.
4. Transtracheal aspirations are usually incubated in an anaerobic atmosphere.
5. Inoculate on tryptic soy agar (TSA) with 10% sheep's blood aerobically, and anaerobically, on chocolate and MacConkey agar and thioglychollate broth.
6. Prepare a sample for Gram stain evaluation.
7. Incubate overnight at 37°C.

LUNG BIOPSIES

1. Physicians will perform this procedure, often at the bedside.
2. Care must be taken to process these specimens with the utmost of care and very thoroughly, as they are taken at great risk to the patient.

3. Inoculate on tryptic soy agar (TSA) with 10% sheep's blood aerobically, and anaerobically, on MacConkey agar and thioglycollate broth.
4. Prepare a sample for Gram stain evaluation.
5. Incubate overnight at 37°C.

URINE CULTURES

Clean Catch

1. Cleanse the periurethral area (tip of penis, labial folds, vulva) with two separate soapings, and rinse with sterile water.
2. Patient urinates a portion of urine into the toilet and stops. The next portion is collected in a sterile container. The last portion of urine is voided into the toilet.
3. Deliver specimen immediately to the lab. Any delay requires refrigeration.
4. Inoculate on tryptic soy agar (TSA) with 10% sheep's blood aerobically and on MacConkey agar using the single-streak method.
5. Incubate overnight at 37°C.

Catheter

1. For an indwelling catheter, disinfect the wall of the catheter at the juncture with the drainage tube.
2. Using a syringe and 21-gauge needle, puncture the cleansed area and aspirate the urine.
3. Transfer the urine to a sterile container and deliver immediately to the lab.
4. Inoculate on tryptic soy agar (TSA) with 10% sheep's blood aerobically and on MacConkey agar using the single-streak method.
5. Incubate overnight at 37°C.

GENITAL SPECIMENS

Urethral

1. In males, the purulent discharge may be collected on a sterile swab and plated directly on the appropriate transport medium (Thayer Martin or Jembec plates). A second swab is saved for a Gram stain smear.
2. *Neisseria gonorrhoeae* is very delicate and can die before the specimen reaches the lab.
3. A small calcium alginate swab may also be gently inserted several centimeters directly into the urethra to obtain a productive sample.
4. Inoculate on tryptic soy agar (TSA) with 10% sheep's blood, MacConkey agar, Columbia (CNA) agar, and thioglycollate broth. Chocolate agar or Thayer Martin agar are also inoculated and incubated with enhanced carbon dioxide.
5. Prepare a sample for Gram stain evaluation.
6. Incubate overnight at 37°C.

Vaginal/Cervical

1. The cervix is the best site for female collections.
2. The physician will use a sterile speculum moistened with warm water so as not to kill the gonococcus.
3. The cervical mucous plug is removed with a cotton ball and forceps.
4. A sterile swab is then inserted into the cervix, rotated, and allowed to remain for several seconds before removing.
5. Plate immediately to a transport medium (Thayer Martin or Jembec plates) and send an additional swab to the laboratory for a Gram stain.
6. Inoculate on tryptic soy agar (TSA) with 10% sheep's blood aerobically. Anaerobically, MacConkey agar, chocolate agar, or Thayer Martin agar, and Columbia agars and thioglycollate broth. The chocolate/Thayer Martin agar is incubated with enhanced carbon dioxide.
7. Prepare a sample for Gram stain evaluation.
8. Incubate overnight at 37°C.

ANAL SPECIMENS

1. Insert a cotton swab about an inch into the anal canal. Move it from side to side to collect a sample from the anal crypts.
2. If fecal material is observed, the swab should be discarded and the procedure performed again.
3. Inoculate on tryptic soy agar (TSA) with 10% sheep's blood aerobically, and MacConkey agar, Hektoen (HE) agar, xylose lysine desoxycholate (XLD) agar, Campylobacter (Campy) agar and gram-negative broth. A Thayer Martin agar may also be inoculated.
4. Prepare a sample for Gram stain evaluation.
5. Incubate overnight at 37°C.

STOOL SPECIMENS

1. Collect stool in a bedpan.
2. Select portions that have blood or mucus and transfer to a plastic stool container.
3. Deliver to laboratory immediately, as the pH changes when the temperature of stool drops, decreasing the recovery potential of pathogens.
4. Rectal swabs may also be collected by inserting a cotton swab beyond the rectal sphincter, rotating the swab and withdrawing it carefully.
5. Inoculate on tryptic soy agar (TSA) with 10% sheep's blood aerobically, and MacConkey, Hektoen (HE) agar, xylose lysine desoxycholate (XLD) agar, Campylobacter (Campy) agar, and gram-negative broth.
6. Incubate overnight at 37°C.

CEREBROSPINAL FLUID (CSF)

1. Usually, three sterile tubes are collected by the physician using a needle and syringe. The first tube filled is labeled #3 (as it was last to be withdrawn), the second tube is labeled #2, and the last tube filled is labeled #1.
2. The tubes are delivered first to the microbiology lab, where cultures are taken off first using tube #3.
3. A portion is prepared for direct fungal and bacterial examination.
4. The CSF is then delivered to other laboratory departments for cell counts and chemistry studies.
5. Inoculate on tryptic soy agar (TSA) with 10% sheep's blood aerobically, and anaerobically, MacConkey agar and thioglycollate broth. A chocolate agar is also inoculated.
6. Prepare a sample for Gram stain evaluation.
7. Incubate overnight at 37°C.

BODY FLUID ASPIRATIONS (JOINT, PLEURA, ETC.)

1. The skin areas around the aspiration site must be well disinfected so as not to introduce bacteria into the site or contaminate the specimen.
2. The aspirate is collected by a physician, the needle corked, and the sample promptly delivered to the lab.
3. If the syringe was washed with sterile heparin before the aspiration, the fluid will not clot.
4. Inoculate on tryptic soy agar (TSA) with 10% sheep's blood aerobically and anaerobically. MacConkey agar, thioglycollate broth, and chocolate agar are also inoculated.
5. Prepare a sample for Gram stain evaluation.
6. Incubate overnight at 37°C.

WOUND CULTURES

1. Aerobic and anaerobic cultures should be taken. Follow the anaerobic collection procedures described on the culturette package.
2. Care must be taken not to contaminate the specimen with skin flora or airborne organisms.
3. If material is aspiratable this technique is preferred so as to avoid cross contamination.
4. Collect the sample by carefully touching the swab end to the area being tested. Rotate the swab around the area to get a good representation of the material.
5. In all cases, make sure the cotton tip of the swab is well saturated with material.
6. Immediately replace the swab back in the holder without touching the cue stick.
7. Break the fluid capsule and let the material soak the end of the swab. This will keep the microorganisms viable until cultures can be set up.

8. Label the swabs with all pertinent information, such as patient name, identification number, date specimen taken, source of specimen, and physician name.
9. Deliver the specimens to the laboratory as soon as possible.
10. Inoculate on tryptic soy agar (TSA) with 10% sheep's blood aerobically, and anaerobically, on MacConkey agar and thioglycollate broth.
11. Prepare a sample for Gram stain evaluation.
12. Incubate overnight at 37°C.

ANAEROBIC CULTURES

1. Special anaerobic collection kits are available and should be used for maximum recovery of anaerobes.
2. Peel open the anaerobic culture package.
3. Without removing the culturette from the inside plastic bag, grasp the culturette.
4. Remove the metal bar and set nearby.
5. Using the cap holder, remove the swab from the container bag (leave the container inside the plastic bag).
6. Using aseptic technique, collect the specimen, being careful not to touch the cue stick.
7. Carefully replace the cap with swab attached into the plastic canister inside the plastic container bag.
8. Push the whole swab, cap, and canister all the way into the plastic container bag (past the marked line).
9. Insert the top of the container bag into the metal closure and fold over at least three to five times until the metal closure approaches the tip of the swab inside the bag.
10. Bend metal closure end in the opposite direction to seal the bag.
11. Turn kit upside down so that the cap is toward the floor.
12. Double check that the plastic protective sleeve (which is about 4 inches long) is over the ampule.
13. Break the ampule nearest the swab tip by squeezing on the glass ampule, and allow the transport media to saturate the swab.
14. Invert the swab again and break the bottom ampule.
15. Keep upright until the tablet is dissolved.
16. When ready to inoculate culture media, use scissors to cut the bag open.
17. Some laboratories will have anaerobic glove boxes in which all anaerobic work is conducted, including the inoculation of the culture media.
18. For laboratories that do not use a glove box it is important to get the samples inoculated onto the TSA culture media as soon as possible and then placed in an anaerobic environment immediately. The anaerobic jar employing the gas pack system is convenient and easy to use. The TSA plates are placed in the jar along with an indicator strip. The gas package is opened from one corner, and 10 ml of water are added to the pack. The pack is then inserted into the jar and the jar is immediately sealed, and incubated at 37°C overnight.
19. Significant anaerobes include *Clostridia* and *Bacteroides* species.

CARBON DIOXIDE–ENHANCED GROWTH

1. Carbon dioxide incubators are usually found in larger microbiology laboratories.
2. For the smaller laboratories the candle jar works well in obtaining the right atmosphere for the growth of the *Neisseria* species.
3. Any large jar (a pickle jar is ideal) with a neck opening large enough to pass the petri dish through will work. The inoculated plates are placed on the floor of the jar upside down and a votive candle placed on the lid of a petri dish is lighted and carefully slipped into the candle jar. The lid is secured, and the jar is placed in the incubator without disturbing the seal for 24 to 48 hours. By the time the candle goes out an atmosphere of about 5% to 10% carbon dioxide has been added.
4. Individual sealed CO_2 baggies are also available commercially.

UNACCEPTABLE SPECIMENS

Laboratory results are only as valid as the quality of the specimen obtained. Therefore, it is essential that strict adherence to laboratory protocol be followed when collecting microbiological specimens. The following are guidelines that all microbiology laboratories will, as a minimum, reject.

1. Upper respiratory tract
   a. Throat/nose swabs
      - any swab received dry
   b. Sputum
      - those consisting of saliva only (percentages of white blood cells and epithelial cells will be evaluated using Gram stain techniques)
      - any received in nonsterile containers
2. Lower respiratory tract
   - bronchial washings received in nonsterile containers
   - transtracheal aspirations delivered in an aerobic environment unsuitable for anaerobic culture.
   - any received in nonsterile containers
3. Urine
   - any received in nonsterile containers
   - a delay or more than 1 hour between collection and delivery to the lab.
   - specimens that have not been refrigerated while awaiting delivery to the lab
4. Genital specimens
   - any received on a dry swab
   - any delayed more than 10 minutes (unless in a transport medium designed to hold or preserve organisms causing genital infections, especially gonorrhoea, chylamydia, and herpes)
   - a delay of more than 30 minutes for delivery of Thayer Martin plates for gonorrhoea
   - dehydrating transport media

5. Stool specimens
   - enema-induced specimens
   - stools that have been refrigerated
   - prolonged delay in plating the specimen
6. Body fluids, including cerebrospinal fluids
   - NEVER rejected
   - note time received and condition of specimen on the final report
7. Tissue samples
   - any received in fixatives, formalin, alcohol, etc.

APPENDIX B—METRIC CONVERSIONS

Power of 10	Decimal Equivalent	Prefix	Symbol
10^{12}	1,000,000,000,000	tera	T
10^{9}	1,000,000,000	giga	G
10^{6}	1,000,000	mega	M
10^{3}	1,000	kilo	k
10^{2}	100	hecto	h
10^{1} or 10	10	deka	da
10^{0}	1	this is the base unit*	
10^{-1}	0.1	deci	d
10^{-2}	0.01	centi	c
10^{-3}	0.001	milli	m
10^{-6}	0.000001	micro	u
10^{-9}	0.000000001	nano	n
10^{-12}	0.000000000001	pico	p

*Base units are: length—meter (m), volume—liter (1), and mass—gram (g).

1 kilogram (kg) = 1000 grams (g)
1 gram (g) = 1000 milligrams (mg)
1 milligram (mg) = 1000 micrograms (μg)
1 microgram (μg) = 1000 nanograms (ng)
1 nanogram (ng) = 1000 picograms (pg)
1 picogram (pg) = 10^{-12} grams (g)
1 gram (g) = 10^{-3} kilogram (kg)
1 milligram (mg) = 10^{-3} gram (g)
1 microgram (μg) = 10^{-3} milligram (mg)
1 nanogram (ng) = 10^{-3} microgram (μg)
1 picogram (pg) = 10^{-3} nanogram (ng)
1 gram (g) = 10^{12} picograms (pg)

Temperature: Centigrade $= \frac{5}{9}(F - 32)$. Fahrenheit $= \frac{9}{5}C + 32$

SOME IMPORTANT CONVERSIONS

Length

1 cm (centimeter) = 2.54 inches
1 km (kilometer) = 0.6 miles

1 mi (mile) = 1.62 km
1 meter (m) = 1.1 yards (yd) = 3.3 feet (ft)
1 meter (m) = 39 inches (in)

Volume

1 cubic centimeter (cc) = 1 milliliter (ml)
1 pint (pt) = 474 milliliters (ml) = 0.474 liter (l)
1 fluid ounce (fl oz) = 30 milliliters (ml)
1 liter (l) = 1.06 quarts (qt)
1 quart (qt) = 0.95 liters (l)
1 teaspoon (tsp) = 5 milliliters (ml)
1 gallon (gal) = 3.8 liters (l)

Mass

1 ounce (oz) = 28 grams (g)
1 gram (g) = 0.035 ounces (oz)
1 kilogram (kg) = 2.2 pounds (lb)
1 pound (lb) = 450 grams (g) = 0.45 kilograms (kg)

UNIT CONVERSION METHOD

To convert from one unit to another, use the unit cancellation method. For example, how many seconds are there in 4 days?

1. Start with the "given"—4 days.
2. Convert days to hours.
3. Convert hours to minutes.
4. Convert minutes to seconds.
5. Answer

$$\underset{1.}{4 \text{ days}} \times \underset{2.}{\frac{24 \text{ hours}}{(1 \text{ day})}} \times \underset{3.}{\frac{60 \text{ minutes}}{(1 \text{ hour})}} \times \underset{4.}{\frac{60 \text{ seconds}}{(1 \text{ minute})}} = \underset{5.}{345{,}600 \text{ seconds}}$$

PERCENT COMPOSITION

Many laboratory results are expressed in grams per deciliter (g/dl).

1 deciliter (dl) = 0.1 liter (l) = 100 milliliters (ml),

therefore, g/dl is also = g/100 ml.

Percent composition is expressed as the number of grams per 100 units. Therefore, laboratory results may be expressed as a percent concentration.

SPECIFIC GRAVITY

Specific gravity is the density of a liquid, or the number of times heavier the liquid is than water. The specific gravity of distilled water = 1.000. The density of distilled water is 1.000 g/l or 1.000 mg/ml.

The specific gravity of urine is often measured to determine the concentration of dissolved solids. Normal specific gravities for urine are: first morning sample—1.015 to 1.025; after much water and no food—1.005 or less.

APPENDIX C—OSHA'S BLOODBORNE PATHOGEN RULE (Effective March 6, 1992)* (*Federal Register,* December 6, 1991)

To whom does it apply?

All health care workers, service employees, etc., who may be occupationally exposed to blood or other potentially infectious materials.

Why was the rule established?

To reduce occupational exposure of employees and to reduce workplace exposures to bloodborne pathogens.

The exposure control plan:

1. The employer must develop a written control plan, citing who may be exposed and how, how to evaluate exposure incidents, and a schedule for implementing the standards.
2. The plan must be reviewed and updated annually.
3. All employees must be given information and training at no cost to the employee at their initial hire and annually thereafter.
4. Hepatitis B vaccination must be made available to all employees at no cost to them within 10 days of initial hire. Employees who decline the service will sign a declination acknowledging continued risk of exposure.
5. Universal precautions must be practiced by all employees, whereby *all* human blood and human body fluids are considered infectious for HIV, HBV, HCV, or other bloodborne pathogens.
6. Methods of control include:
   a. establish engineering control to minimize hazards and reduce employee exposure—e.g., puncture-resistant containers to hold sharps, self-sheathing needles, resuscitation bags, and ventilation bags.
   b. establish workplace controls, including restrictions for eating, drinking, smoking, applying cosmetics or lip balm, handling contact lenses, prohibition of mouth pipetting, food storage, use of handwashing facilities, and

*Reprinted from Occupational Exposure to Bloodborne Pathogen, U.S. Department of Labor, OSHA, OSHA pamphlet no. 3127.

decontamination of equipment. Also, frequent handwashing, even after removal of rubber gloves, and prohibiting bending, breaking, or recapping needles.

c. use personal protective equipment to prevent exposure or contamination, including gloves, gowns, lab coats, face shield, masks, and eye protection that is not permeable to blood or other potentially hazardous infectious materials. Such protection may not be able to pass through protective covering onto street clothes, undergarments, skin, eyes, mouth, etc.
d. employer must provide personal protective equipment at no cost to the employee, and the employee must wear this equipment whenever occupational exposure may occur.
e. employer must ensure that employees remove all protective equipment before leaving the work area and after it becomes contaminated.
f. employer must provide laundry service for cleaning of personal protective equipment and disposal of contaminated equipment.
g. employer must ensure that employees wear all personal protective clothing and gear whenever the potential for contamination exists and see that disposable gloves are not washed for reuse.

7. Employer must maintain a clean work environment for employees and establish appropriate decontamination methods for employees to follow. Cleaning standards will apply to the environment, equipment, and work spaces. Spills must be cleaned as follows:
   a. use tongs, dustpan, etc. to pick up broken glass.
   b. place contaminated glass in sharps container.
   c. spray area with 10% bleach solution (10 parts water to 1 part bleach), then clean with paper towels.
   d. discard all contaminated cleaning rags in a biohazards container.
8. Label all containers holding biological materials with the fluorescent orange warning labels. Make sure the warning label is readily visible on all collection containers designated to hold contaminated or infectious waste or materials for use.

Essentials for laboratory workers:

1. Gloves must be worn at all times when handling all body fluid material.
2. Sharps as well as broken glass must be disposed of in hard-walled, sharps containers. Such containers will be strategically placed and readily available for use.
3. Employers must provide nonpermeable protective clothing for those at risk of contamination by potentially hazardous body fluids.
4. Employers must make available hepatitis B vaccinations, at no cost to the employee. Employees may decline but are required to sign a waiver of liability. Employees do have the right to request the vaccination at a later date without cost to them.
5. Employers must provide education and training for their employees.
6. To clean a biohazardous spill, a 3% to 10% bleach solution is poured over the site, allowed to sit, then cleaned up with disposable towels.
7. Spills on instrumentation are also cleaned with bleach. Equipment sent for repair will be sprayed with a disinfectant bleach before being serviced.

8. Biohazardous trash will be properly disposed of according to weight and volume generated by a facility. Generally, biohazardous waste generated under 50 pounds is exempt from removal by a biohazardous waste management company.
9. Clothing worn on duty by health care personnel will not be worn outside the workplace, even to and from work.

Table C–1 Summary of References for Federal Health and Safety Guidelines

Guidelines	Issuing Agency	Purpose
Standard Precautions	Centers for Disease Control and Prevention (CDC), United States Public Health Department, Atlanta, Georgia	Issued in 1996 to augment and synthesize universal precautions and techniques known as body substance isolation (BSI). Standard precautions contain measures intended to protect all health care providers, patients, and visitors from infectious diseases.
Transmission-based Precautions	CDC	Designed to reduce the risk of airborne, droplet, and contact transmission of pathogens. These are used in addition to standard precautions and are intended for specific categories of patients.
Universal Blood and Body Fluid Precautions (Universal Precautions)	CDC	Released in 1985 to assist health care providers to greatly reduce the risk of contracting or transmitting infectious diseases, particularly AIDS and hepatitis B.
Clinical Laboratory Amendments of 1988 (CLIA '88)	Health Care Financing Administration (HCFA), United States Department of Health and Human Services (HHS)	Safeguards the public by regulating all testing of specimens taken from the body.
Occupational Safety and Health Administration (OSHA) Guidelines	OSHA, United States Department of Labor	Requires employers to ensure employee safety in regard to occupational exposure to potentially harmful substances.

Table C-2 Standard Precautions

STANDARD PRECAUTIONS
FOR INFECTION CONTROL
CDC 1996

Wash Hands (Plain soap)
Wash after touching **blood, body fluids, secretions, excretions** and **contaminated items.**
Wash immediately **after gloves are removed** and **between patient contacts.**
Avoid transfer of microorganisms to other patients or environments.

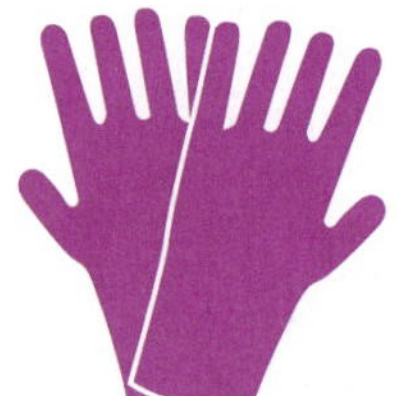

Wear Gloves
Wear when touching **blood, body fluids, secretions, excretions** and **contaminated items.**
Put on **clean** gloves just **before touching mucous membranes** and **nonintact skin.**
Change gloves between tasks and procedures on the same patient after contact with material that may contain high concentrations of microorganisms. Remove gloves promptly after use, before touching noncontaminated items and environmental surfaces, and before going to another patient, and wash hands immediately to avoid transfer of microorganisms to other patients or environments.

Wear Mask and Eye Protection or Face Shield
Protect mucous membranes of the eyes, nose and mouth during procedures and patient-care activities that are likely to generate **splashes** or **sprays of blood, body fluids, secretions,** or **excretions.**

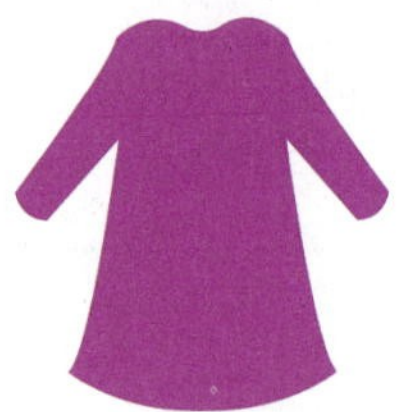

Wear Gown
Protect skin and prevent soiling of clothing during procedures that are likely to generate **splashes** or **sprays** of **blood, body fluids, secretions,** or **excretions.** Remove a soiled gown as promptly as possible and wash hands to avoid transfer of microorganisms to other patients or environments.

Patient-Care Equipment
Handle used patient-care equipment soiled with **blood, body fluids, secretions,** or **excretions** in a manner that prevents skin and mucous membrane exposures, contamination of clothing, and transfer of microorganisms to other patients and environments. Ensure that reusable equipment is not used for the care of another patient until it has been appropriately cleaned and reprocessed and single use items are properly discarded.

Table C–2 Continued

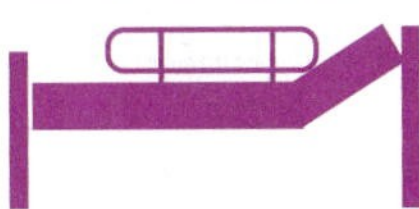

Environmental Control
Follow hospital procedures for routine care, cleaning, and disinfection of environmental surfaces, beds, bedrails, bedside equipment and other frequently touched surfaces.

Linen
Handle, transport, and process used linen soiled with **blood, body fluids, secretions,** or **excretions** in a manner that prevents exposures and contamination of clothing, and avoids transfer of microorganisms to other patients and environments.

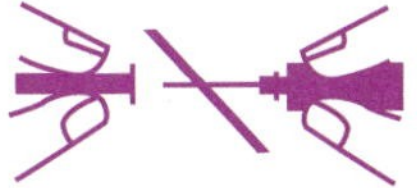

Occupational Health and Bloodborne Pathogens
Prevent injuries when using needles, scalpels, and other sharp instruments or devices; when handling sharp instruments after procedures; when cleaning used instruments; and when disposing of used needles.

Never recap used needles using both hands or any other technique that involves directing the point of a needle toward any part of the body; rather, use either a one-handed "scoop" technique or a mechanical device designed for holding the needle sheath.

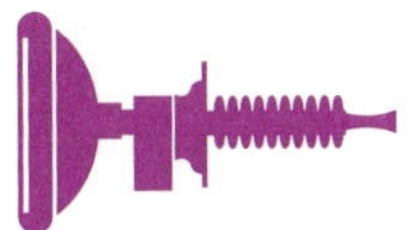

Do not remove used needles from disposable syringes by hand, and do not bend, break, or otherwise manipulate used needles by hand. Place used disposable syringes and needles, scalpel blades and other sharp items in puncture-resistant sharps containers located as close as practical to the area in which the items were used, and place reusable syringes and needles in a puncture resistant container for transport to the reprocessing area.

Use **resuscitation devices** as an alternative to mouth-to-mouth resuscitation.

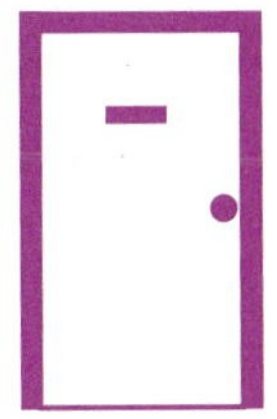

Patient Placement
Use a **private room** for a patient who contaminates the environment or who does not (or cannot be expected to) assist in maintaining appropriate hygiene or environmental control. Consult Infection Control if a private room is not available.

Table C–3 Airborne Precautions, One Category of Transmission-Based Precautions (*Courtesy of Brevis Corp.*)

AIRBORNE PRECAUTIONS
(in addition to Standard Precautions)

VISITORS: Report to nurse before entering.

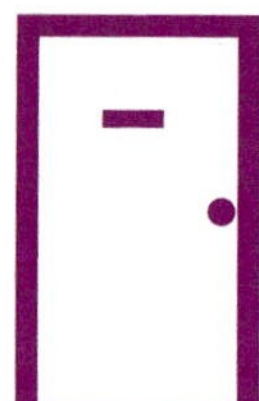

Patient Placement
Use **private room** that has:
Monitored negative air pressure,
6 to 12 air changes per hour,
Discharge of air outdoors or HEPA filtration if recirculated.
Keep room door closed and patient in room.

Respiratory Protection
Wear an **N95 respirator** when entering the room of a patient with known or suspected infectious pulmonary **tuberculosis**.
Susceptible persons should not enter the room of patients known or suspected to have **measles** (rubeola) or **varicella** (chickenpox) if other immune caregivers are available. If susceptible persons must enter, they should wear an **N95 respirator**. (Respirator or surgical mask not required if immune to measles and varicella.)

Patient Transport
Limit transport of patient from room to essential purposes only.
Use **surgical mask** on patient during transport.

Table C–4 Contact Precautions, One Category of Transmission-Based Precautions (*Courtesy of Brevis Corp.*)

CONTACT PRECAUTIONS
(in addition to Standard Precautions)

VISITORS: Report to nurse before entering.

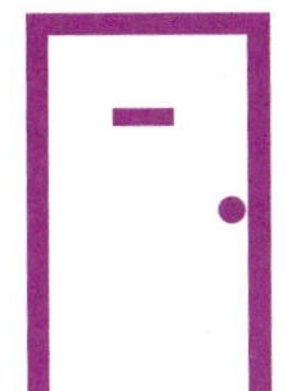

Patient Placement
Private room, if possible. Cohort if private room is not available.

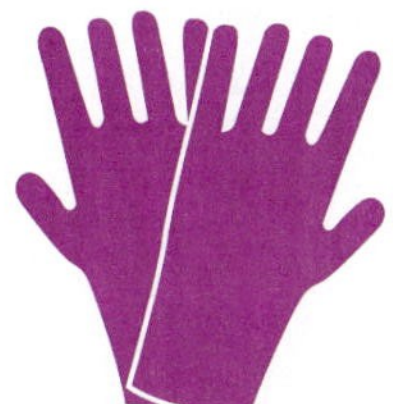

Gloves
Wear gloves when entering patient room.
Change gloves after having contact with infective material that may contain high concentrations of microrganisms **(fecal** material and **wound drainage).**
Remove gloves before leaving patient room.

Wash
Wash hands with an **antimicrobial** agent immediately after glove removal. After glove removal and handwashing, ensure that hands do not touch potentially contaminated environmental surfaces or items in the patient's room to avoid transfer of microrganisms to other patients or environments.

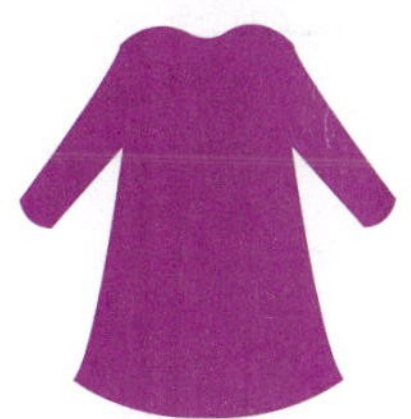

Gown
Wear gown when **entering** patient room if you anticipate that your clothing will have substantial contact with the patient, environmental surfaces, or items in the patient's room, or if the patient is **incontinent**, or has **diarrhea**, an **ileostomy**, a **colostomy**, or **wound drainage** not contained by a dressing. **Remove** gown before leaving the patient's environment and ensure that clothing does not contact potentially contaminated environmental surfaces to avoid transfer of microrganisms to other patients or environments.

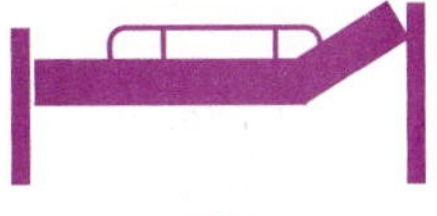

Patient Transport
Limit transport of patient to essential purposes only. During transport, ensure that precautions are maintained to minimize the risk of transmission of microorganisms to other patients and contamination of environmental surfaces and equipment.

Patient-Care Equipment
Dedicate the use of noncritical patient-care equipment to a single patient. If common equipment is used, clean and disinfect between patients.

Table C-5 Droplet Precautions, One Category of Transmission-Based Precautions (*Courtesy of Brevis Corp.*)

DROPLET PRECAUTIONS
(in addition to Standard Precautions)

VISITORS: Report to nurse before entering.

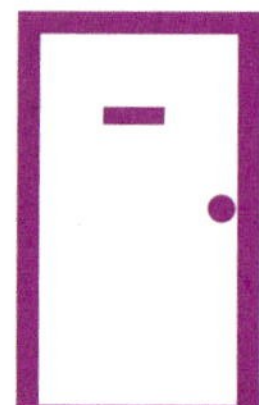

Patient Placement
Private room, if possible. Cohort or maintain spatial separation of **3 feet** from other patients or visitors if private room is not available.

Mask
Wear mask when working within **3 feet** of patient (or upon entering room).

Patient Transport
Limit transport of patient from room to essential purposes only.
Use **surgical mask** on patient during transport.

APPENDIX D—CLINICAL LABORATORY IMPROVEMENT ACT (CLIA 88) (*Federal Register,* February 28, 1992)

I. Personnel Standards—Testing personnel are required to demonstrate their testing skills prior to performing tests on patient samples, and all laboratory personnel are required to meet rigorous responsibility requirements. This section describes who can perform what category of testing.

A. Laboratory director qualifications
   1. Highly complex testing laboratories
      a. licensed pathologist or board certified, licensed Ph.D. clinical laboratory scientist
      b. licensed physician (M.D. or D.O.) with one year of training in the laboratory as a resident and two years of experience supervising highly complex testing
      c. can direct no more than five laboratories
   2. Moderately complex testing laboratories
      a. as in 1. above or
      b. earned a master's degree in any clinical laboratory science and have one year each of laboratory training or work experience and supervisory experience.
      c. earned a bachelor's degree in any clinical laboratory science and have two years each of laboratory training or work experience and supervisory experience.

B. Technical consultant standards
   1. Moderately complex testing laboratories
      a. licensed physician (M.D. or D.O.) with one year of training or experience in the laboratory in the area for which technical responsibilities fall
      b. doctoral or master's degree in a clinical laboratory science and one year training or experience
      c. bachelor's degree in a clinical laboratory science and two years training or experience

C. Clinical consultant qualifications
   1. Highly complex testing laboratories
      a. M.D. or board-certified Ph.D. scientist
   2. Moderately complex testing laboratories
      a. consultant must be qualified as a laboratory director or
      b. be a licensed doctor of medicine or licensed doctor of osteopathy

D. Technical supervisor qualifications
   1. Highly complex testing laboratories
      a. licensed pathologist or
      b. licensed physician (M.D. or D.O.) with one year of training or experience in microbiology performing highly complex procedures
      c. Ph.D. and M.D. (nonpathologist) with one year of experience

d. M.S. with two years of experience
e. B.S. degree with four years of specialty experience
f. need not be on site daily, but must be available

E. General supervisor qualifications
   1. Moderately complex testing laboratories
      a. minimum of an associate degree plus two years of training or experience
      b. must be on-site if testing is being performed by a high school graduate

F. Testing personnel—no differentiation between medical technologist and medical laboratory technician. Until September 1997, high school graduates with documented training and experience could perform all levels of testing under the supervision of a general supervisor.
   1. Highly complex testing laboratories
      a. effective September 1997, all persons conducting high complexity testing must have at least an associate degree in laboratory science or medical laboratory technology
   2. Moderately complex testing laboratories
      a. since September 1997, high school graduates with training and experience have been limited to performing tests in the moderately complex category under a general supervisor
      b. must complete an official military medical laboratory procedures course of at least 50 weeks' duration
      c. receives semiannual evaluations during first year of employment then annually thereafter

II. Testing Standards—Test performance requirements are based on test complexity and risk factors related to erroneous test results. Testing is divided into three categories: (1) waived tests, (2) moderately complex tests, and (3) highly complex tests. Categorization of laboratory tests is based on several criteria, including knowledge needed to perform the test; training and experience; reagent preparation complexity; troubleshooting and maintenance required; characteristics of the operational steps, calibrations, quality control, and proficiency testing materials; and the degree of interpretation and judgment required.

A. Waived tests—Erroneous results are very unlikely in this category and unlikely to cause reasonable risk if reported incorrectly.
   1. dipstick or tablet urinalysis procedures
   2. spun microhematocrit
   3. fecal occult blood
   4. urine pregnancy tests
   5. erythrocyte sedimentation rate (ESR)
   6. copper sulfate hemoglobin tests
   7. blood glucose screens performed using FDA-cleared home testing devices
   8. ovulation test kits

Laboratories performing waived tests are subject to application fees and random inspections. They are not subject to routine inspections, personnel requirements, proficiency testing requirements, quality control/quality assurance requirements, and patient test management requirements.

B. Moderately complex tests—There may be reasonable risk of harm to the patient if these tests are performed incorrectly. Although risk may be present, it is minimized because methods are not complex. Test performance does involve some independent knowledge and judgment of method, instrumentation, and data interpretation to a limited degree. Moderately complex tests comprise over 80% of all laboratory test procedures and include:
   1. Bacteriology
      a. primary inoculation of cultures
      b. urine culture and colony count kits
      c. microscopic examination of direct wet-mount preparations
      d. isolation, presumptive and/or confirmatory identification of aerobic bacteria from throat, urine, or genital specimens
      e. Gram stain
      f. darkfield examination for *Treponema pallidum*
      g. procedures for simple reagent preparations
      h. manual screening devices for urine infections
      i. automated procedures that do not require operator intervention during the analytic process
      j. acid-fast stain
   2. Mycology
      a. primary inoculation of cultures
      b. yeast isolations and identifications limited to *Candida albicans*
      c. examination of direct wet-mount preparations
      d. microscopic evaluation of potassium hydroxide (KOH) preparations
      e. tests using selective mediums for the presence or absence of dermatophyte infections
      f. manual procedures with limited numbers of steps
      g. automated mycology procedures that do not require operator intervention during the analytic process
   3. Parasitology
      a. pinworm preparations and microscopic evaluations
      b. *Trichomonas vaginalis* evaluations
      c. microscopic evaluations of direct wet-mount preparations for the presence or absence of parasites
      d. manual procedures with limited numbers of steps
      e. culture devices indicating presence or absence of *Trichomonas vaginalis*
   4. Virology
      a. manual procedures with limited numbers of steps
      b. automated procedures that do not require operator intervention during the analytic process
C. Highly complex tests
   1. Bacteriology
      a. isolation and identification of aerobic and anaerobic specimens not listed in moderately complex tests
      b. automated or semiautomated procedures requiring operator intervention during the analytic process

   c. serotyping
   d. antigen or toxin test and kit procedures requiring microscopic evaluations
   e. manual procedures with multiple steps in the analytic process
   f. semiautomated nonculture urine screening devices that predict urine infections
   g. concentration, smear, and primary culture inoculations for mycobacteria
   h. all other mycobacteria procedures
2. Mycology
   a. isolation and identification of fungi
   b. automated or semiautomated mycology procedures requiring operator intervention during the analytic process
   c. manual procedures with multiple steps in the analytic process
   d. identification techniques requiring interpretive skills
3. Parasitology
   a. identification techniques requiring interpretive skills
   b. concentration and differential staining techniques
   c. antigen test and kit procedures requiring microscopic evaluations
   d. manual procedures with multiple steps in the analytic process
4. Virology
   a. isolation and identification techniques
   b. antigen test and kit procedures requiring microscopic evaluations
   c. manual procedures with multiple steps in the analytic process
   d. automated or semiautomated virology procedures requiring operator intervention during the analytic process

III. Quality Assurance Requirements—Each laboratory performing moderate and/or highly complex testing must establish and follow written policies and procedures for a comprehensive quality assurance (QA) program. Laboratories may customize QA activities based on services offered, complexity of testing performed and reported, as well as its unique practices.

A. The QA program will
   1. monitor and evaluate the overall quality of the total testing process including the following of specimens from their origin through the testing as well as reporting process
   2. evaluate the effectiveness of its policies and procedures
   3. identify and correct problems
   4. ensure accurate, reliable, and prompt reporting of results
   5. ensure adequacy and competence of staff
B. QA activities will include
   1. patient test management assessment
   2. quality control assessment
   3. proficiency test assessment
   4. comparison of test results
   5. relationship of patient information to patient test results
   6. personnel assessment

7. communications
8. complaint investigations
9. quality assurance review with staff
10. quality assurance records

APPENDIX E—COMMON MEDICAL ABBREVIATIONS

AFB: acid-fast bacilli

AIDS: Acquired immunodeficiency syndrome

alk: alkaline

AKA: also known as

AMA: American Medical Association

AMT: American Medical Technologists

ana: anaerobic

ARC: AIDS-related complex

ASAP: as soon as possible

ASMT: American Society for Medical Technology

ASCLS: American Society for Clinical Laboratory Science (formerly ASMT)

ASCP: American Society of Clinical Pathologists

ASM: American Society for Microbiology

ATCC: American Type Culture Collection

BA: blood agar

BCG: Bacille Calmette–Guérin (attenuated TB for immunization)

BEA: bile esculin agar

BFP: biological false positive

BHI: brain-heart infusion (broth or an agar)

BID: twice a day

BM: bowel movement

BP: blood pressure

BCYE: buffered charcoal yeast extract agar

BS: bismuth sulfite agar, blood sugar

C: centigrade or Celsius

c: with

Ca: calcium

CA: cancer

CBC: complete blood count

CAHEA: Committee on Allied Health Education and Accreditation

CAMPY: *Campylobacter* agar

CAP: College of American Pathologists

CBC: complete blood count

cc: cubic centimeter

CCU: coronary-care unit

CDC: Centers for Disease Control and Prevention

CEO: chief executive officer

CFU: colony-forming unit

CICU: coronary intensive-care unit

CLED: cystine-lactose-electrolyte–deficient agar

CLIA: Clinical Laboratory Improvement Act

cm: centimeter

CM: cooked meat broth

CMI: cell-mediated immunity

CMV: cytomegalovirus

CNA: Columbia colistin–nalidixic acid agar

CNS: central nervous system

CO: carbon monoxide

CO_2: carbon dioxide

C&S: culture and sensitivity

CSF: cerebrospinal fluid

CVA: cerebrovascular accident

D&C: dilation and curettement/curettage

D.O.: doctor of osteopathy

DOB: date of birth

DNA: deoxyribonucleic acid

dx: diagnosis

ΔH_2O: distilled water

ENT: ears, nose, and throat

EENT: eyes, ears, nose, and throat

ELISA: enzyme-linked immunosorbent assay

EMB: Eosin methylene blue agar

EPEC: enteropathogenic *Escherichia coli*
epi: epithelial cells
F: Fahrenheit
FBS: fasting blood sugar
FTA-ABS: fluorescent treponemal antigen–antibody absorption test
FUO: fever of unknown origin
ga: gauge
g, gm: gram
GC: gonorrhea or gonococcus
GN: gram-negative broth
gr: gray
gu: genitourinary
HAA: hepatitis-associated antigen
HAI: hemagglutination inhibition
HAV: hepatitis A virus
HBV: hepatitis B virus
HCFA: Health Care Financing Administration
HE: Hektoen-enteric agar
HEPA: high-efficiency particulate air filter
HIV: human immunodeficiency virus
HPF: high-power field
HPLC: high-pressure liquid chromatography
H_2O: water
ICU: intensive-care unit
ID: infectious disease
IFA: immunofluorescent assay; indirect fluorescent antibody
IM: intramuscular; infectious mononucleosis
IU: international unit
IV: intravenous
K^+: potassium
KB: Kirby-Bauer (antibiotic sensitivity test)
KIA: Klinger's iron agar
KOH: potassium hydroxide
L, l: liter
LPF: low-power field
MAC/Mac: MacConkey culture medium
MAI: *Mycobacterium avium–intracellulare*
MBC: minimal bactericidal concentration
MD: medical doctor
MID: minimum infective dose
MR: methyl red
mg: milligram
MI: myocardial infarction
MIC: minimal inhibitory concentration
ml: milliliter
MLT: medical laboratory technician
MOTT: mycobacteria other than Tuberculosis
MT: medical technologist
Na^+: sodium
NAACLS: National Accrediting Agency for Clinical Laboratory Sciences
NaCL: sodium chloride; salt
NCA: National Certification Agency
NCCLS: National Committee for Clinical Laboratory Standards
neg: negative
nm: nanometer
NPO: nothing by mouth
NYC: New York City agar
OB: obstetrics
OF: oxidation-fermentation medium
oil: oil immersion, or 100X power
ONPG: *o*-nitrophenol-*B*-galactosidase test
OP: outpatient
O&P: ova and parasites
OSHA: Occupational Safety and Health Administration
path: pathology
PEA: phenylethyl alcohol agar
pH: relative acidity or alkalinity of a solution
PID: pelvic inflammatory disease
PKU: phenylketonuria
PPD: purified protein derivative (a skin test for TB)
PPLO: pleuropneumonia-like organisms
PPNG: penicillinase-producing *Neisseria gonorrhoeae*
PRAS: prereduced, anaerobically sterilized medium
PRN: as needed

PSP: phenolsulfonphthalein

QA: quality assurance

QC: quality control

QD: every day

QH: every hour

QNS: quantity not sufficient

QUAL: qualitative

QUANT: quantitative

RIA: radioimmunoassay

RIPA: radioimmunoprecipitation assay

RBC: red blood cell

RNA: ribonucleic acid

RPR: rapid plasma reagin (a screening test for syphilis)

RPM: revolutions per minute

SCACM: South Central Association of Clinical Microbiologists

sm: small

sp. gr.: specific gravity

SS: *Salmonella-Shigella* agar

Staph.: staphylococcus

STAT: immediately

STD: sexually transmitted disease

Strep.: streptococcus

TB: tuberculosis

TDM: therapeutic drug monitoring

Thio: thioglycollate broth

TID: three times a day

TORCH AGENTS: include *Toxoplasma gondii*, rubella, cytomegalovirus, and herpes simplex agents.

TM: Thayer Martin

TPI: *Treponema pallidum* immobilization test

TSI/TSIA: triple sugar iron agar

TSS: toxic shock syndrome

Trich.: *Trichomonas vaginalis*

TTA: transtracheal aspiration

UA: urinalysis

URI: upper respiratory infection

UTI: urinary-tract infection

VD: venereal disease

VDRL: Venereal Disease Research Laboratory, a screening test for syphilis

VP: Voges-Proskauer

VPI: Virginia Polytechnical Institute

WBC: white blood cell

wte: white

XLD: xylose lysine deoxycholate agar

$>$: greater than

$<$: less than

$=$: equal to

♀: female

♂: male

GLOSSARY

Abiogenesis (a'bio-gen-e-sis): spontaneous generation, the theory that living organisms originated from lifeless matter.

Absolute zero (ab-se-lut' zee'ro): zero degrees Kelvin—the temperature at which heat is absent, and no heat for performance of work or energy can be derived. In Celsius this temperature is –273°, or –460° F.

Accole (a-kol'l)e: early ring form of *Plasmodium falciparum* that is found at the margin of circulating red blood cells.

Acid (as'id): a substance with a pH (relating to the hydrogen ion concentration) of less than 7. Acids are corrosive, sour/bitter, and react with bases or alkalis to produce a salt and water.

Acquired immunodeficiency syndrome (AIDS) (ah-kwird' im"u-no-de-fish'en-se sin'drom) (a'dz): a severe immunodeficiency disease caused by the human immunodeficiency virus, which attacks the T-helper lymphocytes, leaving the patient vulnerable to any number of opportunistic infections that ultimately lead to the patient's death.

Acquired immunity (a-qwi'yrd i-mew'ni-tee): specific immunity that has built up antibodies due to previous exposure to a foreign antigen, such as an infectious microorganism.

Actinomyces (ak'tin-o-mi-seez): a group of filamentous gram-positive bacillary rods that tend to have moldlike or fungal appearances and characteristics.

Active acquired immunity (ak'tiv a-qwi'yrd i-mew'ni-tee): specific immunity attributable to the presence of an antibody formed in response to an antigenic stimulus. One can obtain active immunity by having the disease or by receiving modified or attenuated pathogens or toxoids, as in a vaccination.

Active site (ak'tiv sit): location on a chemical substance, chemical reaction or on a cell in which another substance reacts to produce a change.

Active transport (ak'tiv tranz'port): movement of substances across the cell membrane from an area of lower concentration to an area of higher concentration.

Adenosine triphosphate (ATP) (ah-den'o-seen tri-fos'fate): a high energy compound found in cells that performs an important function in energy storage and transfer.

Adenovirus group (ad"e-no-vi'rus grup): any of a large group of viruses causing disease of the upper respiratory tract and conjunctiva.

Aedes (a-e'dez): a genus of mosquitoes that causes yellow fever.

Aedes aegypti (a-e'dez a-e-gyp'ti): a species of mosquito that transmits the causative organisms of yellow fever and dengue fever.

Aerial mycelium (a"er-el mi-se'le-um): a mass of threadlike hyphae projecting into the air from the fungal thallus.

Aerobe (a'er-ob): microorganisms that live and grow in the presence of oxygen.

Aerobic bacteria (a'er-o-bic bak-te're-ah): single-celled, prokaryotic microorganism that lives and grows in the presence of free oxygen.

Aerosol (air'o-sol): atomized particles suspended in the air; solution of compressed gas containing a chemical substance that will destroy airborne microbes.

Afflictions (ah-flik'shunz): conditions that cause pain or suffering.

Aflatoxin (af-luh-tok'sin): a toxin secreted by certain strains of the fungus *Aspergillus flavus.* It is found mostly on moldy peanuts.

Agar (a'gur): a gelatinous substance used as a culture medium for bacterial growth.

Agglutinins (ah-gloo'ti-nins): protein substances that cause agglutination, or clumping together of cells.

AIDS (a′dz): See Acquired immunodeficiency syndrome.

Algae (al′jee): a group of lower marine plants that contain chlorophyll, a green pigment that helps to manufacture food.

Alkali (al′kah-li): a substance with a pH (relating to the hydrogen ion concentration) of more than 7. Alkalis have basic properties and may contain hydroxide or carbonate groups such as lye, caustic soda, sodium hydroxide, and sodium carbonate.

Allergen (al′er-jen): a substance that causes an allergic response.

Ameba, amoeba (a-mee′buh): one-celled microorganism that moves by cytoplasmic extensions that are projected and retracted in response to external stimuli.

Amebal, amoebal (amoeboid) movement (a-me′bal mu-ve-ment): moving like an amoeba.

Ameboid, amoeboid (a-mee′boyd): resembling an amoeba in form or in movement.

Amino acid (ah-mee′no as′id): class of organic compounds containing amino (NH_2) and carboxyl (COOH) groups that occurs naturally in plant and animal tissues and forms the main constituent of proteins.

Amino group (ah-mee′no groop): consists of the NH_2 molecule.

Anaerobe (an-a′er-ob): microorganisms that live and grow in the absence of oxygen.

Anaerobic bacteria (an-a′er-ob-ik bak-te′re-ah): single-celled, prokaryotic microorganisms that can live and grow in the absence of free oxygen.

Anaphylactic shock (an-uh-fi-lak′tik shock): a severe allergic response to an injected antigen; may be fatal.

Anaphylaxis (an-uh-fi-lak′sis): see Anaphylactic shock.

Animalcules (ah′ne-mal-kules): name given to tiny living microscopic organisms as seen by early microbiologists of the eighteenth century.

Animalia (ah′ne-mal-yah): a major classification group for all animals. All living matter is classified into one of three kingdoms: plantae, animalia, and protista.

Anopheles (ah-nof′e-lez): a genus of mosquito that carries the parasite causing malaria.

Antibiosis (an″ti-bi-o′sis): an association between two organisms that is detrimental to one of them. One of the organisms produces an antibiotic that is harmful to the other.

Antibiotics (an″ti-bi-ot′iks): chemotherapeutic substances of microbial origin that are capable of inhibiting or killing bacteria and other microorganisms.

Antibiotic sensitivity test (an″ti-bi-ot′ik sen″si-tiv′i-tee test): a test in which chemical substances capable of killing or inhibiting the growth of microorganisms are added to suspensions of the intended microorganism and allowed to grow overnight to determine the bactericidal or bacteriostatic effect of the chemical substance.

Antibody (an′ti-bod-ee) (pl. antibodies): a protein produced by the plasma cells, T-lymphocytes, and released into the blood in response to the presence of a foreign antigen.

Antigen (an′ti-jen): a foreign substance that, when introduced into an animal body, stimulates the production of a specific antibody.

Antigen-antibody response (an″ti-jen an′ti-bod-ee re-spon-se): when a foreign antigen (microorganism) enters the body, the immune system activates the plasma cells to make specific proteins to destroy the foreign invader.

Antimicrobial agent (an-tee-mi-kro′bee-yul a′gent): any biological or chemical substance able to destroy microorganisms.

Antiseptic (an″ti-sep′tik): a chemical compound that can inhibit or stop the growth of bacteria without necessarily killing them.

Antiserum (an-ti-se′rum): serum containing antibodies, usually taken from humans or animals that have been subjected to the action of an antigen.

Antitoxin (an′tee-tok-sin): antibody capable of neutralizing a specific toxin.

Apoenzyme (ap″o-en′zim): the protein part of an enzyme pair that requires a coenzyme (additional enzyme) to form an active enzyme system to react with a specific substance.

Arachnids (a-rak′neds): members of the class arthropods that include spiders and mites. They characteristically have four pairs of walking legs and no wings.

Arbovirus group (ar″bo-vi′rus): viruses that are transmitted to humans by mosquitoes and ticks, including yellow fever and equine encephalitis.

Arthropods (ar-thro′podz): members of the phylum Arthropoda. They are characterized by segmented bodies, jointed limbs, and chitinous shells that are molted from time to time.

Artificial acquired immunity (art-i-fish-al a-qwi′yrd i-mew′ni-tee): specific immunity obtained by a deliberate exposure to an antigen, such as a vaccine.

Ascaris (as-kar′is): one of the genera of roundworms that cause intestinal disorder in humans.

Aspergillus (as″per-jil′us): a genus of fungi, commonly found in the air, on peanuts, on spoiling foods, and sometimes in lung or pulmonary infections. Some are opportunistic pathogens.

Asepsis (ay-sep′sis): the exclusion of microorganisms.

Aseptic (a-sep′tik): exclusion of the presence of infectious pathogens.

Aseptic method (a-sep′tik meth′ud): a system of laboratory techniques and practices designed to exclude the presence of all infectious pathogens.

Asymptomatic infection (ay″simp″tuh-ma′tik in-fek′shun): an infection showing no symptoms.

Ataxia (e′taksea): a symptom, not a specific disease or diagnosis. Ataxia means clumsiness, or loss of coordination. Ataxia may affect the fingers and hands, the arms or legs, the body, speech or eye movements. This loss of coordination may be caused by a number of different medical or neurological conditions.

Atom (at′om): the smallest particle of an element that has all the properties of the element and can take part in a chemical reaction.

ATP: See Adenosine triphosphate.

Attenuate (ah-ten′u-ate): to weaken or dilute the pathogenicity of a virus or other pathogen by exposing it to air, heat, chemicals, light, or excessive culturing. To slow the growth of bacteria without necessarily killing them.

Attenuated (ah-ten′u-a″ted): thinning, weakening, or diluting the degree of pathogenicity of a pathogen by exposing it to heat, chemicals, light, or through repeated subculture.

Autoclave (aw′to-klav): self-locking apparatus for the sterilization of materials by steam under pressure. Autoclaving is one of the most effective methods for the destruction of all types of microorganisms.

Autogenous vaccine (aw″to-jen′us vak′seen): a vaccine produced from a culture of bacteria taken from a patient who is to be treated with that vaccine.

Autoimmune disease (aw″to-i-mun′): disease due to immunologic action of one's own cells or antibodies on complements of the body.

Autoimmunity or autoimmune disorder (aw″to-i-mu′ni-te): a condition that occurs when the body forms antibodies against its own tissues.

Autolysis (aw-tol′i-sis): destruction or disintegration of cells or tissues by enzymes produced from within the organism.

Autotrophic (aw″to-trof′ik): the ability of an organism to synthesize nutrients if water, carbon dioxide, inorganic salts, and an energy source are available.

Bacillary dysentery (ba′sil-er-ee dis′in-ter-ee): inflammation of the colon caused by a species of the genus *Shigella.*

Bacillus (ba′sil-us): 1. a genus of gram-positive, rod-shaped bacteria characterized by their large rectangular rod shape and their requirement for oxygen for growth. 2. (pl. bacilli) rod-shaped bacteria; may be rectangular, club shaped, long, thin, or tiny.

Bacillus anthracis (bah-sil′us an-thra′sus): a gram-positive obligate aerobic rod-shaped bacillus that causes anthrax in cattle.

Bacillus cereus (bah-sil′us sir′eus): a gram-positive obligate aerobic rod-shaped bacillus commonly found in soil as a saprophyte. Can also cause food poisoning.

Bacillus subtilis (bah-sil′us sut′lus): a gram-positive obligate aerobic rod-shaped bacillus commonly found in air, soil, and water as a saprophyte.

Bacteremia (bak″te-ree′mee-uh): presence of living bacteria in the blood, with or without significant response on the part of the host.

Bacteria (bak-teer′ee-uh): microscopic, unicellular plantlike organisms belonging to the Protista kingdom. Some bacteria are disease producing, and some are essential to humans.

Bacterial chromosome (bak-teer′ee-yul kro′mo-som): structure within a bacterium that contains a linear strand deoxyribonucleic (DNA) that transmits genetic information.

Bactericides (bak-ter′i-sidz): agents that destroy (kill) bacteria.

Bactericidal (bak-ter″i-si′dal): destructive to bacteria.

Bacteriologist (bak-teer-ee-ol′o-gist): one who studies or does research with bacteria.

Bacteriophage (bak-te″re-o-faj″): a virus that infects bacterial cells, sometimes lysing the cell.

Bacteriostatic (bak-te″re-o-stat′ik): arresting or stopping the growth or multiplication of bacteria; an agent that also stops bacterial growth.

Balantidium coli (bal″an-ti-di′e-um co′li): ciliated protozoan common in swine and rarely causes dysentery in humans.

Basal body (bay′sal bod′ee): microscopic granule found at the base of a cilia or flagella.

Base (base): (See also alkali.) substance that combines with acids to form salts.

Binocular microscope (bin-ok′u-lar mi′kro-skop): a microscope with two eyepieces, permitting the use of both eyes simultaneously.

Binomial nomenclature (bi-no′me-al no′-min-klay″tur): botanical or zoological (scientific) name consisting of two terms, the first being the genus (a proper name) and the second the species (a common name)—e.g., *Homo sapien.*

Biochemist (bi′o-kem′ist): a scientist specializing in the chemical reactions of the body.

Biogenesis (bi″o-jen′e-sis): theory that opposed that living matter always arises from preexisting matter, spontaneous generation.

Biohazard (bi″o-haz-erd): dangerous to living persons. Material that is potentially contaminated with microorganisms.

Biologist (bi″olo-o-gest): a scientist who specializes in the study of biology.

Biology (bi-ol′o-jee): study of the functions of living organisms, including plants and animals.

Blastomyces (blas″to-mi-sez): a genus of pathogenic dimorphic fungi that grow as mycelial forms at room temperature and as yeastlike forms at room temperature. They cause respiratory infections and are found all over North America.

Booster (boo′-str): a subsequent repeat immunization given at a later date to enhance the antibody levels of the primary immunization.

Borrelia burgdorferi (bo-rel′e-ah burg-dor′fer-i): the species of a gram-negative aerobic bacterium that causes Lyme disease. The bacteria is transmitted to humans by the bite of ticks.

Botanist (bot′a-nist): a scientist who specializes in the study of plants and plant life.

Botulism (bot′yoo-lizm): food poisoning due to the toxins secreted by *Clostridium botulinum,* acquired by eating improperly canned or preserved food.

Bovine tuberculosis (bo′vine tew-bur-kew-lo′sis): a form of tuberculosis found in cattle. It can be transmitted to humans through the raw milk of an infected cow.

Branhamella catarrhalis (bran′hah-mel-ah kat-a-ray′lus): a gram-negative coccus commonly found to inhabit the upper respiratory tract (formerly, *Neisseria catarrhalis*).

Brightfield microscope (brit′feeld mi′kro-skop): a microscope that receives its light such that the details appear dark against a light background.

Broad-spectrum antibiotics (brawd spek′trum an″ti-bi-ot′ikz): chemotherapeutic substances of microbial origin that are capable of inhibiting or killing both gram-negative and gram-positive bacteria.

Brownian movement (brown′e-en moo′ve-ment): random movement of microscopic particles and bacteria when suspended in a liquid. The movement is due to molecular impact of the particles with the molecules of the liquid rather than actual motility of the microorganism.

Brucellosis (broo-se-lo′sis): a disease caused by the bacteria of the genus *Brucella.* It is transmitted from animal to animal, and from animal to human. Hogs, cattle, and goats are the major sources of infection. Also called Malta fever, undulant fever.

Budding (bud′ing): asexual reproduction in which a portion of the cell body is thrust out and then separates to become a new cell.

Buffer (buf′er): a substance that, by its presence in a solution, increases the amount of acid or alkali necessary to restore the hydrogen ion concentration to a neutral pH.

Campylobacter (kam″pi-lo-bak′ter): a genus of gram-negative enteric rods that causes gastroenteritis.

Candida (kan′di-duh): a genus of yeastlike molds that include disease producing members as well as members that are essential or helpful to humans.

Candidiasis (kan′di-dye′uh-sis): infection caused by the fungus *Candida albicans.* It can infect mouth, bronchi, lungs, nail, skin, vagina, and digestive tract. Also called thrush.

Candida albicans (kan′di-dah al′bi-kanz): a yeastlike pathogenic fungus that causes a variety of infections, including thrush and moniliasis.

Capsid (kap′sid): a protein shell that protects the nucleic acid of a virus.

Capsule (kap′sul): a gelatinous layer surrounding the cell wall of certain microorganisms, also called "slime layer."

Carcinogen (kar-sin′o-jen): any substance that can cause cancer.

Carbohydrate (kar″bo-hi′drate): a compound containing carbon, hydrogen, and oxygen in the proportions $(CH_2O)n$. Important source of energy for the body. Found primarily in sugars and starches.

Carboxyl group (kar-bok′sil): a monovalent group COOH found in organic acids called carboxylic acids, such as formic, acetic, and benzoic acids.

Carbuncle (kar′bung-k′l): a collection of boils, usually caused by pus-forming *Staphylococcus aureus,* that infects deep into the subcutaneous tissue.

Caries (kair′eez): decay and rotting of bones or teeth.

Carotene (kar′o-teen): plant pigment, red or purple, that helps in the formation of vitamin A.

Carrier (car′ree-er): person who harbors a microorganism without showing any disease symptoms.

While appearing to be in good health, the infected individual can transmit the microorganism to others.

Cell (sel): basic structural unit of living organisms.

Cell envelope (sel en′va-lop): the collective layers around the prokaryotic cell. The structure and composition of the cell envelope differs between gram-positive and gram-negative bacteria.

Cell membrane (sel mem′brane): a thin layer of plasmalike material that surrounds the cytoplasm and organelles. It is located between the cell wall and the protoplasm of the cell and allows molecules to pass in and out of the cell.

Cell wall (sel wahl): a structure found surrounding eukaryotic cells such as plant cells, algae, and fungi. It is basically composed of cellulose and provides rigidity and protection for eukaryotes.

Cellular respiration (sel′u-lar res-per-a-shun): all of the chemical reactions that release energy for the support of cell life.

Centrioles (sen′tree-oles): minute bodies (organelles), rods, or granules found in the centrosome; they play an important role in mitosis or cell division.

Centrosome (sen′tro-sohm): a specialized area of condensed cytoplasm located near the nucleus, containing the centrioles, to which the chromosomes are attracted during mitosis.

Cervicitis (ser″vi-si′tis): inflammation of the cervix uteri.

Cestode (ses′tod): includes the tapeworms, a class of parasites characterized by long, flat, ribbonlike body segments.

Chemotherapeutic agent (keem-o-ther-uh-pew′tik a′jent): drug or chemical used to prevent or treat infections by inhibiting or killing microbes in the living body.

Chemotherapy (kem-o-ther′uh-pee): treatment of infectious diseases as well as malignancies by the use of chemicals, some of which may be very toxic, especially those used to treat cancers.

Chitin (ki′tin): a chemical composing the cell walls of some fungi. It is a polymer made up of n-acetyl glucosamine.

Chlamydia psittaci (klah-mid′e-ah si-ta′ki): gram-negative, nonmotile bacteria that is an obligate intracellular parasite (cannot grow outside the host). It causes psittacosis (parrot fever).

Chlamydia trachomatis (klah-mid′e-ah tra-ko′ma-tis): gram-negative, nonmotile bacteria that is an obligate intracellular parasite (cannot grow outside the host). It causes trachoma, conjunctivitis, lymphogranuloma venereum, and a number of other genital infections. It is one of the most prevalent sexually transmitted diseases.

Chlamydospores (klam′i-do-sporz″): large thick-walled terminal asexual spores formed by the rounding to a fungal cell. They are not shed.

Chlorination (klor-e-na′shen): process of treating with chlorine or a chlorine compound to disinfect sewage or drinking water.

Cholera (kol′er-a): an acute, infectious, often fatal epidemic disease caused by *Vibrio colerae*. It is characterized by watery diarrhea, rice-water stools, muscular cramps, suppressed urination, vomiting, and collapse.

Chromatin (kro′mah-tin): substance of the chromosomes, composed of DNA and basic proteins. Material in the nucleus that stains with basic dyes.

Chromosomes (kro′mo-somz): main structures in the nucleus of the cell. Contains linear threads of DNA, which carry genetic information transmitted during mitosis or meiosis. Humans have 23 pairs (or 46) chromosomes in every cell nucleus.

Cilia (sil′ee-uh): hairlike cytoplasmic projections on certain cells. Their rhythmic beating causes movement on certain aquatic organisms or movement of fluids over surfaces of ciliated cells.

Ciliates (sil′ee-atez): microorganisms possessing cilia.

Cladosporium (klad″o—spo′re-um): a genus of fungi that produces black spots on meat and vegetables.

Clostridium (klo-strid′e-um): a genus of gram-positive obligate anaerobic rod-shaped bacteria whose members cause diseases as lockjaw and gangrene.

Clostridium botulinum (klo-strid′e-um botu′li-num): a genus of gram-positive obligate anaerobic spore-forming bacterial rods common in sewage, feces, and soil that causes the food poisoning botulism.

Clostridium difficile (klo-strid′e-um dif-i-seel): a genus of gram-positive obligate anaerobic spore-forming bacterial rods common in sewage, feces, and soil that causes colitis in infants.

Clostridium perfringens (klo-strid′e-um per-fringe′ins): a genus of gram-positive obligate anaerobic spore forming bacterial rods common in sewage, feces, and soil that causes gas gangrene.

Clostridium tetani (klo-strid′e-um tet′ani): genus of gram-positive obligate anaerobic spore-forming bacterial rods. Common in horse feces and soil. It causes lockjaw or tetanus.

Coagulase (ko-ag′u-las): bacterial enzyme produced by *Staphylococcus aureus* and *Yersinia pestis* that reacts with a cofactor found in blood plasma. A coagulase test can be used as a diagnostic tool for the presence of these organisms.

Coagulate (ko-ag′u-lat): to clot or clump together.

Coagulation (ko-ag′u-la-shun): formation of a soft, semisolid, or solid mass.

Coccidiodes (kok-sis″e-oi′dez): genus of pathogenic fungi found mostly in hot dry climates that causes coccidiodomycosis, a pulmonary infection.

Coccus (kok′us): (pl. cocci) spherical bacterium.

Coenzyme (ko-en′-zime): nonprotein part of an enzyme pair, often containing phosphorus and some vitamins, that unites with an apoenzyme to form a functioning enzyme system found in the metabolism of fats, carbohydrates, and some amino acids.

Cold autoagglutinins (kold aw-to-a-glu′ti-ninz): antibodies developed to self that are apparent only at refrigerated temperatures.

Colostrum (ko-los′trum): the first milk secreted from a mother's breast after giving birth. It contains the mother's antibodies, which the baby will naturally passively acquire during breast-feeding.

Commensal (ko-men′sal): an organism living in or on another without harming its host. Normal flora.

Competitive inhibition (cum′pet-i-tiv in″hibish′un): the blockage of bacterial metabolism by an agent that mimics a nutrient needed by the bacteria.

Complement (comp′le-ment): a series of proteins that react with one another and the antigen to form a complex that then allows the antibody to bind to the antigen-complement complex to then destroy the antigen.

Compound (kom′pownd): a substance made up of two or more atoms or molecules chemically bonded together in definite proportions; for example, salt (sodium chloride)-NaCl and sulfuric acid-H_2SO_4.

Compound microscope (kom′pwond mi′kro-skop): a microscope that consists of two lens systems—the eyepiece lens and the objectives lens—that magnify the object.

Concentrate (kon′sen-trate): solution that contains a large amount of solute (dissolved particles). The more solute the stronger the concentration.

Conidia (ko-nid′i-ah): asexual spores produced by budding or septation from the tip of an aerial hypha.

Conjugation (kon-juh-gay′shun): mating process in lower organisms, characterized by the temporary union of two mating organisms.

Contagious (kon-ta′jus): capable of being transmitted from one individual to another.

Contractile vacuole (kon-trak′til vak′u-ol): a hole or opening in the protoplasm of a cell that contracts.

Corynebacterium diphtheriae (ko-ri″ne-bak-te′re-um dip-the′re-ii): a gram-positive, nonmotile rod-shaped bacteria that infects the throat and causes diphtheria.

Counterstain (kown′ter-stan): 1. stain applied to make the effects of the primary stain more visible; e.g., methylene blue is added after the material has been stained with carbol fuschin to aid in seeing the red tubercule rods against a blue background. 2. second stain added to dye the remaining material on the slide once it has been stained and decolorized, as in the Gram stain. Safranin is a red counterstain added after the crystal violet has been applied and washed off.

Cristae (kris′tee): ridges or folded crests of the membranes of the mitochondria.

Cryptococcus (krip″to-kok′us): a genus of yeastlike fungi that can cause lung diseases and encephalitis.

Cryptococcus neoformans (krip″to-kok′us ne-o-for′manz): a yeastlike organism that causes meningitis. The organism is often carried in with pigeon excreta.

Culex (ku′leks): genus of mosquitos that carry the microfilariae of several parasitic diseases.

Cyclosis (si-klo′sis): movement of the cytoplasm within the cell without any external force.

Cyst (sist): stage in the life cycle of a parasite in which they are enveloped in a protective wall.

Cytochrome (si′to-krom): one of several iron-containing cellular pigments found in mitochondria. They are needed for the process of cellular respiration, which produces energy for cell functions.

Cytologist (si-tol′o-jist): one who specializes in the study of cells—their origin, structure, function, and pathology.

Cytoplasm (si′to-plazm): gel-like protoplasm of a cell that surrounds the nucleus. It is bound by the cell membrane and holds the organelles in place.

Darkfield microscope (dark′feeld mi′kro-skop): a microscope that receives its light from the side of the field such that the details appear light against a dark background.

Daughter cell (daw′ter sel): cell arising from cell division, as in mitosis.

Definitive host (de′fin-i-tiv host): host in which the sexual reproduction of a parasite takes place.

Degeneration (de-gen″e-ra′shun): deterioration or breakdown from a higher to a lower form with less functioning ability. When tissue degenerates, chemical changes occur, and it no longer is able to function.

Degranulation (dee-gran-yoo-lay′shun): process that occurs in a white blood cell whereby a lysosome containing digestive enzymes digests an entraped bacterium.

Dehydration synthesis (de″hi-dra′shun sin′the-sis): a chemical reaction in which water is removed from smaller molecules to synthesize or make one larger molecule.

Dehydrogenase (de-hi′dro-jen-asz): an enzyme that catalyzes the oxidation of a specific compound by removing a hydrogen atom.

Dementia (de′mencha): being in a deteriorated state of mentality, demonstrated by a marked decline of the patient's formal intellectual level and general emotional apathy.

Denitrifying bacteria (dee-ni′tri-fi-ying bak-tee′re-ah): group of bacteria found in soil that remove nitrogen from nitrates and ammonia, freeing nitrogen into the air.

Dermatophytes (der′mah-to-fitz): group of fungal infections that attack the skin.

Diatoms (di′a-tomz): class of algae that produces silica. These algae are harvested for their commercial value.

Diatomaceous earth (dye-uh-to-may′shus urth): sedimentary rock consisting of empty silaceous shells of diatoms, used as a filtering agent.

Differential staining (dif″er-en-shul sta′ning): adding two or more dyes to differentiate various structures within a substance.

Differentiate (dif-ur-en′shee-ate): the process of making different; an organism's increase in complexity and organization of cells during development.

Diffusion (di-fu′zhun): process of spreading out or movement of molecules through a substance. The larger the molecules the slower the movement. Molecules of a solution of a high concentration move more rapidly toward molecules of a lesser concentration. Temperature and the size of the material holding the substances also influence the rate of movement.

Digenea (di-jen′eah): subclass of the trematode parasites that have two stages of reproduction—one sexual in the mature form and one asexual in the larval form.

Dilute (di′lut): small amount of solute dissolved in a solvent.

Dimorphism (di-mor′fizm): ability to exist in two forms, as in some fungi—at room temperature they grow as molds, with hyphae and mycelium, and at body temperature, they grow as yeasts.

Diphtheria (dif-theer′ee-uh): acute infectious disease caused by the bacterium *Corynebacterium diphtheriae.*

Diphyllobothrium (di-fil″o-both′re-um): genus of large tapeworms. *D. latum* is the fish tapeworm.

Diplobacilli (dip-lo-ba-sil′i): two bacilli joined together end to end as a result of incomplete fission.

Diplococci (dip′lo-cok-si): spherical or coffee bean-shaped cocci occurring in pairs.

Diploid (dip′loid): pair of or two similar chromosomes—2N.

Dipylidium caninum (di-fil′a″de-um ka′nee-yum): tapeworm infecting dogs.

Disaccharide (di-sak′ah-ride): a double sugar formed from two simple sugars or monosaccharides.

Disinfect (dis-in-fekt′): to kill pathogens by chemical or physical means.

Disinfectant (dis″in-fek′tant): any agent or chemical compound that kills pathogens or prevents microorganisms from causing a disease.

Disinfection (dis″in-fek′shun): process of killing pathogenic organisms by chemical or physical means.

Dormant (dor′munt): inactive, quiescent.

DPT vaccine (DPT vak-seen′): a combination vaccine derived from the toxoids of diphtheria, pertussus (whooping cough), and tetanus.

Droplet infection (drop′let in-fek′shun): infection due to the inhaling of respiratory pathogens suspended on liquid particles exhaled by someone who is already infected.

Droplet nuclei (drop′let nuk-le′i): tiny evaporated drops carried in the air containing microorganisms.

Echinococcus (e-ki″no-kok′us): genus of small tapeworms found mostly in dogs and foxes.

Eclipse period (e-klips′pe′ri-od): time or period of darkness without activity.

Ectoplasm (ek″to′plazm): the outer, rigid, relatively granule-free layer of the cytoplasm.

Edematous (e-dem′a-tus): excessive accumulation of fluid in the body tissues, which causes swelling.

Electron microscope (e-lek′tron mi′kro-skop): a microscope in which an electron beam instead of light forms the image for viewing, thus allowing far greater (up to a million times) magnification of the object.

Element (el′e-ment): substance containing only one kind of atom.

Emerging pathogens (e′mer-ging path′-o-jens): microorganisms once not considered to be pathogenic, or cause disease, but are now found to be infectious and cause disease.

Encapsulate (en-kap′sue-late): to surround a part with a capsule.

Endolimax nana (en-do′li-max na′na): a protozoan causing intestinal disorders in humans.

Endoplasm (en-do′plazm): inner, relatively fluid layer of the cytoplasm.

Endoplasmic reticulum (en-do′plaz-mik re′tik-u-lum): network of folded membranes in the cytoplasm of a cell that transport materials throughout the cell.

Endoscope (en′do-skop): instrument used for the visual examination of the interior of a body cavity.

Endospore (en′do-spor): spore formed within the parent cell.

Endotoxin (endo′toxsin): a toxin or poison of lipopoly saccharide found in the cell wall of bacteria, especially gram-negative bacteria. It is thought to play a significant role in many disease complications, especially shock. This type of toxin is released into the body by bacteria already present in the body.

Entamoeba (en″ta′mee-bah): a genus of unicellular amoeba that can parasitize the gastrointestinal tract.

Entamoeba coli (en-ta′me-bah co′li): protozoan that causes intestinal disorders in humans.

Entamoeba hartmanni (en-ta′me-bah hart′man-i): protozoan that causes intestinal disorders in humans.

Entamoeba histolytica (en-ta′me-bah his-to′lit-i-ka): protozoan that causes intestinal disorders in humans.

Enteric (en-ter′ik): pertaining to the small intestine.

Enterobacter aerogenes (en″ter-o-bak′ter air′rah-jen-eez): a species of gram-negative facultative anaerobic rod-shaped enteric bacteria that frequently causes upper respiratory, urinary, and nosocomial infections.

Enterobacteriaceae (en″ter-o-bak-ter″e-a′se-e): family of gram-negative facultative anaerobic rod-shaped bacilli that inhabit the large intestine as well as soil, water, and plants. Several species can be opportunistic or nosocomial pathogens and some cause urinary and respiratory infections.

Enterobius vermicularis (en″ter-o′by-us ver′mik-u″layr-is): species of tiny roundworms, called pinworms, that infect primarily children. This parasite inhabits the large intestine, bowel, and especially the appendix. Worms lay their eggs at the anal opening most often during the night.

Enzyme (en′zim): 1. any protein that acts as a catalyst. It increases the rate of a biochemical reaction without being changed in the reaction. Enzymes are necessary for life functions and are very specific in that each enzyme acts on only one compound or substrate. Enzyme names tend to end in *-ase.* 2. Metabolic catalyst that speeds up, slows down, or alters the rate of a biochemical reaction without being changed in the reaction.

Enzyme-Substrate complex (en′zim sub′strate complex): the temporary binding of an enzyme molecule and a substrate molecule, during which time the enzyme activity takes place.

Epidemic (ep″i-dem′ik): pertaining to the outbreak of a disease or diseases that occur in unusually high occurrences during certain times and places.

Epidemiology (ep″i-de″me-ol′o-jee): study of factors surrounding spread, frequency, and distribution of diseases, injury, and other health-related events.

Epidemiologist (ep″i-de″me-ol′o-jist): one who specializes in the study of factors surrounding spread, frequency, and distribution of diseases, injury, and other health-related events.

Epidermophyton (ep′i-der″mof‴i-ton): a genus of fungus that attacks both skin and nails but not hair. It causes athlete's foot.

Equilibrium (e″kwi-lib′re-um): state of balance between two reactions or opposing forces.

Ergot mold (ur′got mold): a mold which grows on the rye plant, and is caused by the fungus Claviceps purpurea.

Erythrocytes (e-rith′ro-sitz): red blood cells.

Escherichia coli (esh″e-rik′e-ah co′li): gram-negative facultative anaerobic rod-shaped bacillus found to be the main inhabitant of the large intestine of humans. Some strains cause severe colitis, especially in young children.

Euglena (yu-glee′nah): genus of unicellular chlorophyll-producing parasites that stagnate fresh water.

Eukaryote (u-kar′e-ot): organisms whose cells have a true nucleus held by a nuclear membrane. It has chromosomes and divides by mitosis.

Exobiology (ek″so-bi-ol′o-je): extraterrestrial biology.

Exbiota (eks′bye-o-tuh): life forms outside of the earth and its atmosphere.

Excrement (ex′cre-ment): fecal waste material discharged from an organism.

Exoenzyme (ek″so-en′zim): enzyme that acts outside the cell that secrets it.

Exotoxin (exo′toxsin): a toxin or poison produced by microorganisms that is released into the surrounding environment, such as in *Clostridium botulinium.* The toxin is released into the food or meat while still in the can. This exotoxin is poisonous when one eats the contaminated food.

Facultative anaerobes (fak′ul-ta″tiv an-a′er-obz): organisms that can live and grow with or without the presence of molecular oxygen.

Fasciola (fah-si′o-lah): genus of flatworms or trematodes, called "flukes" (worms that are flat, fleshy, and leaf shaped), that parasitize the liver.

Fasciolopsis (fas″e-o-lop′sis): a genus of the trematode flukes.

Fastidious (fas-ti′di-us): organisms that are difficult to grow, requiring specialized or enhanced culture media for growth.

Feline (fe′line): pertaining to cats.

Fermentation (fer″men-ta′shun): the decomposition of a carbohydrate in the absence of oxygen.

Fever (fe′ver): abnormally high body temperature. Normal body temperature is 37°C (98.6°F). Normal rectal temperatures are slightly higher, while normal axillary temperatures are slightly lower.

Filamentous (fil-uh-men′tus): threadlike.

Filterable virus (fil′ter-ah-bl vi′rus): a virus capable of passing through the pores of a filter that retains other microorganisms.

Filtrate (fil′trat): liquid that passes through a filter.

Filtration (fil′tra-shun): process of a fluid passing through a filter.

Fimbria: (fim′bree-uh) [pl. fimbriae (fim′bree-ee)]: fringelike protrusion from the outer extremity of the fallopian tube.

Fission (fish′un): asexual reproduction common in bacteria and protozoa in which the cell splits into two or more daughter parts, each of which becomes a new organism.

Fixation (fik-say′shun): chemical process used to kill or preserve cells or tissues for microscopic study.

Fixed phagocytes (fix′d fag-o′sitz): tissue cells that comprise the reticuloendothelial system (RES) and are firmly attached to liver, spleen, bone marrow, and lymph node tissues.

Fixing (fix′ing): process of adhering material to a slide or a stain to material by heating or by the addition of a chemical fixative such as iodine or methanol.

Flagella (flah′jel-la): (s. flagellum) flexible whiplike structure found on cells and microorganisms, used as an organ of locomotion.

Flagellate (flah′gel-ate): one-celled microorganism possessing flagella.

Flagellin (flah′jel-in): a protein subunit from which a bacterial flagellum is made.

Flash method (flash meth′ud): method of pasteurizing milk whereby it is rapidly heated for 30 seconds, then rapidly cooled. Also called "high temperature short-time method."

Flora (flo′ruh): microorganisms present in a given area (e.g., intestinal flora, skin flora, urogenital flora). Flora are not normally considered to be pathogenic.

Fomites (fo′mits) (sing., fomes): inanimate objects or material such as bedding, clothing, or a bedpan upon which disease-producing agents can be spread.

Food vacuole (food vak′u-ol): hole or opening in the protoplasm of a cell that gathers food for the organism.

Formula (for′mu-lah): chemical symbols used to describe compounds. Formulas by definition describe the proportion of each element present in a compound. For example, $CaCl_2$ has one calcium atom for every two chloride atoms.

Fungi (fun-ji′) (sing., fungus): low form of eukaryotic microscopic plant life lacking chlorophyll; may be filamentous (mold) or unicellular (yeast).

Fusarium (fu-sa′re-um): genus of fungi found everywhere in nature and on decaying foods.

Gametocyte (gah-met′o-sit): sexual stage of the malarial parasite that can produce one of the two sex cells or gametes.

Gamma globulin (gam′ah glah-bu′lun): a class of protein composed almost entirely of immunoglobulins, the proteins that make the antibodies.

Gastritis (gas-tri′tis): inflammation of the stomach lining. It may be bacterial, viral, parasitic, or chemical.

Gene (jen): one of the biological units of heredity found on chromosomes. Genes make up segments of the DNA molecule. There are thousands of genes in the chromosomes of each cell nucleus.

General infection (gen′e-ral in′fek-shun): infection that has spread to many parts of the body.

Geneticist: (je-net′i-sist): scientist specializing in the study of genes and chromosomes.

Germicide (jer′mi-sid): agent that destroys pathogenic microorganisms.

Germicidal (jer″mi-si′dal): destructive to pathogenic microorganisms.

Germinate (jur′mi-nate): to start growth in a seed or spore.

Germ (jerm) **theory:** belief that living microorganisms cause disease.

Giardia (je-ar′de-ah): genus of flagellate protozoa spread by contaminated food and water and found in the intestine of humans that causes diarrhea, weight loss, and gastrointestinal discomfort.

Giardia intestinalis (je-ar′de-ah in-test′in-al-is): flagellate protozoa that causes intestinal disorders in humans.

Giardia lamblia (je-ar′de-ah lam′bleah): flagellate protozoa that causes intestinal disorders in humans.

Glucan (glu′kan): a polymer of glucose subunits that when joined together form a cell wall of glucan in some fungi.

Glycoalyx (gly-ko-kal′ix): a type of bacterial capsule that enables the bacteria to stick to environmental surfaces.

Golgi apparatus (gol′je ap″ah-ra′tus): organelle in cells that packages and wraps proteins (enzymes, hormones, etc.) for export out of the cell.

Gram stain (gram stan): standardized procedure for staining bacteria according to their ability to accept and retain dyes based on certain characteristics in the composition of their cell walls. The gram characteristics are used as the starting point in the identification process for all bacteria. Gram-positive bacteria retain the initial crystal violet stain due to the peptidoglycan and teichoic acid in the cell wall that resist dissolution by the acid-alcohol decolorizer. Gram-negative bacteria lose their outer lipoprotein and lipopolysaccharide layer in the decolorizing process, leaving the now naked peptidoglycan layer to accept the safranin counterstain.

Gram-variable (gram ve′re-abl): sometimes older bacterial cultures, although gram positive will show borderline or variable reaction because they fail to retain the crystal violet stain. Additionally, bacteria grown on acid media may also show this gram-variable reaction.

Haemophilus (he-mof′i-lus): genus of gram-negative cocco-bacillary, facultative anaerobic bacteria that can cause pink eye, meningitis, and ear and respiratory infections. Often requires chocolate agar, among other nutrients, for optimal growth.

Haploid (hap′loid): single chromosome number, or half the diploid number. N numbers of chromosomes, or one of each type, is found in each cell.

Helix (hel′iks): coiled or spiraled structure winding around a uniform tube in a staircase manner.

Helminths (hel′minthz): parasitic worm; a nematode (roundworm) or trematode (fluke).

Hemolysin (hee-mo-lye′sin): a substance that frees hemoglobin from the red blood cells by breaking them open or destroying the cells.

Hemolyze (also hem′ol-liz) (he′mo-liz): the rupture of red blood cells releasing the hemoglobin.

HEPA (high-efficiency particulate air): filters that can deliver clean air to an enclosure, such as a cubicle or a room.

Hepatitis B (hep″ah-ti′tis): a viral infection attacking the liver, transmitted to humans via blood, tears, saliva, semen and contaminated needles. It is easily transmitted to health care workers through needle-stick injuries and improper handling of specimens.

Hepatomegaly (hep″ah-to-meg′ah-le): enlargement of the liver.

Herpesvirus group (her′pez-vi′rus grup): any of a large group of viruses, including herpes simplex I and II viruses, herpes zoster (shingles), and varicella (chicken pox).

Heterotrophic (het″er-o-trof′ik): type of nutrition in which an organism requires for its growth a source of carbon much more complex than is carbon dioxide.

High-temperature short-time (HTST) method: a method of pasteurizing milk. See also flash method.

Histiocytes (his′-te-o-sites): a name sometimes given to macrophages located in tissues.

Histoplasma (his″to-plaz′mah): a genus of pathogenic fungi that usually begins in the lungs and often has no symptoms until it begins to spread to other organs. *H. capsulatum* is common in the rural Midwest but is being seen more today as an opportunistic infection of immunocompromised patients.

Histoplasma capsulatum (his-to-plaz-mah cap-sul-at-um): a dimorphic fungus that causes histoplasmosis.

Homogeneous (ho″mo-je′ne-us): of uniform quality, composition, or structure.

Hookworm (hook′wurm): a parasitic roundworm that enters the body through the skin and migrates to the intestine where it attaches itself to the wall of the intestine with its hooklets and sucks blood for its food.

Host (host): plant or animal that harbors and provides sustenance for another organism.

Hydrocarbon (hi″dro-kar′bon): organic compounds containing only hydrogen and carbon.

Hydrolysis (hi-drol′i-sis): splitting of a compound into two parts by addition of water to a substance.

Hydronium ion (hi-dro′ne-um i′on): hydrated proton H_3O^+ as it exists in aqueous solution.

Hydroxide (hi-drok′side): negatively charged ion OH- formed when a base or alkali is dissolved in water.

Hydrophic (hi′dro-fik): substance that is not attracted to water.

Hydrophilic (hi″dro-fil′ik): substance that can readily react with or combine with water.

Hydrophobic (hi″dro-fo′bik): insoluble in water, does not absorb water.

Hydrotrophic (hi″dro-tro′fik): a nonmotile organism that demonstrates a growth response in the presence of water or moisture.

Hymenolepis (hi″men-ol′e-pis): genus of dwarf tapeworms found in humans.

Hypergammaglobulinemia (hi″per-gam″ah-glob″u-lin-e-me-ah): increase of gamma globulins in the blood.

Hypersensitive (hi″per-sen′si-tiv): exaggerated immune response to certain allergens that causes reactions ranging from hives to anaphylactic shock.

Hypersensitivity (hi″per-sen′si-tiv-i-tee): condition in which the body reacts with an exaggerated immune response to a foreign agent.

Hypertonic solution (hi″per-ton′ik so-loo′shun): solution with an osmotic pressure greater than the one with which it is being compared. If compared with normal or isotonic saline it will have a concentration greater than 0.85%.

Hypha (hi′fa): (pl. hyphae) one of the filamentous threads or filaments composing the mycelium of a fungus.

Hypotonic solution (hi″po-ton′ik so-loo′shun): solution with an osmotic pressure less than the one with which it is being compared. If compared with normal or isotonic saline it will have a concentration less than 0.85%.

Hypothesis (hi-poth′e-sis): educated guess based on reasonable experimentation to explain a group of phenomena.

Immiscible (i-mis′i-b′l): not susceptible to being mixed.

Immune (i-mun′): to have resistance to, to overcome disease, or be protected from infection by the presence of antibodies.

Immune serum (i-mun′ ser′um): protein substance such as gamma globulin or another serum with antibodies present that is injected to produce a passive immunity.

Immunity (i-mu′ni-te): condition brought about by the immune system to give protection from an infectious agent.

Immunization (im″u-ni-za′shun): process of making one immune or protected from a disease by injecting a vaccine. Also called an "inoculation" or "vaccination."

Immunocompromised (im″u-no-kom′pro-mizd): having the immune system weakened by the administration of immunosuppressive drugs, irradiation, malnutrition, and by certain disease processes, such as AIDS.

Immunoglobulin (im″u-no-glob′u-lin): any of several proteins of animal origin with a known antibody activity.

Immunology (im″u-nol′o-je): study of the structure and function of the immune system.

Immunosuppression (im″u-no-su′presh′un): inhibition of the formation of antibodies to antigens that may be present. It may be induced as part of therapy (as after organ transplantation), or it may be a result of clinical symptoms. See also Immunocompromised.

Impetigo (im″pe-ti′go): a highly contagious skin infection caused by group A streptococci marked by pustular vesicles that rupture and form yellow crusts. It is common in children and is easily spread.

Incubation period (in″ku-ba′shun peer′ee-ud): time required for development, as in symptoms of disease after infection.

Infection (in-fek′shun): invasion and multiplication of microorganisms in body tissues.

Infection control practitioner (ICP) (in-fek′shun con′trol prak-tish′un-er): an individual who practices prevention of disease, such as an infection control officer.

Infectious hepatitis (in-fek′shus hep-e-ti′tis): inflammation of the liver characterized by jaundice and fever; hepatitis A virus (HAV).

Infestation (in-fes-tay′shun): living on or within the skin of the host by animal parasites, usually insects.

Inflammation (in″flah-ma′shun): localized protective response to an injury, or destruction of the surrounding tissues in which the area swells, heats up, and reddens due to the increased blood flow to the site.

Infusion (in-fu′zhun): steeping of a substance in water to obtain its soluble principles. Infusion flows by gravity.

Inoculating loop (i-nok′u-late-ing lup): a specially adapted long thin holder with a wire loop attached for plating bacteria onto culture media. Plastic disposable loops are also available.

Insoluble (in-sol′u-b′l): unable to be dissolved.

Interferon (in″ter-fer′on): a natural glycoprotein released by cells that are invaded by viruses, rickettsias, and even some bacteria. Interferon initiates noninfected cells to produce another protein with antiviral characteristics. It has great promise as a cancer treatment.

Intracellular (in″trah-sel-u-lar): within or inside a cell.

Intradermal (in″trah-der′mal): within the dermis layer of the skin.

In vitro (in vee′tro): "in glass"; refers to biological experiments done in petri dishes or test tubes.

In vivo (in vee′vo): "in the living"; refers to laboratory experiments testing chemical agents in a living organism.

Ionize (i″on-i-z): dissociation or separation of a substance in solution to ions or charged particles.

Isomer (i′so-mer): compounds that have the same molecular formula but have different structural arrangements of the molecules.

Isotonic solution (i″so-ton′ik so-loo′shun): solution with the same tonicity as the one with which it is being compared. A solution in which body cells can be bathed without a net loss of water on either side of the semipermeable membrane.

Ixodes dammini (ik-so′dez dam′mi-ni): species of hard-bodied ticks found in the Midwest and eastern parts of the United States that are carriers of the bacterium that causes Lyme disease.

Ixodes pacificus (ik-so′dez pa′si-fi-kus): species of hard-bodied ticks found in California and along the western coast of the United States that are carriers of the bacterium that causes Lyme disease.

Kaposi's sarcoma (kap′o-sez sar-ko-′mah): a metastasizing malignant sarcoma of the skin. It is an opportunistic neoplasm most often associated with AIDS.

Koch's postulates (koks pos′tu-lats): a set of rules or criteria set down by Robert Koch that must be met in order for a microorganism to be established as the cause of a given disease.

Labile (la′bil): chemically unstable, susceptible to heat.

Laminar airflow (lam′i-nur aer-flo): flow of air currents in which streams do not intermingle; air moves along parallel flow lines.

Latent (la′tent): dormant, an inactive period.

Leukocidin (lew-ko-sigh′din): a toxic substance that kills white blood cells.

Leukocytes (lew′ko-sitz): white blood cells, some of which are ameboid in shape and can destroy invading pathogens.

Leukopenia (loo″ko-pe′ne-ah): a decrease in the number of white blood cells.

Lipid (lip′id): group of substances, including fats, greases, oils, and waxes, that are insoluble in water and soluble in nonpolar solvents as ether, hexane, and chloroform. Lipids may be simple, as in triglycerides, or neutral fats or compound lipids, as the phospholipids in lecithin, and fatty acids, as in cholesterol.

Lipoprotein (lip″o-pro′teen): large macromolecular structures containing a simple protein and a lipid—the form in which lipids are transported in the blood. There are four such classes: (1) Chylomicrons transport lipids after a meal from the intestine to the tissues; (2) VLDL (very-low-density lipoproteins) produced by the liver; (3) HDL (high-density lipoproteins) also produced by the liver; (4) LDL (low-density lipoproteins) produced by the metabolism of VLDL.

Local infection (lo′kal in′fek-shun): infection that is restricted to one area of the body.

Lockjaw (lok′jaw): common name for the disease tetanus.

Low-temperature holding (LTH) method: a method of pasteurizing milk in which it is chilled immediately upon collection then later heated for 30 minutes and finally rapidly cooled.

Lustrous (lus′trus): shiny, a characteristic attributed to metals.

Lymphadenopathy (lim-fad″e-nop′ah-thee): disease that enlarges the lymph nodes.

Lymphoma (lim-fo′mah): any neoplastic (malignant) disorder of the lymphoid tissue, as Hodgkin's disease.

Lymphopenia (lim″fo-pe′ne-ah): decrease in the number of lymphocytes in the blood.

Lyophilization (li-of″i-li-za′shun): preparation of a stable biological substance by rapid freezing and dehydration of the frozen product under a high vacuum.

Lyse (lize): to destroy, break open, or to cause a disruption or dissolution of cells, bacteria, or tissue.

Lysin (li′sin): antibody that causes complement-dependent lysis or destruction of cells.

Lysosome (li′so-som): one of the cell organelles that aid in the digestion of proteins by secreting digestive enzymes.

Lysozyme (li′so-zim): a protein enzyme present in saliva, tears, and many animal fluids that functions as an antibacterial agent. It is secreted from the lysosome organelle of a cell to digest dying parts of the cell.

Macroconidia (mak-ro′ko-nid′i-ah): very large conidia.

Macromolecule (mak″ro-mol′e-kul): very large molecule such as those in proteins, polysaccharides, or rubber.

Macronucleus (mak-ro-new′klee-us): the larger of two nuclei found in the paramecium. Its metabolic control functions.

Macrophage (mak-ro′faj): large mononuclear leukocytes that originate in the bone marrow and are released into circulation as immature monocytes en route to the tissues. In the tissues, they become macrophages waiting to participate in the immune process to function as phagocytes.

Mastigophora (mas″ti-gof′o-rah): a subphylum of protozoa that have one or more flagella and a centrally located nucleus.

Meiosis (mee-o′sis): a process of cell division in which reproductive cells or gametes are formed. At the completion of the two phases four daughter cells are formed and gamete will contain N numbers of chromosomes.

Meningitis (men-″in-ji′tis): inflammation of the membranes covering the brain and spinal cord and associated with acute febrile illness usually caused by the presence of a virus, bacterium, or a fungus.

Mesosome (mez′o-sohm): invagination or inpocketing of the bacterial cell membrane important in cell wall synthesis.

Microaerophilic (mi″kro-a″er-o-fil′ik): organisms that require less than the normal amount of oxygen to grow. Prefers a reduced oxygen atmosphere for growth.

Microbes (mi′krobs): organisms that can be seen only with the aid of a microscope.

Microbiology (mi″kro-bi-ol′o-je): the study of organisms that can be seen only through a microscope including, bacteria, fungi, viruses, parasites, and rickettsia.

Micrococcus tetragenus (mi-kro-kok′us te-tradj′e-nus): gram-positive coccus found in soil and air and also in the sputum of tuberculosis patients.

Microconidia (mik-ro′ko-nid′i-ah): tiny or very small conidia.

Microfilament (mi″kro′fil-a-ment): microscopic threadlike structures that provide for ameboid motility in eukaryotic cells.

Microfilaria (mi″kro′fi-la″re-ah): prelarval stage of the Filariodea family that are found in the blood of humans and in the tissues of the vector.

Micrometer (mi-krom′e-ter): a unit of length equal to one millionth of a meter used to measure microscopic distances and sizes.

Micronucleus (mi-kro-new′klee-us): the smaller of the two nuclei found in the paramecium. It controls reproductive activities.

Microorganisms (mi″kro-or′gah-nizmz): organisms that can be seen only with the aid of a microscope.

Microscope (mi′kro-skop): instrument containing a light source and a magnifying lens that enlarges minute particles.

Microsporum (mi″kro-spo′rum): a genus of fungi that causes diseases of the skin and hair.

Microtubule (mi″kro′tube-yule): eukaryotic cell organelle needed for cellular support and secretion.

Milliliter (mil′i-le-ter): one one-thousandth part of a liter, which is the base unit for volume in the metric system. Abbreviation is ml.

Millimeter (mil′i-me-ter): one one-thousandth part of a meter, which is the base unit for length in the metric system. Abbreviation is mm.

Miscible (mis′i-bl): able to be mixed in a solution.

Mitochondria (mi″to-kon′dre-ah): rod-shaped organelle of cells that is responsible for cellular respiration and energy production.

Mitosis (mi-to′sis): process of cell division in which the nucleus divides to form two new cells. Each daughter cell will contain 2N chromosomes.

Mixture (miks′tur): substance containing different types of molecules that may be physically but not chemically combined.

Mobile phagocytes (mo′bil fag′o-cites): white blood cells that wander or rove about to find the injured site.

Mold (mold): common name given to fungi that produce long filaments.

Molecule (mol′e-kule): joining together of two or more atoms to function as a unit; For example, OH=hydroxide and H_2O=water.

Monera (mo-ne′rah): a kingdom of unicellular organisms without true nuclei; prokaryotes including bacteria, blue-green algae, actinomyces, and viruses.

Monocular microscope (mon-ok′u-lar mi′kro-skop): microscope with only one eyepiece.

Monosaccharide (mon″o-sak′ah-ride): A simple sugar that cannot be further broken down into simpler substances by hydrolysis.

Moraxella catarrhalis (mor′ ex-ah lla kat-a-ray′lus): a gram-negative coccus commonly found to inhabit the upper respiratory tract (formerly *Branhamella catarrhalis* and *Neisseria catarrhalis*).

Morphology (mor″fol′o-je): form, structure, and shape of organism.

Mucor (mu′kor): a genus of saprophytic fungi found in nature and on rotting food.

Multicellular (mul″ti-sel′u-lar): many cells together to form a plant or animal. Composed of many cells.

Mutagenic (mu″tah-jen′ik): a change in the genetic structure of an organism that eventually changes its characteristics.

Mutate (mu′tate): to change the genetic material, which can eventually lead to a change in the characteristics of an organism.

Mycelium (mi-se′le-um): mass of threadlike hyphae.

Mycobacteria (mi″ko-bak-te′re-ah): a genus of gram-positive aerobic acid-fast rodlike bacteria. Notable members cause tuberculosis and leprosy. Many previously thought to be saprophytic strains are found as opportunistic infections in immunocompromised patients.

Mycoplasma (mi″ko-plaz′mah): a genus of highly pleomorphic gram-negative aerobic bacteria that lack cell walls, including the pleuropneumonialike organisms (PPLO).

Mycoplasma pneumoniae (mi″ko-plaz′mah nu-mo′ne-ay): cause of primary atypical pneumonia chiefly among young people under 30.

Mycoses (mi-ko′ses): any disease caused by a fungus.

Myxovirus group (mik″so-vi′rus): any of a group of RNA viruses, including influenza, parainfluenza, mumps, and Newcastle disease. Myxoviruses characteristically cause red blood cells in chickens to agglutinate.

Narrow-spectrum antibiotics (na-row′ spek′trum an″ti-bi-ot′ikz): chemotherapeutic substances of microbial origin that are capable of inhibiting or killing either gram-negative or gram-positive bacteria, but not both types.

Natural acquired immunity (na′tur-al a-kyi′yerd i-mu′ni-te): presence of antibodies that results with-out having had the disease, but that have built up over time.

Natural immunity (na′tur-al i-mu′ni-te): immunity attributed to antibodies present without any obvious stimulus. It may result from one's genetic inherited traits. It is frequently found in newborns and tends to decrease to a low concentration in infancy and later rises to moderate levels during childhood.

Necator (ne-ka′tor): a genus of hookworms found primarily in the Americas that cause intestinal disorders.

Neisseria (ni-se′re-ah): genus of gram-negative aerobic or facultative anaerobic cocci. Members may be normal flora of the respiratory tract or they may cause genital infections (gonorrhea) or central nervous system infections (meningitis).

Neisseria gonorrhoeae (ni-se′re-ah kat-a-rai′lus): gram-negative intracellular facultative anaerobic diplococcus that causes gonorrhea, a sexually transmitted disease.

Neisseria meningitidis (ni-se′re-ah kat-a-rai′lus): gram-negative facultative anaerobic coccus that causes meningitis.

Nematode (nem′ah-tod): roundworm

Neurodegenerative (nyer′o de′gen er-ativ): the degeneration or breakdown of nervous tissue including brain cells.

Neurospora (nu-ros′po-rah): genus of fungi including the pink bread molds.

Neutralism (nu′tral-izm): relationship between two organisms in which neither one affects the other.

Neutralization (nu′tra-liz-a-shun): process of making the pH of a substance neutral—neither basic nor acidic.

Nitrifying bacteria (ni′tri-fi-ying bak-tee′re-ah): group of bacteria that convert the nitrogen of ammonia (NH_3) to nitrates (NO_3^-) and nitrites (NO_2^-).

Nitrites (ni′tritz): salt of nitrous acid. Organic nitrites are produced by certain bacteria.

Nitrogen-fixing bacteria (ni-tro′jen fix′ing bak-tee′re-ah): soil bacteria that convert free atmospheric nitrogen (N_2) into ammonia (NH_3).

Nonencapsulated (non″en-kap′sue-la-ted): not enclosed in a capsule or sheath covering.

Nonpathogenic bacteria (non-path-o′je-nik bak-tee′re-ah): bacteria that do not cause disease.

Normal flora (nor′mal flo′rah): specific microorganisms that live in a specific area of a host without causing disease. The upper respiratory tract has several microorganisms present that do not cause disease. The mouth, skin, and bowel are also sites for these commensals.

Nosocomial (nos″o-ko′me-al): pertaining to or originating in a hospital.

Nosocomial infection (nos″o-ko′me-al in-fek′shun): infection or disease not carried by the patient but that originated from within a hospital environment.

Nuclear membrane (nu′kle-er mem′brain): thin covering that surrounds the nucleus of a cell.

Nucleic acid (nu-kle′ik asid): organic compounds of either DNA or RNA, containing carbon, hydrogen, nitrogen, and phosphorus.

Nucleoid (nu′klee-oid): small area found in prokaryotic cells containing genetic material. It is not a true nucleus because it is not surrounded by a nuclear membrane. Resembling a nucleus.

Nucleotide (nu′kle-o-tide): subunits of nucleic acids composed of three repeating molecular groups—a five-carbon sugar, a nitrogen base, and a phosphate group.

Nucleus (nu′kle-us): control center for all cell activity. Contains the chromosomes and DNA.

Nucleolus (nu-kle′o-lus): a rounded body in the nucleus of most cells that is the site of ribosomal RNA synthesis.

Nutrient agar (nu′tre-ent ah-ger′): gelatinlike culture media that is solid at room temperature and provides the basic foods needed to grow bacteria.

Nutrient broth (nu′tre-ent broth): liquid culture media that is liquid at room temperature and provides the basic foods needed to grow bacteria.

Objective lens (ob-jek′tiv lenz): lens or lens system in a microscope located nearest the object being viewed. In a compound microscope they are usually mounted on a revolving nosepiece or turret.

Obligate anaerobe (ob′li-gate an-a′er-ob): microorganism that can live and grow only in the absence of molecular oxygen.

Obligate intracellular parasites: (ob′li-gate in′trah-sel-u-lar par-a-site): parasites that can exist only inside cellular material.

Ocular lens (ok′u-lar lenz): eyepiece lens in a microscope.

Oil-immersion objective (oil i-mer′zhun ob-jek′tiv): objective lens that requires a drop of clear oil to clarify the object being viewed. It is usually the 100X magnification objective lens.

Opportunistic (op″or-too-nis′tik): refers to an organism that does not normally cause disease but can become pathogenic under certain conditions.

Opportunistic pathogen (op″or-too-n is′tik path-o′jen): organism that does not normally cause disease in a healthy person but does become pathogenic under certain conditions, especially when the host is immunocompromised or immunosuppressed.

Opportunistic infection (op″or-too-n is′tik in-fek′shun): infection that does not pose a threat to a person with a normal healthy immune system but seizes the opportunity to infect those with a weakened immune system.

Opsonin (op-so′nin): antibody that renders bacteria and other foreign cells susceptible to phagocytes.

Optics (op′tiks): pertaining to the eye or the eyepiece of the microscope.

Optimal temperature (op′ti-mal tem-per′a-chur): ideal or best temperature for growth.

Oral hairy leukoplakia (luko′plak ya): An infection of the mouth similar to thrush (which is caused by a yeast infection). Despite having similar symptoms, its cause is not known.

Organic compound (or-gan′ik kom′pownd): a chemical substance derived from living organisms consisting of carbon, hydrogen, and nitrogen.

Organelle (or-gah-nel′): specialized structures found with the cytoplasm of cells, each with a specific function.

OSHA: Occupational Safety and Health Administration.

Osmolality (oz″mo-lal′i-te): the concentration of a solution in terms of moles of solute per kilogram of solvent.

Osmosis (oz-mo′sis): passage of a solvent's molecules (such as water) through a selective permeable (meaning only the solvent's molecules, not the solute molecules can pass through) membrane from a solution of lesser solute concentration to a solution of greater solute concentration.

Osmotic pressure (os-mah′tik presh′ur): pressure exerted by water molecules within the selective permeable membrane, expressed in millimeters of mercury (mm Hg).

Oxidation (ok″si-da′shun): combining of a compound with oxygen to result in an increase of positive charges (protons) or a loss of negative charges (electrons).

Papovavirus group (pap″o-vah-vi′rus): a group of small DNA viruses including the papilloma viruses and warts. Many are potentially carcinogenic.

Paragonimus (par″ah-gon′i-mus): genus of the trematode parasites with two invertebrate hosts, the snail and the crab or crayfish. *P. westermani* is a liver fluke common in Asia.

Paramecium (par″ah-me′she-um): genus of ciliated protozoans found in fresh water that do not usually infect humans.

Para-aminobenzoic acid (PABA) (pa′ra-ah-meen′o-ben-zo′ik asid): an organic acid that helps some bacteria to form folic acid, a substance required for growth.

Paramyxovirus group (par″ah-mik″so-vi′rus): subgroup of the myxovirus group that are larger, including mumps and measles viruses.

Parasites (par′ah-sitz): organisms that live on or within another living organism at whose expense it obtains some advantage.

Parasitism (par′a-sit-izm): 1. Condition that exists in which one organism living off another adversely affects that organism, but the affected organism cannot live without the parasitizing organism. 2. To be infected or infested with parasites.

Paratyphoid fever (par-e-tye′foid fee′vur): an acute intestinal disease, caused by *Salmonella schottmuelleri* and *Salmonella cholerasuis,* similar to typhoid fever, but less severe.

Parfocal (par-fo′kal): microscopes that have their objective lens mounted such that when they are rotated the focus of the microscope is not changed.

Passive acquired immunity (pas′siv a-qwi′yrd i-mew′ni-tee): immunity that results from having received antibodies from another source. This immunity is short-lived. The transfer of mother's antibodies to baby in utero as well as through breast milk (especially colostrum); lasts several months until the infant can begin making its own antibodies.

Pasteurization (pas″ter-i-za′shun): a heating process originally developed by Louis Pasteur to destroy pathogenic bacteria in beer and wine and later used also for milk.

Pathogen (path′o-jen): disease-causing microorganism.

Pathogenic bacteria (path-o′jen-ik bak-tee′re-ah): bacteria that are capable of producing disease.

Pathogenicity (path″o-je-nis′i-te): ability of an organism to cause disease.

Pathologist (pah-thol′-o-jist): a medical doctor who specializes in the study of disease.

Pediculus (pe-dik′u-lus): genus of lice. *P. humnanus* or *P. capitis* is head lice.

Pellicle (pel′i-kul): a surface cell membrane surrounding the paramecium.

Penicillium (pen″i-sil-i′um): a genus of fungi consisting of the blue molds found on moist foods as fruit or bread. The antibiotic penicillin is derived from this mold.

Penicillium notatum (pen″i-sil-i′um no-tat′um): bluish mold found on bread and in cheese. It is the species used to produce penicillin, a common antibiotic.

Peptide bond (pep′tide bond): carbon-nitrogen (C-N) bond formed between amino acids.

Peristalis (perr-i-stal′sis): rhythmic and wavelike contractions of the digestive tract which push food through the tract.

Petri dish counter (pe′tri dish cown′ter): a magnifying device scored into squares and used to count colonies of bacteria growing in culture media. Bacterial cell counts are most often performed in public health testing of milk and water.

pH (pee aich): negative logarithm of the hydrogen ion concentration. Values greater than 7 are acidic and values less than 7 are basic or alkaline.

Phage (faj): a virus of bacteria; a bacteriophage.

Phagocyte (fag″o-site): certain white blood cells capable of engulfing microorganisms or other cells and foreign materials.

Phagocytosis (fag″o-si-to′sis): engulfing and digestion of microorganisms or other cells and foreign materials by certain white blood cells capable of this phenomenon.

Phagolysosome (fag″o-lye′so-som): organelle formed by the fusion of a lysosome with a phagosome in a white blood cell.

Phagosome (fag′o-som): a single membrane body found in a white blood cell. It is formed when two pseudopods fuse to entrap a bacterium.

Phase (faz): pertains to the states of matter—solid, liquid, or gas.

Phase-contrast microscopy (faz kon′trast mi-kros′ko-pee): ability of a microscope to alter the phase relationships of the light passing through so that the parts and shadings of an object can be seen without the aid of stains or other special preparations.

Phenol coefficient (fe′nol ko′e-fish-unt): killing power of a germicide toward a test organism as compared with that of phenol against the same organism.

Photosynthesis (fo″to-sin′the-sis): process in green plants by which carbohydrates for energy are formed from carbon dioxide, water, chlorophyll, and the action of light.

Phospholipid bilayer (fos″fo-lip′id bye′lay-ur): term applied to the composition of the cell membrane. A phospholipid is a lipid compound containing a form of phosphoric acid, a fatty acid, an alcohol, and a nitrogenous base. Embedded within the phospholipid bilayer (double layer) are large protein molecules.

Phthirus (thir′us): genus of lice. *P. pubis* is the pubic or crab louse.

Picornavirus group (pi-kor″nah-vi′rus): a group of extremely small RNA viruses, including the enteroviruses (polio) and the rhinovirus (common cold) groups.

Pili (pi′li): (sing., pi′lus) fine, slender, hairlike structures arising from the basal bodies in the cytoplasmic membrane of many bacterial cells.

Pilus bridge (pi′lus brij): a genetic transfer mechanism in which a bridge consisting of a pilus (pl. pili) links tow bacteria together allowing genetic information to be passed from one bacterium to another.

Pinocytic vesicle (pin′o-sit-ik ves′i-cl): pockets or folds in the cell membrane that allow large molecules such as proteins and lipids to be taken into the cell.

Pinocytosis (pin″o-si-to′sis): mechanism by which cells can ingest large molecules from extracellular fluids by forming invaginations in the cell membrane that close and break off to form fluid-filled vacuoles in the cytoplasm.

Placenta (pla-sen′tah): organ on the uterine wall to which the embryo is attached by way of the umbilical cord.

Plantae (plan′tay): major classification group for all plants. All living matter is classified into one of three kingdoms: plantae, animalia and protista.

Plaque (plak): patch or an abnormal flat area on any external or internal body surface.

Plasmid (plaz′mid): small section of DNA from a donor organism that can be inserted into the DNA of a recipient bacterium.

Plasmodium (plaz-mo′dee-um): genus of sporozoa parasites that attacks blood cells, causing malaria.

Plasmodium falciparum (plaz-mo′dee-um fal-sip′a-rum): species of sporozoa parasites that attacks blood cells, causing malaria.

Plasmodium malariae (plaz-mo′dee-um ma-lar′ee-uh): species of sporozoa parasites that attacks blood cells, causing malaria.

Plasmodium ovale (plaz-mo′dee-um o-val-′ee): species of sporozoa parasites that attacks blood cells, causing malaria.

Plasmodium vivax (plaz-mo′dee-um vi′vaks): species of sporozoa parasites that attacks blood cells, causing malaria.

Plate count (plat cownt): the counting of bacterial colonies on a culture media plate.

Pleomorphic (ple″o-mor″fik): having no definite shape.

Plomaines (plo′manez): products of decomposition of foods which are so badly spoiled that no human could eat them.

Pneumocystis carinii (nu-mo-sis′tis ca-ri′nee-i): microorganism that causes a severe pulmonary pneumonia in patients associated with AIDS and other immunosuppressive diseases. Its classification is still uncertain although most references place it with the protozoa. However some consider it to be a yeastlike fungus because of its genetic characteristics and its ability to take up silver stain.

Polymer (pol′i-mer): collection of repeating molecules forming large molecules, such as starch, cellulose, and plastics.

Polypeptide (pol″e-pep′tide): series of many amino acids linked together by carbon-nitrogen (C-N) bonds.

Polyribosome (pol″ee-rye′bo-som): collection of ribosomes.

Polysaccharide (pol″e-sak′ah-ride): large complex molecules made up of many sugar molecules bonded together in long chains.

Post mortem (post mor′tem): a surgical examination or autopsy performed on the deceased in order to determine the cause of death.

Potable (po′tah-bl): fit to drink.

Poxvirus group (poks-vi′rus): group of similar viruses that produce eruptive pustular diseases, including cowpox (vaccinia), smallpox, and chicken pox.

PPLO: pleuropneumonialike organisms.

Precipitin (pre-sip′i-tin): antibody that reacts with an antigen to give a visible precipitate reaction.

Precipitate (n) (pre′sip-i-tat): resultant production of solid particles when two liquid chemicals are reacted or when two liquids are reacted, such as in antigen-antibody reaction.

Precipitate (adj) (pre′sip-i-tat): to cause a substance to separate into an insoluble form.

Primordial (pri-mor′dee-yul): since the beginning of time.

Prion (pry′on): an infectious agent composed only of a protein substance that is now believed to be the cause of certain neurological degenerative diseases that result in dementia and death.

Proglottid (pro-glot′id): individual body segments that make up a tapeworm. Each section can be regenerated and contains all reproductive capabilities. Eggs are released from the proglottids.

Prognosis (prog-no′sis): forecast of the possible outcome of disease.

Prokaryote (pro-kar′e-ot): unicellular organism lacking a true nucleus and nuclear membrane. Its genetic material consists of a single loop of DNA and no chromosomes.

Property (pra′per-tee): characteristic of a substance.

Protein (pro′teen): 1. large complex organic compounds of amino acids that contain carbon, hydrogen, oxygen, nitrogen, and sometimes sulfur or phosphorus and made up from one or more polypeptides, that are amino acids joined by peptide bonds. 2. Food products that are rich in protein, the building blocks of life, including meat, eggs, fish, cheese and milk.

Protist (pro′tist): a member of the kingdom Protista.

Protista (pro′tis-tah): a kingdom of unicellular organisms having distinct nuclei including protozoa and some algae.

Protozoa (pro″to-zo-ah): subkingdom including unicellular eukaryotic organisms.

Protoplasm (pro′to-plazm): jellylike substance found in living cells. It holds the organelles in place.

Pseudomonas aeruginosa (soo″do-mo′nas a-rig′i-no-sa): gram-negative obligate aerobic rod-shaped bacillus that produces a greenish-blue pigment (cyanin) and fluorescein. It is a major cause of severe, often fatal, nosocomial infections as well as being associated as a secondary infection in patients with severe burns.

Pseudopodia (sue-do-po′dee-uh): temporary projection of the cytoplasm on an ameboid cell that helps it to move or to trap small particles.

Ptomaine (to′mayn): nitrogenous compound formed by microbes from the decay of proteins or dead animal material.

purification (pewr-e-fi-ka′shun): the process of making clean or pure.

Puerperal sepsis (pu-er′per-al sep′sis): infection resulting from an infection (usually streptococcal) originating in the birth canal and spreading from the endometrium throughout the body into the bloodstream. In the mid-nineteenth century this dreaded disease would spread through an entire maternity ward, killing most of the new mothers.

Purulent (pewr′yoo-lunt): to contain, consist of, or form pus.

Pustule (pus′tule): small, rounded raised swelling of the skin containing pus.

Pus (pus): protein-rich liquid inflammation product made up of white cells, cellular debris, and a thin fluid, as in serum.

Putrefactive bacteria (pu″tre-fak′tiv bak-tee′re-ah): bacteria that produce a foul, rotten odor upon their decay.

Pyogenic bacteria (pye-o-jen′ik bak-te′ree-uh): bacteria that produce pus.

Reagent (ree-ay′junt): any substance involved in a chemical reaction or used to detect or determine the presence or characteristics of another substance.

Recipients (re-sip′e-ent): persons who receive something, for example, blood transfusions.

Refractive (re-frak′tiv): capable of bending back.

Resolution (rez″oh-loo′shun): ability of a microscope's lens to make fine distinctions between two very close objects. The greater the resolution, the closer the objects can be and still be viewed as two separate objects.

Reticuloendothelial system (RES) (re-tik′u-lo-en″do-the′le-yal sis′tim): network of cells found throughout the body especially in the blood, connective tissue, spleen, liver, bone marrow, and lymph nodes that aid in the production as well as destruction of blood cells.

Retrovirus (ret″ro-vi′rus): RNA virus capable of replicating or making a DNA virus.

Retting (ret-ing): soaking or exposing fibers to moisture. Also, rotting by being left exposed to moisture.

Rhabdovirus group (rab″do-vi′rus): group of morphologically similar bullet-shaped viruses, including rabies.

Rheumatic fever (roo-mat′ik fee′vur): disease affecting the heart, caused by repeated infections with beta hemolytic group A streptococcus pathogen. It is characterized by inflammation of the heart, blood vessels, connective tissue, and joints.

Rhizoids (rhiz′oid): rootlike structures of a vegetative mycelium that form runners to root a new mold of the *Rhizopus* family.

Rhizopus (ri″zo′pus): genus of fungus found on bread.

Ribose (ri′bos): five-carbon sugar structured in a pentagon.

Ribosome (ri-bo′som): grainy structures attached to the endoplasmic reticulum that contain enzymes to control protein synthesis.

Rickettsia (ri-ket′se-ah): genus of minute-sized bacteria, that stain as gram-negative coccobacilli, often pleomorphic. Unlike other bacteria, they can multiply only in host cells.

Rickettsia prowazekii (ri-ket′se-ah pro-wa-ze′kii): causative organism of scrub typhus. It is spread to humans by lice and fleas.

Rickettsia typhi (ri-ket′se-ah ti-fe′): causative organism of murine typhus. It is spread to humans by rat fleas.

RPR: rapid plasma reagin. A screening test for syphilis.

Saccharomyces cerevisiae (sak-a-ro′mi-ses ser va′si-i): saprophytic yeast used in the fermentation process of beer and wine and in baking bread.

Salmonella (sal″mo-nel′ah): genus of gram-negative facultative anaerobic rod-shaped enteric bacilli whose members cause intestinal disorders, food poisoning, and typhoid fever.

Salt (sawlt): sodium chloride (common table salt), or any compound formed by the reaction of an acid and a base.

Saprophyte (sap′ro-fite): organism that obtains its nutrition from dead or decaying organic matter.

Saprophytic (sap′ro-fit-ik): organism that obtains its nutrition from dead or decaying matter.

Sarcina (sahr′si-nuh): gram-positive cocci arranged in a cuboidal structure.

Sarcina lutea (sahr′si-nuh lew′tee-uh): non-pathogenic species of *Sarcina* commonly found in dust.

Sarcoptes (sar-kop′tez): genus of mites including *S. scabiei,* which causes scabies (a sexually transmitted disease) in humans and the mange in animals.

Saturated (sach′e-rat-ed): containing the maximum amount of solute that can be dissolved by a solvent.

Schistosoma (shis″to-so′mah): genus of trematodes, found in Africa, the far east, and South America, known as "blood flukes" which enter the skin through contaminated water. Snails are intermediate hosts.

Schizont (skiz′ont): asexual stage of development of the malarial parasite in which the nucleus of the trophozoite divides into many smaller nuclei.

Scrapie (scrap′ee): a disease of sheep caused by prions that result in the sheep scraping their fur off.

Sebaceous gland (see-bay′shus gland): gland that produces fat or sebum.

Sedimentation (sed-e-men-ta′shen): process that produces a deposit at the bottom of a liquid.

Septic sore throat (sep′tik sore throte): inflammation of the pharynx and/or the tonsils due to bacteria or their toxins.

Selective permeable membrane (se′lek-tiv per-me′abl mem′brane): membrane through which only the solvent's molecules, not the solute molecules, can pass. In this one-way passage the molecules move from the side of lower concentration to the side of higher solute concentration.

Sepsis (septicemia) (sep′sis) (sep″ti-se′me-ah): systemic disease associated with the presence of pathogenic microorganisms or their toxins in the blood.

Seroconversion (sero-con-ver-shun): the production of detectable antibodies following infection with a foreign antigen. This may take anywhere from a few days to years, as in HIV antibodies.

Sheath (sheeth): tubular case or envelope.

Shigella (shi-gel′ah): genus of gram-negative facultative anaerobic rod-shaped enteric bacilli whose members cause dysentery.

Silica (sil′i-kah): silicon dioxide occurring in nature as sand or quartz. It has many uses, ranging from glass and gems to computer parts.

Simple staining (sim′pl stan′ing): use of only one dye to visualize the bacteria.

Slime layer (slime la′yer): sticky outer covering secreted by some bacterial cells, also called a "capsule."

Slough (sluf): to shed or cast off dead tissue from living tissue.

Sodium hypochlorite (so-di′yum hi-po′clor-ite): $NaHClO_4$, mild bleach solution effective in killing microorganism.

Soluble (sol′u-bul): able to be dissolved.

Solute (sol′ut): substance dissolved in a liquid to form a solution.

Solution (so-loo′shun): mixture formed when one substance is readily dissolved in another.

Solvent (sol′vent): substance, usually a liquid in which another substance (the solute) is dissolved.

Species chromosome number (spe′chez kro′mo-som num′ber): given or standard number of chromosomes found in every cell of that species. Humans have 46 chromosomes in each diploid cell.

Spindle-fiber apparatus (spin′dl fi′br a-per′a-tus): structure formed during metaphase of mitosis in which the chromosomes line up closely to form a spindle between each centriole, thus permitting equal distribution of genetic material to the newly formed daughter cells.

Spirilla (spye-ril′uh): spiral-shaped bacteria.

Spirochetes (spi′ro-keetz): highly coiled bacteria; a general term given to members of the Spirochaeta family. *Treponema pallidum,* the cause of syphilis, is the most notable spirochete.

Splenomegaly (sple″no-meg′ah-le): enlargement of the spleen.

Sphagnum moss (′sfagnem): a moss-like fungus that resembles a fern. It grows close to wet acid areas such as on wet rock.

Spongiform encephalopathies (spun′gee form en sef fal opa thees): spongelike appearance of brain tissue that results in a pathological disease, namely dementia.

Sporangia (spor′an-giah): sacks or casings in which the spores of a fungus are produced or borne.

Spores (sporz): 1. the reproductive element of the lower organisms as fungi, algae, or protozoa. 2. a refractile oval body formed within a bacteria, especially *Bacillus* and *Clostridium,* which is a resting stage that allows the bacteria to withstand harsh environments until favorable conditions are again present. They are resistant to heat, drying and toxic chemicals.

Sporogenesis (spo″ro-jen′e-sis): production of spores.

Sporothrix (spo″ro-triks): genus of dimorphic fungi, found on living or dead vegetation, that causes sporotrichosis, a nodular infection of the skin often transmitted by a thorn or splinters.

Sporozoa (spo-ruh-zo′uh): class of parasitic protozoa with both sexual and asexual phases.

Stain (stayn): dye used to color tissues or cells so that they can be seen better microscopically.

Staphylococci (staf″i-lo-kok′i): (sing. staphylococcus), spherical-shaped gram-positive bacteria arranged in grapelike clusters.

Staphylococcus (staf ″i-lo-kok′us): genus of gram-positive obligate anaerobic bacteria appearing in clusters that are commonly found on the skin and may cause boils, carbuncles, and nosocomial infections.

Staphylococcus aureus (staf″i-lo-kok′us o-re′us): gram-positive facultative anaerobic coccus. It usually appears in clusters and causes upper respiratory infections, boils, nosocomial hospital infections, and food poisoning. Many people are carriers of this organism.

Staphylococcus epidermidis (staf″i-lo-kok′us e-pi-der″mi-dis): gram-positive facultative anaerobic coccus. It usually appears in clusters and is found to inhabit the skin and upper respiratory tract.

Sterilization (ster-il-i-zay′shun): process used to kill all contaminating microorganisms.

Steam sterilizer (steem ster′i-liz″er): apparatus that employs steam to get rid of or kill microorganisms.

Streptobacilli (strep-to-ba-sil′i): type of rod-shaped bacillus forming long chains.

Streptococci (strep-to-kok′i): (sing. streptococcus) spherical gram-positive bacteria arranged in chains or pairs.

Streptococcus (strep″to′kok-us): a genus of gram-positive obligate anaerobic bacteria appearing in pairs or chains. Several stains are infectious, causing strep throat, pneumonia, and septicemia.

Streptococcus pneumoniae (strep″to-kok′us new-mon′e-ae): gram-positive facultative aerobic coccus, usually in pairs or chains. Causes pneumonia.

Streptococcus pyogenes (strep″to-kok′us pye odj′e-neez): gram-positive facultative aerobic coccus, usually in pairs or chains. Causes strep throat, scarlet fever, and rheumatic fever. Also known as group A streptococcus.

Streptococcus viridans (strep″to-kok′us vir′i-denz): gram-positive facultative aerobic coccus, usually in pairs or chains, found as a normal inhabitant of the upper respiratory tract. Causes bacterial endocarditis and septicemia.

Strongyloides (stron″ji-loi′dez): genus of nematode parasites that cause intestinal disorders.

Substrate (sub′strate): any substance that acts upon an enzyme.

Svedberg unit (sved′burg yu′nit): rate of sedimentation of deposition of a large molecule, in a specified medium, of 10^{-13} cm per second under a centrifugal force.

Symbiosis (sim″bi-o′sis): mutually beneficial relationship between two or more organisms of different species.

Taenia (te′ne-ah): genus of the cestode or tapeworm family. Well known are the beef (*T. saginata*) and the pork (*T. solium*) tapeworms that lodge in the intestines of humans and animals.

Tapeworm (taip′wurm): parasitic cestode worm that has a flattened ribbonlike body.

Taxonomy (tax-on′-uh-mee): science of classifying organisms.

Tetanus (tet′ah-nus): lockjaw. Disease caused by *Clostridium tetani* that induces painful muscular contractions of the neck and jaw.

Tetrad (tet′rad): group of four.

Thermal death point (thur′mal deth point): See Thermal death time.

Thermal death time (thur′mal deth time): length of time needed to kill microorganisms kept at a specific temperature.

Thermolabile (thur-molay′bil): sensitive to or killed by heat.

Thoracic (tho-ras′ik): pertaining to the thorax or chest area.

Thyroiditis (thigh-royd-eye′tis): inflammation of the thyroid gland.

Tincture (tingk′tur): alcoholic or hydroalcoholic solution prepared from a chemical substance or an animal or vegetable drug.

Titer (ti′ter): process of serial or doubling dilutions of a substance to determine the least amount of that substance that can react with another substance.

T-lymphocyte (lim′fo-sit): one of the white blood cells that is particularly involved in immunity and destroyed by HIV.

Toxin (tok′sin): poisonous substance produced by animal or plant cells.

Toxoid (tok′soid): toxin weakened by treatment with heat or chemicals without destroying its ability to stimulate antitoxin or produce antibodies.

Toxoplasma (tok″so-plaz′mah): genus of sporozoan parasites that attack the lungs, liver, heart, skin, muscle, and brain. *T. gondii* is transmitted to humans by infected cat feces, raw mutton, pork, and goat meat. It is also an opportunistic infection of immunocompromised patients.

Toxoplasma gondii (tok″so-plaz′mah gon′dii): species of sporozoan parasites transmitted to humans in raw meats and by cat feces. It can be transmitted from an infected mother to her infant in utero.

Transverse binary fission (trans′vurs bye′n erry fish′un): asexual method of reproduction occurring in bacteria in which a cell wall develops around the bacterium before it divides in two.

Trematode (trem′ah-tod): a class of flatworms called flukes that are broad and leaf shaped.

Trichina (trik-i′nah): organism of the genus Trichinella, a roundworm which is transmitted to humans via infected uncooked pork.

Trichocyst (trik-o′sist): cysts of the Trichinella roundworm.

Trichomonads (trik″o-mo′nad): parasites of the genus Trichomonas.

Trichomonas (trik″o-mo′nas): genus of a flagellate protozoa parasites found in humans.

Trichomonas buccalis (trik″o-mo′nas bu-kal′is): a species of flagellate protozoa parasites found in the mouth and gums.

Trichomonas hominis (trik″o-mo′nas hah-min′is): a species of flagellate protozoa parasites found in the mouth and intestines.

Trichomonas vaginalis (trik″o-mo′nas vaj-i-nal′is): sexually transmitted disease found in men and women.

Trichophyton (tri-kof′i-ton): genus of fungi that causes various infections of the skin, hair, and nails.

Trichuris (trik-u′ris): genus of nematodes parasites in the intestines that includes the whipworm *Trichuris trichiura.*

Trophozoite (trof″o-zo-′it): the active motile feeding stage of a sporozoan parasite.

Trypanosoma cruzi (tri″pan-a-so′mah cru-zi): species of protozoa parasites transmitted to the blood of humans by the tsetse fly. *T. cruzi* causes Chagas' disease.

Trypanosoma gambiense (tri″pan-a-so′mah gam-beyn′zi): species of protozoa parasites transmitted to the blood of humans by the tsetse fly. *T. gambiense* causes African sleeping sickness.

Trypanosoma rhodesiense (tri″pan-a-so′mah rho-de-yen′zi): species of protozoa parasites transmitted to the blood of humans by the tsetse fly. *T. rhodesiense* also causes African sleeping sickness.

Turbid (tur′bid): cloudy state of a solution or substance.

Turret (ter′et): revolving device attached to the tube of a microscope to hold the objective lens.

Typhoid fever (ti′foid fe′ver): bacterial infection transmitted to humans by *Salmonella typhii,* a virulent organism that attacks the intestinal tract and the blood.

Unicellular (u″ni-sel′u-lar): single-celled organism such as bacteria.

Unit membrane (yoo′nit mem′bran): chemical structure of the plasma or cytoplasmic membrane consisting of a protein and lipid layer.

Universal precautions (u″ni-ver-sal pre′kaw-shuns): standardized set of safety measures taken by health care workers to protect themselves as well as patients from transmitting potential pathogens. Instead of having different criteria for different types of infectious diseases, similar criteria to cover all possible situations have been developed to protect the patient's right to privacy.

Unsaturated (un-sat′-u-rat″ed): solution not containing its maximum amount of solute before being unable to be dissolve any more.

Urethritis (u′re-thri′tis): inflammation of the urethra.

Urogenital (yur-o-jen′i-tal): pertaining to the urinary and genital organs.

Vaccination (vak″si-na′shun): injection of antigens or pathogens to produce immunity in a person. Originally, the term was in reference to the injection of attenuated cow (Latin *vacca*) pox virus as in smallpox vaccination. Today, the term is synonymous with immunization.

Vaccine (vak′sen): preparation made from a suspension of living or dead pathogens or a solution of bacterial, viral, or pollen antigens, which can stimulate antibody formation when injected.

Vaccinia (vak-sin′e-ah): viral disease of cattle caused by the cowpox virus. Antigenically it is quite similar to the smallpox virus. When vaccinated with the cowpox virus, a single cowpox lesion forms at the site of inoculation and soon immunity to the disease smallpox occurs.

Variola (vah-ri′o-lah): smallpox.

Vacuole (vak′u-ol): space or cavity in the protoplasm of a cell.

Vaporization (va″por-i-za′shun): conversion of a liquid, usually water to steam or vapor.

VDRL: Venereal Disease Research Laboratory. A screening test for syphilis.

Vector (vek′tor): arthropod or other agent that carries microorganisms from one infected individual to another.

Virulence (vir′u-lens): degree of pathogenicity or disease-producing ability of an organism.

Viruses (vi′rus-z): (sing. virus) submicroscopic infectious organisms that are composed of deoxyribonucleic acid (DNA) or ribonucleic acid (RNA) surrounded by a protective protein coat. Viruses are unable to maintain their own life; they must parasitize a healthy cell. Viruses will feed off the cell and use the cell's reproductive ability to produce new viral particles.

Virologist (vi′rol-o-gist): scientist specializing in the study of viruses and diseases they cause.

Vital stain (vye′tul stain): dye used for staining living organisms or tissues.

Volvox (val′vox): genus of green flagellates found in pond water.

Wandering phagocyte (wan-der′ing fag″o-site): white blood cells that are able to search out foreign matter by moving about through the blood and tissues to engulf microorganisms or other cells and foreign materials.

Wuchereria bancrofti (voo′ker-e′re-ah ban-crof′tee): species of filarial nematode worms transmitted to the blood of humans by insect bites.

Yeast (yest): general term use to describe unicellular, nucleated rounded fungi that reproduce by budding. *Candida albicans,* which causes thrush or moniliasis, and *Saccharomyces cerevisae,* a yeast used in baking and in making beer and wine, are notable.

Yield (yeeld): to produce or give off.

INDEX